24.00

Surgery of the Neonate

Surgery of the Neonate

Arnold G. Coran, M.D.
Professor of Surgery and Head, Section of Pediatric Surgery,
University of Michigan Medical School, Ann Arbor

Douglas M. Behrendt, M.D.
Professor of Surgery, Section of Thoracic Surgery,
University of Michigan Medical School, Ann Arbor

William H. Weintraub, M.D.
Associate Professor of Surgery, Section of Pediatric Surgery,
University of Michigan Medical School, Ann Arbor

Denis C. Lee
Medical Illustrator and Associate Professor of Art and
Postgraduate Medicine, University of Michigan
Medical School, Ann Arbor

Little, Brown and Company
Boston

First Edition

Library of Congress Catalog Card No. 78-50614

ISBN 0-316-15635-3

Printed in the United States of America

Preface

The specialty of pediatric surgery has developed during the past 25 years to the point at which it is now recognized as a separate subspecialty of surgery with board certification status. Within the specialty of pediatric surgery there has developed a subspecialty of neonatal and infant surgery with its own diagnostic and therapeutic peculiarities. Several comprehensive textbooks and atlases of pediatric surgery have been published. Few of them, however, include a detailed description of the operative techniques. Furthermore, a number of those textbooks have many authors and fail to reflect a consistent management philosophy.

Surgery of the Neonate is an attempt to discuss in detail the diagnosis, preoperative preparation, and minute details of the operative procedures as performed in one institution that treats a large volume of major neonatal and infant surgical diseases. Not every abnormality encountered in the newborn and infant is outlined in this book; rather, the more common anomalies that most surgeons are called upon to treat are described in detail. We have made no effort to catalog all the operative procedures available for each surgical entity or to review the literature extensively; we have instead elected to describe our personal approach, which we believe has been successful. We hope, therefore, that surgeons who care for infants will find this book to be a practical guide providing specific emphasis on those technical details that make such operations regularly successful.

A. G. C.
D. M. B.
W. H. W.

Contents

Surgery of the Neonate

1

Anesthesia of the Neonate

Jordan Waldman and Keith Liedling

The anesthetic care of the neonate and infant begins at the time of the anesthetist's preoperative evaluation. Although the patient is often only hours old, considerable information has already been accumulated that is useful for operative management. Most of these patients are treated in neonatal units where there are daily flow sheets upon which much of the pertinent data concerning the patient's course is recorded. These flow sheets, in addition to the history and physical examination, are an important source of information.

Preoperative Evaluation

Restrictions

During the review of the chart and the flow sheet of the intensive care unit (ICU), a special point to check is the presence of the permission of the parents or the guardian for surgery and anesthesia. Also, any restrictions concerning administration of drugs or blood should be clearly stated here, as well as the extent of surgery permitted.

Nurses' Records

A check should be mandatory of the nurses' notes for the trend and status of blood pressure, pulse, temperature, intake and output, and body weight. Specific notes should be made on the anesthetic record or in the patient's chart concerning abnormal laboratory values, the level of the preoperative hemoglobin or hematocrit, and the presence of drugs that will affect the course of the anesthetic, for example, steroids, aminoglycoside antibiotics, and sedative drugs. Special attention should be given to the possibility of hypocalcemia and hypoglycemia in the premature infant and in infants of diabetic mothers. Tetany may exist at total serum calcium levels lower than 7 mg per 100 ml. Decreased myocardial contractility resulting from low levels of free calcium ion can be detected clinically by the presence on the electrocardiogram (ECG) of a prolonged QT interval. Hypoglycemia is a constant risk in any newborn who has an abnormal perinatal period, but especially in infants of diabetic mothers. All infants should have their blood glucose level maintained at levels higher than 30 mg per 100 ml. Care should always be taken to ascertain whether hypoglycemia is a cause of neurologic or circulatory depression. Serum glucose estimations are made intraoperatively with Dextrostix.

Records of Respiratory Therapists

The records of respiratory therapists contain information concerning oxygen and ventilatory support. To help prevent retrolental fibroplasia, every attempt is made to keep the arterial oxygen (Po_2) below 100 mm Hg. The infant has usually been stabilized in the neonatal intensive care unit at an inspiratory oxygen concentration that provides a Po_2 between 60 and 80 mm Hg if there is no cyanotic congenital heart disease. In the presence of cyanotic congenital heart disease one should attempt to maintain the Po_2 greater than 30 mm Hg.

Physical Examination

On physical examination an appraisal is made of the patient's general condition and of the condition of the cardiovascular and respiratory systems. In the neonate assessment of pulmonary function is often difficult. Color can be deceptive, especially with the normal presence in the newborn of peripheral cyanosis. The color of the mucous membranes is a better indication of cyanosis than is the color of the extremities. Any one of the following should be a warning of the onset or the presence of acute respiratory failure: tachypnea, chest wall retractions, nasal flaring, grunting, and apnea. Clinical impressions should be supported by testing arterial blood gases if the clinical situation permits. Arterialized capillary samples are often inaccurate in critically ill infants. Many of these patients will already have umbilical artery catheters in place, to allow for frequent, accurate assessment of blood gases and acid-base status and continuous monitoring of intraarterial blood pressure.

Hydration

The state of hydration is evaluated from simple physical signs and, when possible, changes in accurate measurements of body weight. Poor tissue turgor indicates at least 5 percent dehydration. Poor tissue turgor accompanied by sunken fontanelles indicates a 5 percent to 10 percent dehydration; these signs accompanied by sunken eyeballs indicate 10 percent to 20 percent dehydration. Metabolic acidosis usually accompanies dehydration and hypovolemia. When mild, acidosis can usually be corrected with proper volume replacement. When it is necessary to correct a metabolic acidosis, the calculation of the amount of sodium bicarbonate is based upon the formula 0.3 mEq × weight in kilograms (see page 18). One-half the calculated amount is then given. This is an underestimation of the total amount of bicarbonate necessary to correct the deficit, but often, once correction has been started, further correction will occur spontaneously. Administration of sodium bicarbonate should be by slow infusion, to avoid plasma hypertonicity, sodium excess, and possible cerebral hemorrhage.

Hemoglobin Values

It is expected that all newborn patients who are to have surgery will have a hemoglobin value of at least 12 g per 100 ml. When the hemoglobin value is less than 12 g per 100 ml the neonate should be transfused with packed red blood cells before induction of anesthesia or with whole blood early in the operative period. A rule of thumb for safe transfusion of whole blood when the patient is not actively bleeding is 20 ml per kg. Packed red blood cells can be administered in this circumstance at a rate of 10 ml per kg.

Initial Stabilization

Very few neonatal emergencies require immediate surgical correction without initial stabilization. Neonates who are hypovolemic, acidotic, or otherwise unprepared for anesthesia and operation must be allowed time for specific therapy. Possible exceptions to this are patients with cyanotic congenital heart disease who have a Po_2 of less than 30 mm Hg and who are becoming progressively acidotic, or the patient with a diaphragmatic hernia who is in respiratory failure despite appropriate treatment.

Fasting and Preoperative Medication

All patients should fast at least four hours before surgery. When an upper gastrointestinal radiographic procedure has been performed or when there is bowel obstruction with a distended stomach, a large-bore suction catheter (14 French scale) is passed to empty the stomach.

If an intravenous or arterial line is in place, no preoperative medication is given until the patient arrives in the operating room. Then 0.1 mg of atropine is given by the intravascular route. If there are no intravascular lines in place, atropine is given in the above dose intramuscularly half an hour before the patient is brought to the operating room. Newborn patients are normally deficient in vitamin K, and they should receive 1.0 mg of AquaMEPHYTON intramuscularly or intravascularly as soon as possible before surgery.

The Operation

Transportation to the Operating Room

One of the pitfalls in the anesthetic care of neonates can occur while the patient is being transported to and from the operating room. Because of their size and pathologic condition, many of these patients have treatments in progress that must be continued uninterrupted during transport and during surgery. These include maintenance of temperature, controlled administration of fluids and medications, and continuance of respiratory therapy and monitoring systems.

Ideally, the operating room should be only a short distance from the neonatal intensive care unit. In that instance one of the many isolettes available is satisfactory for transport. Portable, battery-operated ECG and blood pressure monitors can easily be applied. There are many battery-operated infusion pumps to assure accurate, uninterrupted administration of fluids and medications during transport. Devices for sustaining continuous positive airway pressure ventilation (CPPV) are used.

When the transport distance within the hospital is long,

there are available battery-operated isolettes that assist in maintaining neonatal body temperature. It should be remembered that an E-type oxygen cylinder contains 560 liters of gas and, at a flow of 7 liters per minute, the supply will last only 80 minutes. These tanks must be turned off when not in use and, if necessary, replaced while surgery is being performed. Also, isolettes should be attached to a power source in the wall and kept warm during surgery, so that there is a warm transport system to return the patient to the intensive care unit. The length of time it takes for a high Po_2 to produce retrolental fibroplasia in a premature infant is still not known. Consequently, an air-oxygen blender should be available on the isolette and during transport for control of inspired oxygen concentration.

Emergencies

It is necessary to anticipate and prepare for neonatal emergencies to avoid being forced by crisis to gather all equipment and personnel in a rushed, haphazard manner. A neonatal surgical crisis is no moment for improvisation. The equipment necessary to anesthetize a neonate for any surgical problem should be available for immediate use at all times. Before the neonate arrives in the operating room, extensive preparations must be made.

Temperature

The temperature of the operating room is adjusted to 21 C (70 F) or greater. The operating table normally used for older children is removed and replaced with an open-care unit (Figure 1-1) modified for use as an operating table. This unit allows the neonate to be cared for on an open surface of adjustable height and tilt with overhead radiant heating, which is servo-controlled by a skin temperature probe. The unit also incorporates fluorescent lighting and an overhead portal to allow access for operating room lights and x-ray machines. During surgery much of the radiant heat is screened from the infant by surgical drapes; therefore a small water mattress is used to supplement the radiant warmers. In addition to the servo-control skin temperature probe, a rectal or esophageal temperature probe is also used. Rectal temperature is maintained between 36.5 C and 37 C. Skin temperature should be maintained 1 C to 1.5 C lower than rectal temperature.

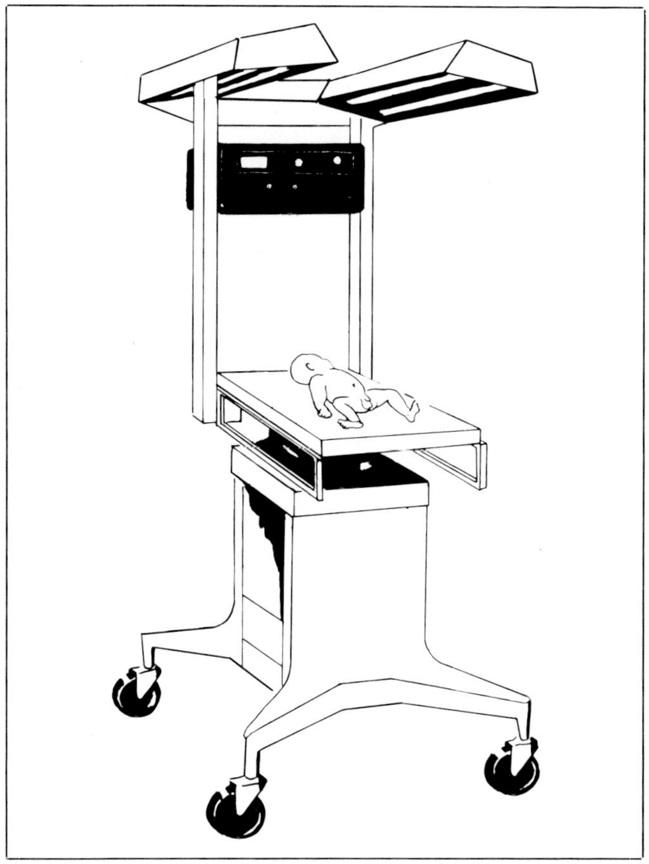

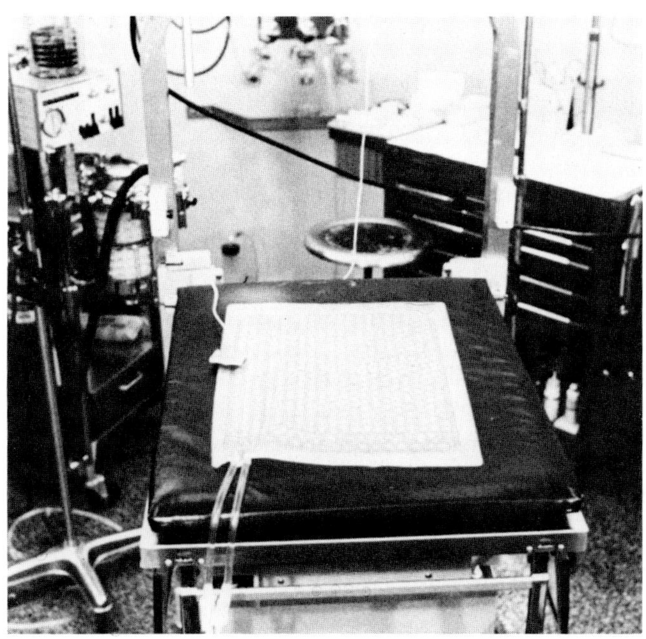

1-1. The Ohio bed.

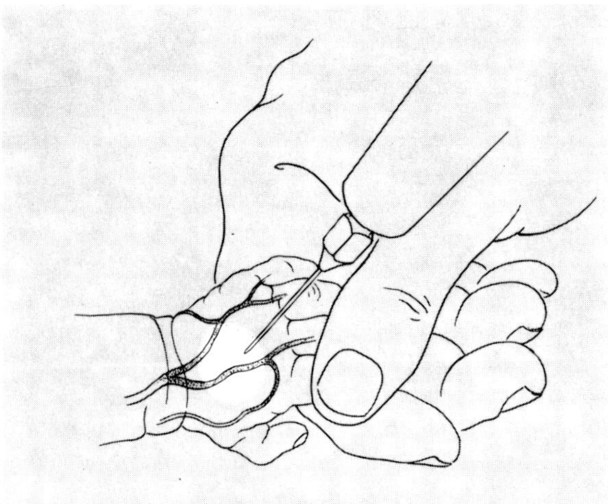

1-3. Cold-light transillumination can be used to locate the vein and insert a cannula.

locating the vein and inserting a cannula (Figure 1-3). When major neonatal surgery is to be performed, an intravenous infusion by needle is not sufficient; if a plastic cannula cannot be inserted percutaneously, a cutdown is performed.

Technique of Saphenous Vein Cutdown

The foot is gently taped to a padded board with the medial side up. After a Betadine preparation, a very small, 3-mm transverse incision is made just anterior and superior to the medial malleolus (Figure 1-4). A small curved hemostat is inserted straight down to the bone (Figure 1-5) and then is scraped along the bone and all the tissue is scooped up and brought out through the incision (Figure 1-6). The clamp will uniformly bring up the easily recognized saphenous vein. The accompanying nerve and subcutaneous tissue are cleaned off and the vein is tied distally with 4-0 Dexon. Silk is avoided because the skin in this area is thin, and the black color is visible. The vein is then routinely catheterized. The saphenous vein is surprisingly large in this area. Even in a premature, a 20-gauge catheter will fit. If the vein looks too small, it is probably not the saphenous vein. The scooping maneuver should be repeated.

Whether the intravenous line is established by the percutaneous or the cutdown route, it is important to remember that the intravenous line must not be placed in the lower extremity if there is any possibility of major intraabdominal hemorrhage during the surgical procedure.

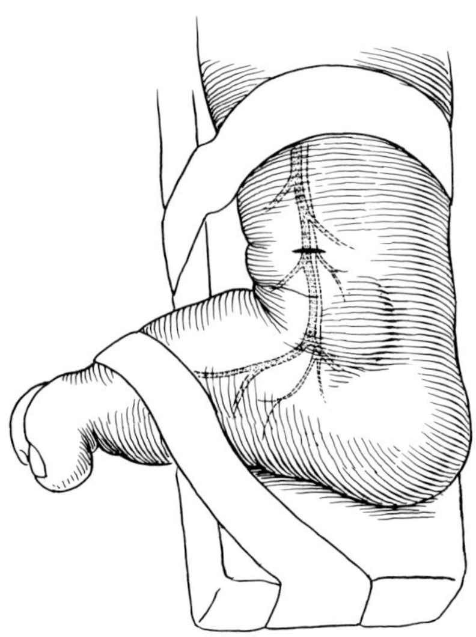

1-4

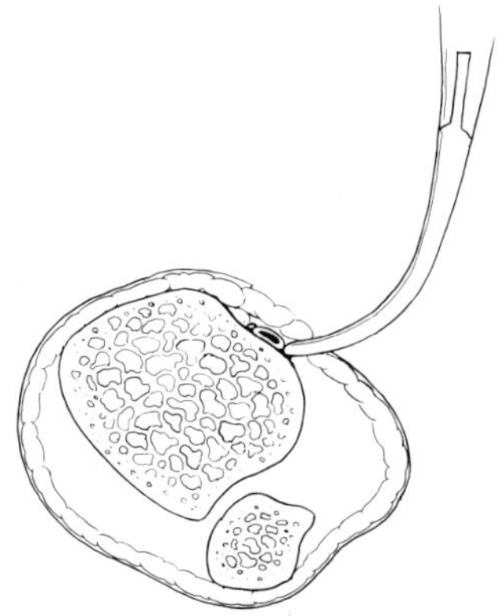

1-5

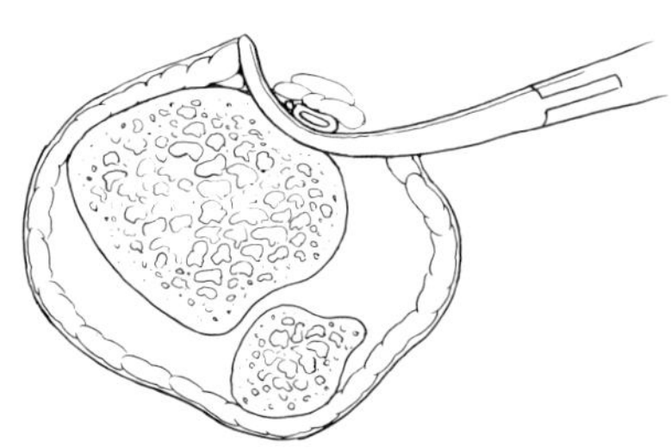

1-6

Intubation

Although the indications for intubation in an awake neonate are not as broad as they once were, certain conditions (such as cystic hygroma involving the base of the tongue and Pierre-Robin syndrome) require that this technique be attempted. With an assistant positioning the head and shoulders properly, intubation is not a difficult procedure in an awake neonate. Intubation in the awake neonate avoids the danger of losing the airway in a situation where the ability to control the airway is questionable.

Following intubation, it is imperative that the tube position be ascertained. Because of the extremely short distance in a neonate from the vocal cord level to the carina, it is easy to perform an inadvertent endobronchial intubation. One technique we have found useful in avoiding this complication is to have an assistant place the tip of his index finger in the suprasternal notch (Figure 1-7). The tip of the endotracheal tube can be palpated as it passes the finger, so that at this point further advancement of the tube is prevented. The chest is then auscultated for equal breath sounds bilaterally.

Adequate fixation of the endotracheal tube is accomplished by placing tincture of benzoin on the skin and then placing adhesive tape on this adhesive surface. It is better to place the tape on the maxillary area of the jaw, to avoid the amount of mobility possible by fixation to the mandibular area.

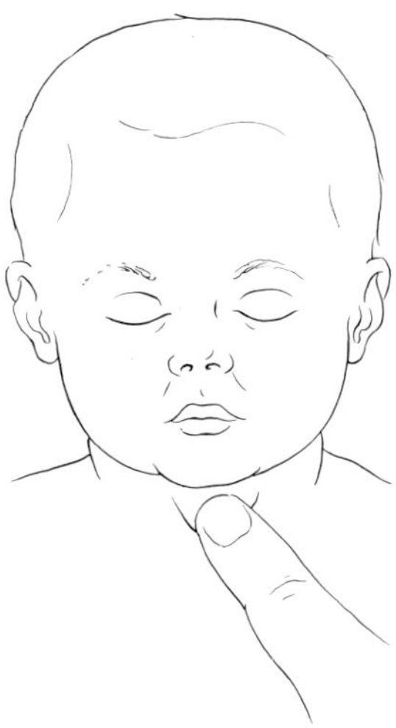

1-7. To prevent endobronchial intubation, an assistant places his index finger in the suprasternal notch, which allows palpation of the tip of the endotracheal tube.

Maintenance Fluids

Although it is necessary to change our technique for certain infants, such as those in congestive heart failure, our general rule for the administration of maintenance fluids is to calculate the maintenance volume from the formula 100 ml per kg of body weight per 24 hours. This is easy to use and is very close to a figure obtained by using the meter-squared method. The choice of fluid is determined by the type and extent of surgery and the metabolic status of the patient. If the procedure is to be of short duration and minimal tissue trauma is expected, 5% to 10% dextrose in 0.2 normal saline solution is administered. When the procedure involves extensive tissue trauma or manipulation of bowel, 5% to 10% dextrose in Ringer's lactate is used. The volume of fluid given is governed by the amount of expected blood loss and the extent of dissection. For short, minor procedures we give only maintenance volumes (4 ml per kg per hour). As the amount of dissection and tissue trauma increases, we will increase the hourly fluids to approximately 18 ml per kg per hour. In the situation where there is evidence of metabolic alkalosis we use 5% to 10% dextrose in normal saline.

Blood Volume

The blood volume changes according to age, although in the small infant it is usually estimated at 80 to 85 ml per kg of body weight. Blood volume is estimated by a method that takes into account the presence of anemia or polycythemia. The plasma volume is first estimated as 5 percent of body weight. This equals 50 ml of plasma per kg of body weight. The blood volume can then be estimated by using the formula:

$$(50 \text{ ml plasma} + \text{hematocrit}) \times \text{body weight in kg} = \text{estimated blood volume}$$

As an example, a 10-kg child with a hematocrit reading of 45 percent would have a blood volume of $(50 + 45) \times 10 = 950$ ml. We usually contemplate blood replacement when the blood loss reaches 5 percent of estimated blood volume and generally give blood when 10 percent loss has been reached or when tachycardia and falling blood pressure indicate that the patient is "asking for blood." Circulating nurses are expected to report frequently the estimated blood loss as determined by freshly weighed sponges and the amount in suction traps. Once blood replacement is instituted, it is warmed and replaced milliliter for milliliter by means of a syringe. If blood loss is continuing, we attempt to stay 5 percent ahead of the estimated blood loss.

Reversal of Anesthesia

Once the surgical procedure has been completed, all neuromuscular blocking agents are reversed unless a deliberate decision has been made to ventilate the neonate mechanically. Atropine (0.03 mg per kg) is used to block the muscarinic effects of neostigmine. Neostigmine is then given in a dose of 0.08 mg per kg of body weight. In most instances, reversal of the neuromuscular block occurs rapidly. If it does not, one must think of the presence of hypothermia, aminoglycoside antibiotics, abnormal pseudocholinesterase, hypoglycemia, or hypocalcemia and treat the cause appropriately. Unfortunately, in some instances, when the above differential diagnosis and appropriate treatment have been carried out, the patient still has not developed an adequate respiratory pattern, and we have had to resort to short-term use of a ventilator.

2

Preoperative and Postoperative Care

Skill in the preoperative and postoperative care of neonates who undergo operation frequently is the key to a successful outcome. Infant patients are more difficult to manage than older children, both because of the technical problems created by small size and because of their unique metabolic needs.

Principles of Intensive Care

Observations on which decisions are made must be quantified whenever possible. The bedside assessment of such signs as color, temperature of the skin, vigor of sucking, and nature of the breathing is very important. This assessment must be supplemented by additional more precise information obtained through modern techniques of patient monitoring. The more ill the patient, the more often such observations are required. For severely ill patients, continuous monitoring is necessary. Figure 2-1 exemplifies the type of flow sheet we have found very helpful in organizing the data essential to caring for critically ill infants.

Infants require proportionately higher doses of most medications than do older patients; therefore age-adjusted dosage schedules must be consulted. A warm, well-fed infant rarely requires sedation. When restlessness occurs, hypoxia or low cardiac output should be suspected. Small doses of morphine (0.1 mg per kg of body weight) and chloral hydrate (14 mg per kg of body weight by mouth or by suppository) are about the only sedatives needed.

The question of preoperative antibiotics is controversial. Our preference is to give antibiotics preoperatively to all infants undergoing major surgery, and for the first five to seven days postoperatively. The coverage is broad-spectrum; we usually use ampicillin (100 mg per kg of body weight per 24 hours) and gentamicin (5 mg per kg per 24 hours).

Metabolic Problems Unique to Infants

Temperature

The small infant placed in a cold environment rapidly loses heat because of having a relatively large surface area and a thin subcutaneous fat layer. Increased metabolic rate and increased oxygen utilization are the normal compensatory mechanisms by which the infant attempts to maintain proper body temperature. Clearly, this is undesirable in a sick neonate. Infants who are septic are especially likely to develop hypothermia. To minimize heat losses resulting from radiation, water evaporation, and convection, incubators were developed. These are excellent for the care of most premature infants, but they provide inadequate access to the very sick baby. Several commercial units are available that allow the infant to be cared for on an open surface of adjustable height with overhead radiant heating, servo-controlled by a temperature probe on the skin (see Figure 1-1). Even with this equipment, it is wise to cover the infant whenever possible and to minimize breezes from surrounding traffic.

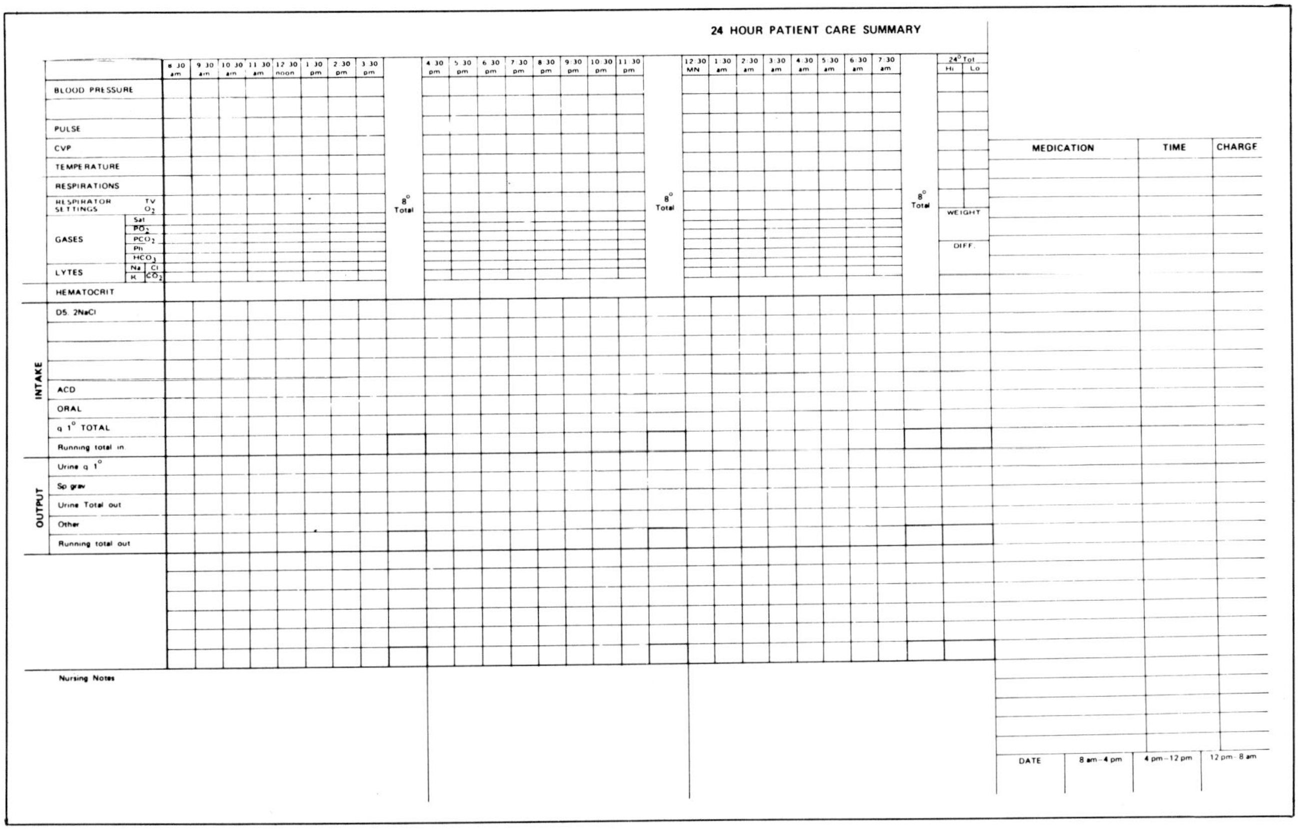

2-1. Example of a flow sheet used in an infant intensive care unit. This sheet maintains an accurate record of hemodynamic variables, intake and output, and blood chemistries.

Disturbances in the Chemical Constituents of the Blood

All newborn infants have poorly developed mechanisms for regulating glucose and calcium levels in the blood. Hepatic glycogen stores are small and are rapidly depleted. Particularly in the newborn subjected to operation, significant hypoglycemia is likely to occur (below 30 mg per 100 ml in full-term infants; below 20 mg per 100 ml in the premature), which leads to convulsions. Fortunately, the blood glucose level can easily be followed on an hourly basis with Dextrostix to supplement the more accurate blood glucose determinations obtained periodically from the laboratory.

Hypoglycemia is treated by slowly administering 1 to 2 ml per kg of body weight of 50% dextrose solution into the central venous cannula, then by increasing the dextrose concentration of the maintenance intravenous fluids to 10% or 15%. Occasionally even this treatment does not suffice, and steroids must be administered (hydrocortisone, 5 mg per kg of body weight every 12 hours). Resumption of oral or gavage feedings usually eliminates this problem, but during the transition intravenous glucose supplementation must be tapered slowly. Not infrequently, the neonate suffering from hemorrhage or septic shock will develop significant hyperglycemia. If the blood glucose remains below 250 mg per 100 ml, no treatment is necessary. Levels above this require insulin therapy.

Hypocalcemia (that is, a calcium concentration less than 7 mg per 100 ml) also tends to occur in newborn infants undergoing operation. Several factors may predispose to this: (1) prematurity, with inadequate calcium stores and underdeveloped parathyroid glands; (2) stress that leads to endogenous steroid production; (3) administration of sodium bicarbonate; and (4) administration of citrate-phosphate-dextrose anticoagulant with transfusion. Hypocalcemia may be manifested by twitching, jitteriness, and convulsions. It can be treated by immediate administration of a 10% calcium gluconate solution given slowly into a central venous line to a total dose of 10 ml for a full-term infant (6 ml for a premature); 1 to 2 g is then added to a 24-hour intravenous maintenance fluid for a day or two. Resumption of oral feeding usually resolves this problem. Most laboratories measure total calcium content, not just the ionized portion that is physiologically important. Thus, when convulsions occur in a setting suggesting hypocalcemia, a therapeutic trial of calcium gluconate may be indicated even when the serum calcium level is reportedly normal.

Hypomagnesemia occasionally coexists with hypocalcemia. Serum magnesium levels less than 1.4 milliequivalents per liter are abnormal in the neonate. Tetany unresponsive to calcium therapy may be treated with 0.2 ml of 50% magnesium sulfate solution given intramuscularly every four hours.

Newborn infants occasionally become jaundiced. Tendency to jaundice is more marked when bilirubin production is excessive; for example, following massive transfusion. The serum bilirubin level should be measured daily after operation in the newborn. Levels over 10 mg per 100 ml require further investigation and prompt therapy to prevent kernicterus.

Infants may be unable to conserve sodium as completely as adults. Therefore they may require some sodium in postoperative intravenous fluids (0.25 normal saline is a reasonable choice if the serum sodium level decreases). The daily requirements for fluids and electrolytes may be estimated from a nomogram. To do this, as is shown in Figure 2-2, (1) find the daily requirements appropriate for the age. Note that this is in milliliters per kilogram of body weight per day. Multiply the daily requirements by the body weight in kilograms to obtain the daily allotment for a normal child. (2) In general, for infants use dilute saline solutions in dextrose given intravenously. (3) As the infant's condition improves, gradually switch from intravenous to oral feedings.

After operations in which cardiopulmonary bypass has been used, one-third of the normal daily fluid requirement is ordered on the first day. This is slowly increased each day according to the signs of congestive heart failure, the serum sodium determination, and the daily body weight. For cyanotic patients who have had systemic-pulmonary shunts, however, a more liberal intravenous regimen is followed (one-half to two-thirds the normal allotment the first day) to prevent increases in blood viscosity leading to shunt thrombosis. Plasma should usually be used to replace blood loss in these patients to reduce the hematocrit. Infants undergoing major abdominal surgery are usually given one and one-half the daily allotment, because of third-space loss into the peritoneal cavity, retroperitoneum, and intestinal lumen. Plasma should be used to replace blood loss, to reduce the normally high hematocrit.

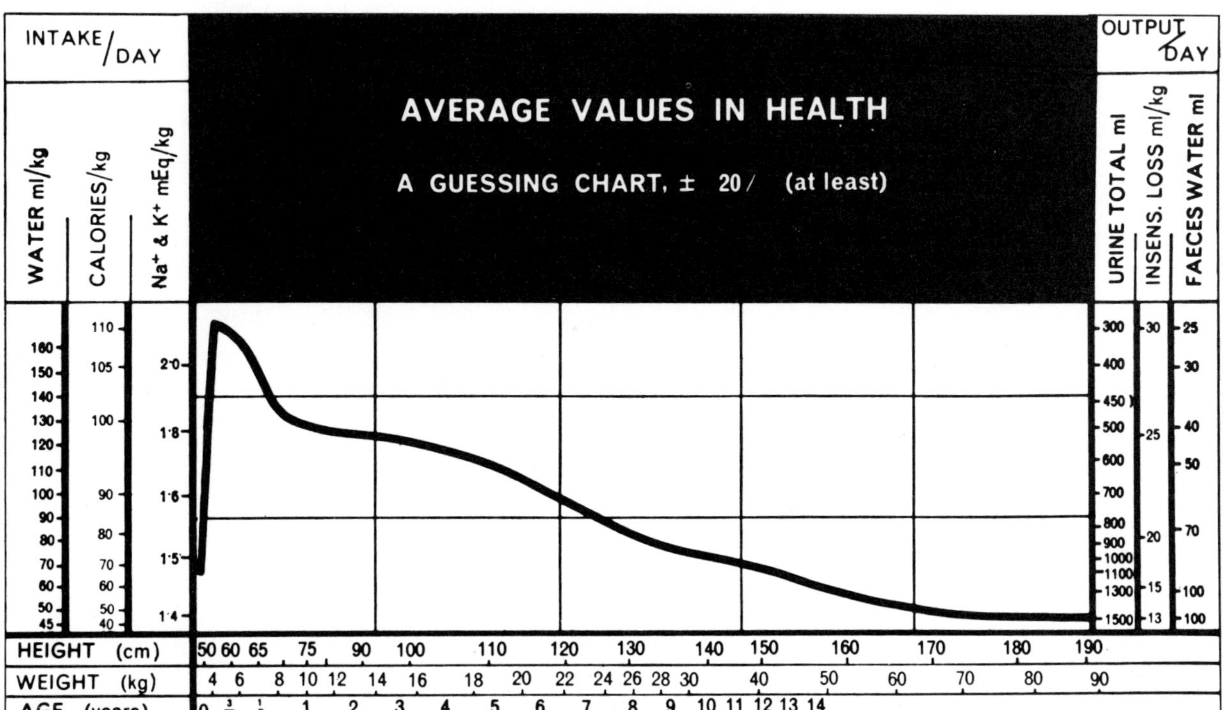

2-2. Nomogram for calculation of fluid requirements and body composition of infants (reproduced by permission of Dr. Eoin Aberdeen).

It is uncommon for children to have cardiac arrhythmias related to potassium depletion or digitalis. Nevertheless, it is wise to determine the serum potassium level several times the first day after cardiac surgery and then at least daily for a few days. Following noncardiac surgery, daily determination of serum potassium should be carried out while the infant is on fluids administered intravenously.

In infants who are profoundly acidotic, some of the excess hydrogen ions are buffered by their movement into cells in exchange for potassium ions. Thus severe intracellular (K^+) depletion develops. After operation, when sodium bicarbonate has been administered to correct the pH and the circulation has been improved, progressive metabolic alkalosis occurs unless intracellular (K^+) is restored by administering potassium chloride in large quantities (for example, 1 milliequivalent per hour) even if the serum (K^+) is normal.

Hyperosmolarity

Sudden increases in an infant's serum osmolarity can result in brain damage and even intracranial hemorrhage from sudden changes in cerebrospinal fluid pressure. It is recommended that no more than a 25-milliosmole (mOsm) increase is safe in any four-hour period. Commonly used hypertonic agents should therefore be administered sparingly and slowly. Sodium bicarbonate, at 3 milliequivalents per kilogram of body weight, will raise the serum osmolarity by 7.5 milliosmoles per kilogram. No more than three doses of this size should be given in a four-hour period. There are 25.2 milliosmoles in 10 milliliters of a 50% glucose solution.

Coagulation Abnormalities

Older infants rarely have serious coagulation abnormalities unless they are severely polycythemic. The newborn is normally deficient in vitamin K, however, and should receive 1 mg intramuscularly before operation. Diffuse intravascular coagulation may be initiated by sepsis or severe hypoxia and should be suspected when troublesome bleeding persists postoperatively.

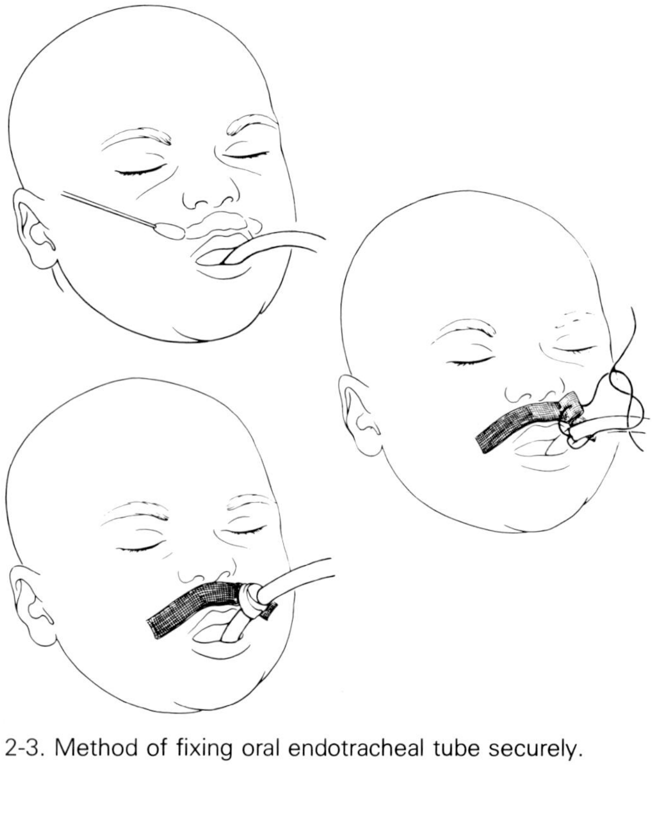

2-3. Method of fixing oral endotracheal tube securely.

Respiratory Care

Provision of proper respiratory support is often the crux of postoperative care in infants who have undergone abdominal or thoracic surgery, just as it is in adults. At the end of operation, a decision must be made about extubation. Vigorous infants who have not had procedures for cardiac conditions or who have had one of the simpler operations for cardiac conditions may be extubated if they were not severely acidotic preoperatively. Most infants who have had major procedures for cardiac conditions should be ventilated postoperatively until fully awake, hemodynamically stable, and free of pulmonary edema. Postoperative ventilation can be carried out satisfactorily for many days through either a nasotracheal tube or an oral endotracheal tube. The nasotracheal tube is somewhat easier to fix in position and is less likely to be dislodged by the infant's chewing it. With proper technique, however, an oral endotracheal tube can be fixed in place securely.

As Figure 2-3 shows, the skin overlying the maxilla is first painted with benzoin. Then a strip of Elastoplast is applied with a fold in the center. A heavy silk ligature is tied around the tube, indenting the wall slightly. The tube is then sutured through the folded Elastoplast. Finally, ½-inch tape is applied over the suture to provide additional stabilization. By this method the tube is secured to the maxilla, which moves relatively little, and saliva will not loosen the fixation.

The tube must be uncuffed and made of nonreactive plastic and, if gas-sterilized, it must be thoroughly aired. To minimize tracheal trauma, it should fit the trachea loosely and not be allowed to slide up and down as the infant moves. The position of the tip must be demonstrated on a chest x-ray film, because it is easy to insert the tube too far. This most commonly results in atelectasis in the upper lobe of the right lung because the tube tends to enter the right bronchus and occlude the upper-lobe branch (Figure 2-4). The nurse caring for the patient should periodically auscultate the chest to be sure both sides are aerating well.

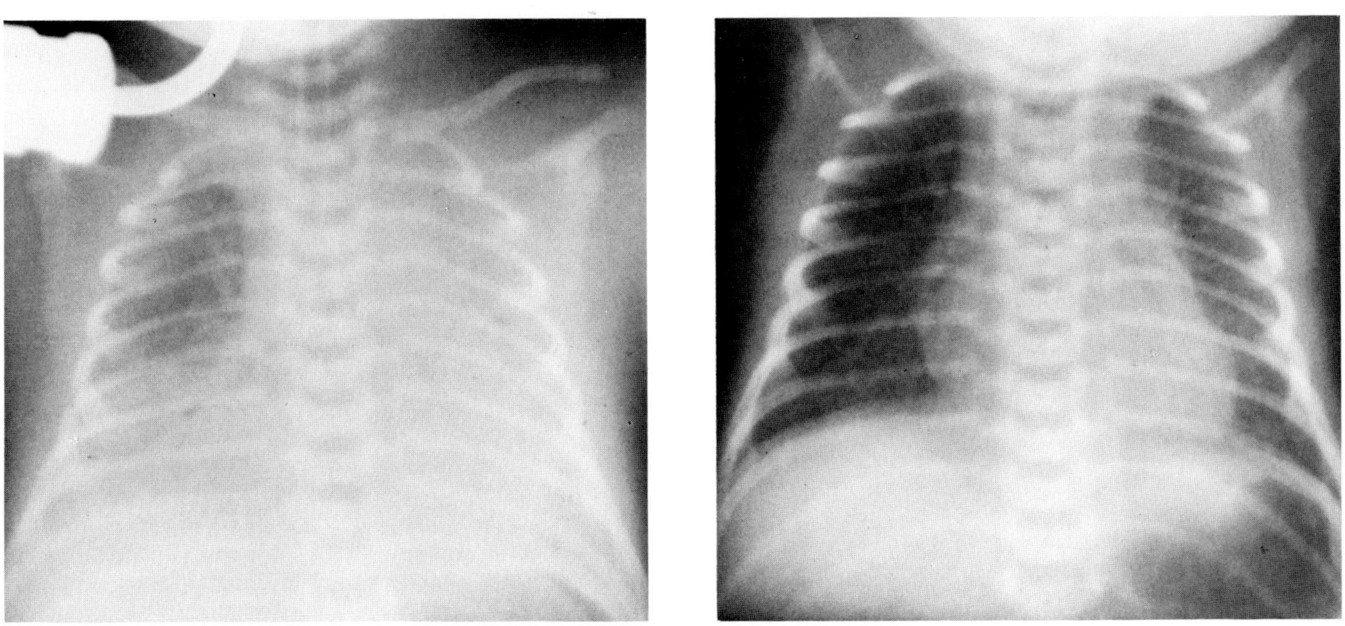

A B

2-4. Chest roentgenograms of an infant illustrating (A) cannulation of right main bronchus by an excessively long endotracheal tube with atelectasis of the left lung. (B) Withdrawal of the tube to the proper position resulted in full expansion of the lung.

The inspired gas must be fully humidified, either through the machine if the patient is being ventilated or by some other means, such as a tent, if he is breathing spontaneously through a tube. The services of skilled chest physiotherapists day and night are important. The airway of an infant is so small that retained secretions will quickly lead to pulmonary collapse if these precautions are not observed. A blocked tube is a certain indictment of inadequate nursing and physical therapy. When there is any suspicion that a tube is becoming plugged, it should be changed immediately.

Perhaps no other information is so useful as that supplied by measurement of arterial gases. These measurements allow accurate assessment of the adequacy of oxygenation, the alveolar ventilation, and the acid-base status. A significantly elevated partial pressure of arterial carbon dioxide ($P\text{CO}_2$) indicates need for intubation and mechanical ventilation. A diminished partial pressure of oxygen ($P\text{O}_2$) may be caused by a ventilation-perfusion imbalance secondary to atelectasis, by pneumonia, by congestive heart failure, or by an obligatory right-to-left cardiac shunt. When the problem is a ventilation-perfusion imbalance, the $P\text{O}_2$ can often be improved by augmenting the inspired oxygen tension ($F\text{IO}_2$) using a tent or incubator. When there is an intracardiac shunt, an operation is usually required to improve oxygenation significantly. From the pH and $P\text{CO}_2$ the base deficit can be determined. From this, the amount of sodium bicarbonate necessary to correct any metabolic acidosis can be calculated. This is illustrated in Figure 2-5, which demonstrates the Siggaard-Andersen curve nomogram.

1. To calculate the base deficit, measure pH and $P\text{CO}_2$. Plot these values on the nomogram, and find the point at which they intersect. Then with a straight edge draw a line through the intersection parallel to the heavy black line. The point at which this line that you are drawing intersects the base-excess curve defines the base excess. To calculate the milliequivalents (mEq) of $NaHCO_3$ required to correct a metabolic acidosis:

$$\text{mEq of HCO}_3 = \frac{\text{Base excess} \times \text{body weight in kg}}{3}$$

For example, a pH of 7.27 with a $P\text{CO}_2$ of 23 gives a base excess of −15. Then, for a 3-kg patient:

$$\text{mEq of HCO}_3 = \frac{15 \times 3}{3} = 15 \text{ mEq}$$

In general, it is good practice to give half the calculated amount, then repeat the blood gas measurements before giving additional bicarbonate.

2. Common patterns of acid-base derangement:

a. Respiratory acidosis: $P\text{CO}_2$ elevated, base excess 0. Treatment: Increase minute ventilation if the patient is on ventilator, or intubate and ventilate if the patient is breathing spontaneously.

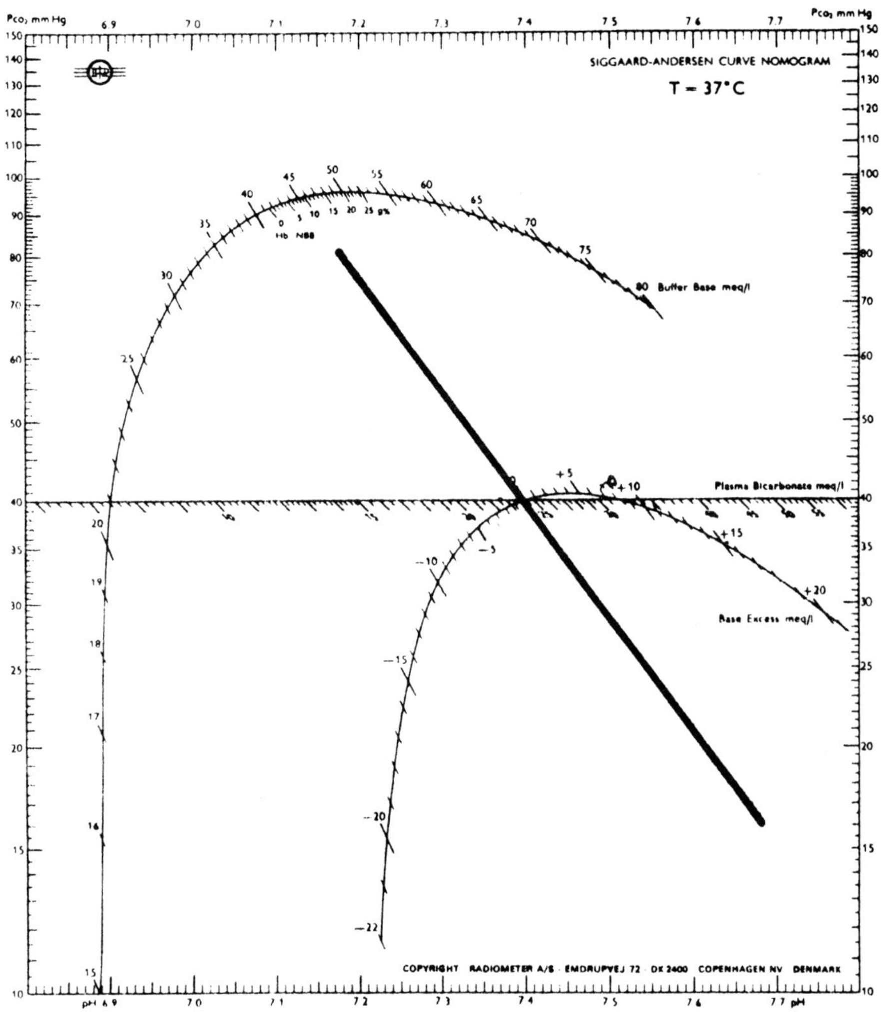

2-5. The Siggaard-Andersen curve nomogram.

b. Metabolic acidosis: P_{CO_2} normal, base excess negative. Treatment: Determine and treat causative problems (for example, poor perfusion), give sodium bicarbonate according to the formula just given.
c. Respiratory alkalosis: P_{CO_2} reduced, base excess 0. Treatment: Reduce minute ventilation if the patient is on ventilator. In general, slight respiratory alkalosis is helpful in reducing respiratory drive of a patient on a ventilator.
d. Metabolic alkalosis: P_{CO_2} normal, base excess positive. Treatment: None, unless pH is elevated significantly (above 7.60). Then give potassium chloride, which will correct the hypokalemia that is usually associated. In severe cases ammonium chloride can be used.

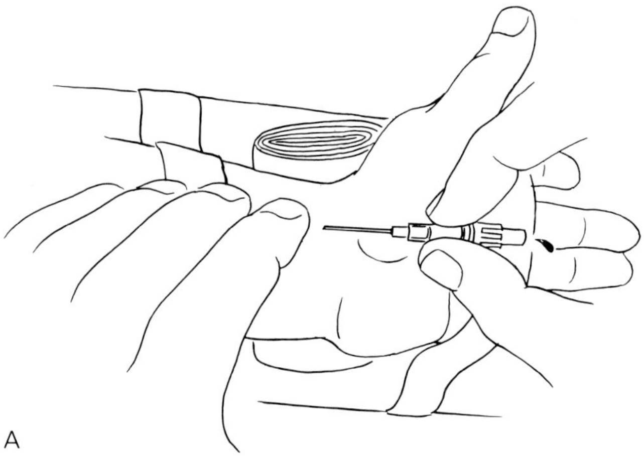
A

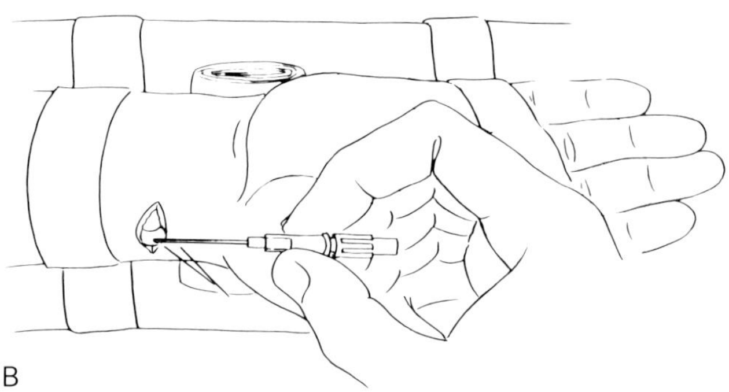
B

2-6. Methods of inserting catheters for monitoring radial artery pressure: (A) percutaneous insertion; (B) insertion under direct vision.

3. Combinations of respiratory and metabolic abnormalities are often encountered. Except in acute situations, it is unusual for pure patterns to persist because normal compensatory mechanisms will intervene to correct the pH. Treatment consists of an appropriate combination of measures, as given in the four parts of paragraph 2.

With practice, repeated arterial punctures can be performed safely in small infants. As in adults, the radial artery is preferred, employing a 2-ml heparinized syringe with a short 22-gauge needle. If precise measurement of Po_2 is not required and if peripheral circulation is good, a capillary sample taken from the infant's (previously heated) heel will give a reasonably accurate estimate of the arterial pH and Pco_2. When frequent blood gas determinations are likely or when a continuous recording of arterial pressure is needed, an arterial catheter is inserted percutaneously or by cutdown.

As illustrated in Figure 2-6, the wrist is extended and fixed to a padded board. (A) To insert catheter percutaneously, first puncture the skin with a number 11 scalpel blade. Then guide an Abbocath-T or similar needle with stylet into the artery by palpation. Once the artery has been entered, be sure to advance the needle into it 1 cm before withdrawing stylet. Rotating the needle 360 degrees as it is advanced helps to guide it up the lumen. (B) To insert catheter under direct vision, dissect artery from its bed on the radial side of the flexor pollicis longus tendon, encircle it with a ligature for countertraction, insert catheter, remove ligature, and suture incision. The catheter must then be secured by sutures and tape in such a way that it cannot be dislodged.

Oxygen toxicity occurs in two forms in infants. First, retrolental fibroplasia is a hazard in premature infants who have been given high concentrations of oxygen. Permanent eye damage has occurred when arterial Po_2 has exceeded 110 mm Hg for longer than one or two hours. Second, bronchopulmonary dysplasia occurs when ventilation with an oxygen concentration of more than 70 percent is carried out for longer than four or five days. Therefore levels of arterial blood gas must be monitored closely and the inspired oxygen concentration reduced as much as possible in infants, especially if they are premature.

Positive End-Expiratory Pressure

Recently it has become evident that patients receiving respiratory assistance tend to accumulate interstitial water in the lungs, which leads to decreased compliance and poor oxygenation. Possible causative factors are: increased water permeability of damaged capillaries; decreased surfactant; diminished plasma oncotic pressure; increased secretion of antidiuretic hormone; the poorly understood effects of homologous blood transfusion; and left atrial hypertension. Increased interstitial water in the lungs may be reflected as an increased alveolar-arterial oxygen gradient (a-ADO_2) and decreased compliance. Vigorous diuresis often results in dramatic improvement in the PO_2 and is one of the mainstays of postoperative respiratory care. With brisk diuresis, the blood volume may decrease, and infusion of salt-poor albumin, plasma, or packed cells may be required to maintain the intravascular space while the extravascular space is dried out.

Another useful adjunct in the treatment of hypoxia is the application of positive end-expiratory pressure (PEEP), which reverses the progressive alveolar collapse that results from constant volume ventilation and which also inhibits the accumulation of interstitial water in the lungs. Positive end-expiratory pressure can be easily applied by connecting a tube to the expiratory port of the respirator and placing the end the desired distance into a container of water, usually starting at a depth of 5 to 10 cm. Most respirators now have a built-in capability to deliver PEEP. In rare instances the cardiac output decreases because of the increase in pulmonary vascular resistance and the decrease in venous return caused by PEEP, which limits the usefulness of PEEP application. Usually, however, application of PEEP results in prompt improvement in arterial PO_2, followed by clearing of edema when edema is evident radiographically.

Continuous Positive Airway Pressure

Positive end-expiratory pressure can also be applied to patients who are breathing spontaneously. This was originally described by Gregory [3] as a way to lower the death rate from hyaline membrane disease in newborn infants and it was called continuous positive airway pressure (CPAP) breathing. We and others have used it principally in infants following cardiac surgery as a compromise between extubation and mechanical ventilation. It is sometimes difficult to ventilate small infants with a volume ventilator because they may breathe out of phase or require heavy sedation. Furthermore, pulmonary dysfunction may be worsened by the combination of mechanical ventilation and oxygen toxicity. CPAP obviates these disadvantages, increases the arterial PO_2 so that the FIO_2 can be reduced, prevents microatelectasis, and counteracts pulmonary edema. Of course, the patients must be sufficiently alert and strong so that they can breathe spontaneously. Although we have applied it postoperatively by means of an indwelling endotracheal tube, it may also be applied with specially designed nasal prongs, a method that takes advantage of the fact that infants breathe exclusively through the nose.

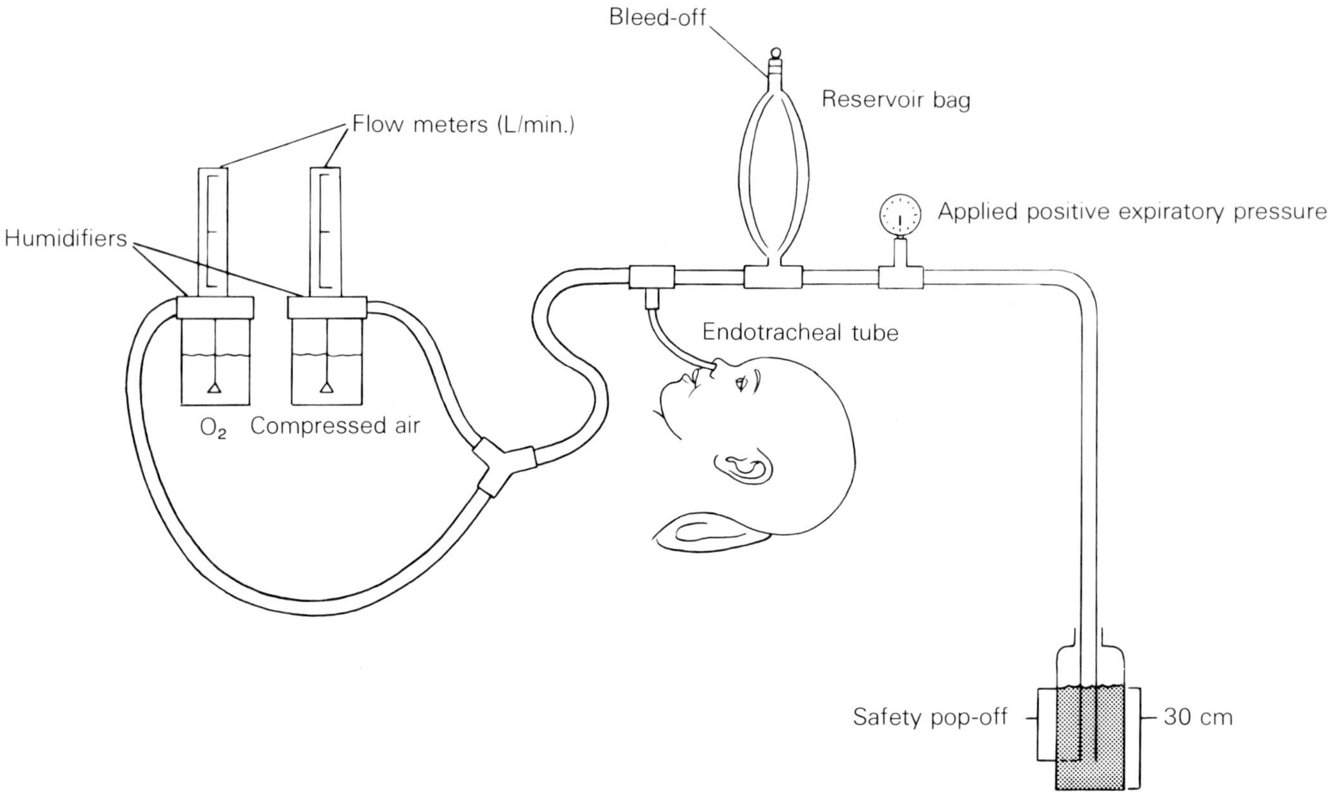

2-7. Continuous positive airway pressure (CPAP) can be administered to spontaneously ventilating patient by systems such as this.

CPAP can be administered to spontaneously ventilating patients by a system such as that illustrated in Figure 2-7. Humidified oxygen and air are mixed to give the desired FI_{O_2}. The total flow rate of gases must be at least 2.5 times the patient's volume per minute to prevent the patient from rebreathing exhaled CO_2. The bleed-off from the reservoir bag is adjusted by a Hofmann clamp to result in a desired reading on the manometer dial (usually 3 to 10 mm Hg), which is the level of CPAP applied to the patient. A water trap provides a safety pop-off in case the pressure in the airway should suddenly rise; for example, if the bleed-off valve should inadvertently become occluded.

One major hazard of PEEP and CPAP at high levels of pressure is their tendency to produce tension pneumothorax. This must be ruled out immediately when the condition of one of these patients deteriorates. We usually do not remove the chest tubes until PEEP has been discontinued.

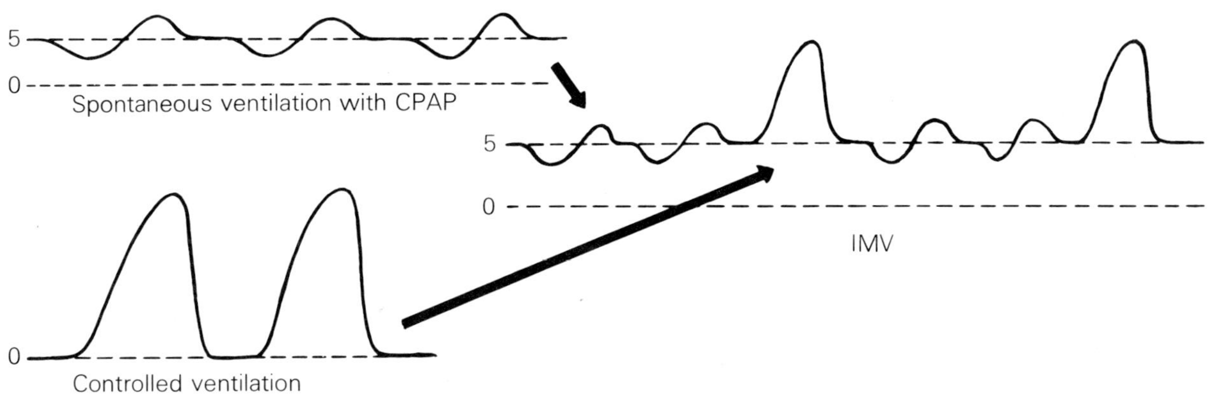

2-8. Intermittent mandatory ventilation (IMV).

Intermittent Mandatory Ventilation

An extremely useful variation of CPAP in infants has been made possible by the recent introduction of a new type of ventilator, exemplified by the "Baby Bird." In this system the patient can breathe humidified gas spontaneously, and the respirator will augment this with periodic "mandatory" breaths at any desired rate. This is called intermittent mandatory ventilation (IMV). As illustrated in Figure 2-8, the CPAP system is modified so that the ventilator can periodically inflate the patient's lungs through a one-way valve, thereby augmenting the patient's spontaneous breathing. This provides a useful compromise between spontaneous ventilation with CPAP (top left) and conventional controlled mechanical ventilation (bottom left). Because it is unnecessary to phase the patient's breathing with the machine, he need not be heavily sedated. The machine's rate can initially be set high, so that the patient's ventilation is effectively taken over. During weaning, the rate can be progressively reduced until the machine is providing only a few breaths per minute. This makes the transition between total ventilatory support and spontaneous breathing smoother and easier than with the older system of switching from machine to T-piece periodically. Furthermore, PEEP can easily be employed with this system by adjusting a dial on the respirator.

Feeding (Enteral and Parenteral)

It is generally agreed (without experimental support) that sucking is a severe exercise tolerance test for an infant. Certainly one of the initial signs of congestive heart failure is poor feeding, and as the infant's condition improves, so does his oral intake.

When the acute hemodynamic problems have subsided and the abdomen is soft (usually two to three days), feeding

Table 2-1. Contents of central infusate (Hyprotigen[a]-dextrose)

Constituent	Content per Liter
Protein hydrolysate	30.0 g
Dextrose (hydrous)	196.6 g
Sodium[b]	15.0 mEq
Potassium[b]	16.0 mEq
Calcium	27.0 mEq
Phosphorus	19.0 mEq
Magnesium	7.6 mEq
Chloride[b]	10.8 mEq
Folic acid	0.5 mg
Multivitamin infusion[c]	5.0 ml
Vitamin K_1	0.2 mg
Vitamin B_{12}	6.6 μg

[a]Casein hydrolysate, McGaw Laboratories, North Irvine, California.
[b]Further adjusted at bedside.
[c]U.S. Vitamin and Pharmaceutical Corporation, New York, New York.
Each liter provides 4.8 grams nitrogen and 800 Calories.

is initiated, orally, through a gastrostomy, or through a nasogastric feeding tube, starting with 5 ml hourly of 5% dextrose in water, then using half-strength then full-strength formula, decreasing the intravenous feedings as the enteral feedings are sequentially increased. It is easiest to specify the 24-hour fluid limit and to allow the nurses to increase the enteral feedings gradually and to decrease the intravenous feedings by equal amounts to meet that amount. If progress is satisfactory, the abdomen should remain soft and bowel movements should begin.

Not infrequently, diarrhea develops with resumption of alimentation. Usually it is sufficient to switch to oral administration of 5% dextrose in water until the diarrhea subsides. Then half-strength feedings and full-strength feedings are sequentially resumed.

The infant may need a pacifier to satisfy his urge to suck. Once he is on full enteral feedings and is sucking well (usually after just a few days), all his feeding is oral with the feeding tube in place. Supplements are given through the tube until he is taking everything by mouth.

If after surgery the infant is unable to feed by way of the alimentary tract within five days, then intravenous nutrition should be initiated. The nutrient solution can be administered into a central venous catheter or into peripheral veins. Our preference is the peripheral route, employing a fat emulsion; if this proves unsuccessful, which is rare, we will then start central venous hyperalimentation.

Solution for Central Hyperalimentation

The composition of the solution for central hyperalimentation is listed in Table 2-1. Half-strength solutions (basic formula diluted in half with 5% dextrose in water) are also prepared by the pharmacy and they are used primarily during the first day or two of therapy. During this period the child is adapting to the very high glucose load, and the high concentration of glucose may produce an osmotic diuresis that will lead to hypertonic dehydration. As the patient's tolerance develops, judged from diminishing glycosuria, full-strength solutions may be used. Administration of insulin is not necessary for nondiabetic children. Iron requirements are met either by weekly intramuscular injections of iron dextran or by blood transfusion. Trace metals are not routinely added to the basic mixture.

Solutions for Peripheral Feeding with Fat

For peripheral feeding with fat, the infusate consists of two separate bottles; one bottle contains only the fat emulsion Intralipid,* and the other bottle contains the amino acids, glucose, electrolytes, and vitamins. Table 2-2 lists the infusate

*Cutter Laboratories, Berkeley, California.

contents for infants. The total number of Calories administered can be increased by infusion of more fat (up to 5 g per kg of body weight per day) or more 10% glucose, or both. The bottle containing the amino acids is prepared aseptically under a laminar flow hood in the hospital pharmacy. Essential fatty acids are present in the Intralipid in large quantities.

Solution for Peripheral Feeding without Fat

A stock solution of 10% Amigen is used to make up the infusate. The mixing is also carried out in the hospital pharmacy under a laminar flow hood. The amino acid solution is diluted with glucose to make up a 2% protein hydrolysate in a 12% glucose solution. The final solution contains 0.56 Calorie per milliliter. Electrolytes are added to the infusate to provide the recommended daily requirements plus additional needs based on the patient's clinical condition. The concentrations of electrolytes and vitamins are essentially the same as those recommended for central feeding and peripheral feeding with fat. Heparin at 0.5 unit per milliliter is added to the solution to reduce phlebitis. In addition, the major portion of the essential fatty acids needed is supplied through daily application of sunflower-seed oil to the skin of the infant's chest. For both peripheral venous methods of feeding, the administration of iron is as described in the central feeding program. Trace metals are given as necessary.

Methods for Central Feeding

Hypertonic infusates must be delivered through a central venous catheter to avoid peripheral venous inflammation and thrombosis. For this purpose, a silicone rubber catheter is passed through the internal or external jugular vein to the superior vena cava. This procedure is best carried out in an operating room or cardiac catheterization laboratory, where adequate exposure, proper instruments, and strict aseptic conditions are available. To minimize bloodstream contamination, the venous catheter is tunneled from the vein entry point to an exit site on the skin that is placed two to four inches away. In the infant it is brought out on the scalp; in the older child the exit site may be the neck or an upper extremity. Central venous intubation by percutaneous puncture of the subclavian vein has also been used. The silicone rubber venous line may be left in place until the completion of therapy unless it becomes accidentally dislodged or septic complications develop.

The central venous catheter can be inserted under local or general anesthesia. The head is turned to the side and the scalp is carefully shaved. A transverse incision, 1 to 2 cm long, is made over the sternocleidomastoid muscle at the junction of the middle and lower thirds of the neck. The external jugular vein is ordinarily preferred and can usually be successfully cannulated, even in the premature infant. If either external jugular vein is unavailable because of previous

Table 2-2. Protocol for peripheral intravenous feeding of infants with fat

Constituent	Volume (ml per kg body wt per 24 hr)	Amount (g per kg body wt per 24 hr)	Calories (kilo-calories)
10% Intralipid	40	4	44
5% Amigen[a] in 5% glucose	80	4 (protein)	32
10% glucose	30	3	12
	—		—
Total volume	150		
Total Calories			88

[a]Manufactured by McGaw Laboratories, North Irvine, California. The crystalline amino acid solution Fre-Amine can be used instead of the protein hydrolysate Amigen.

Table 2-3. Peripheral hyperalimentation without fat

Constituent	Amount per kilogram per 24 hours	
Water	200 to 250	ml
Protein	4 to 5	g
Glucose	24 to 30	g
Calories	112 to 140	Cal
Heparin	100	IU
Sodium	2 to 4	mEq
Potassium	2 to 3	mEq
Chloride	2 to 4	mEq
Magnesium	0.6	mEq
Calcium	1.0	mEq
Phosphate	3.5	mM

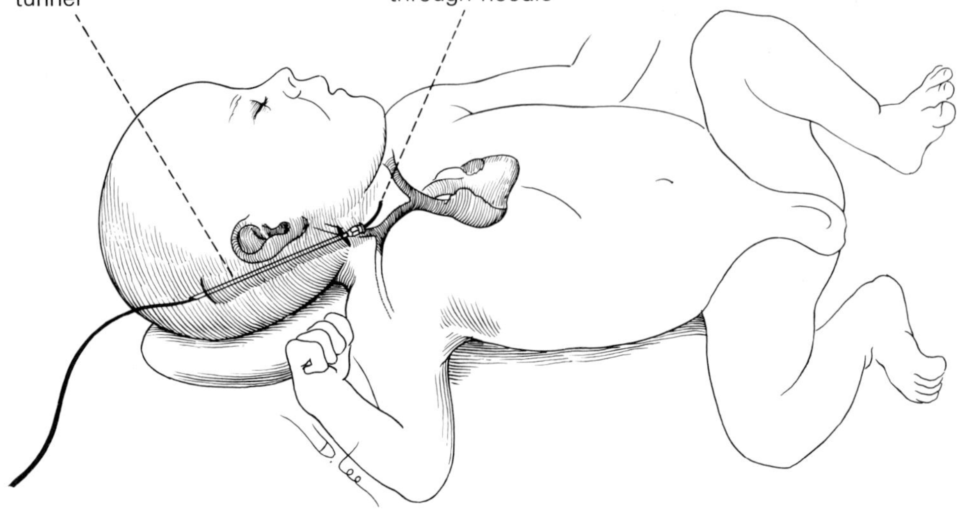

2-9. Insertion and fixation of silicone rubber central venous catheter in an infant.

use or small caliber, however, or if entrance of the catheter from the external jugular vein into the vena cava is not possible, the internal jugular vein can be used for cannulation. A long hollow needle with an obturator in place is passed beneath the skin of the neck from the incision to the scalp (Figure 2-9). If the internal jugular vein is being used, the needle pierces also the belly of the sternocleidomastoid muscle. After the obturator is removed, the silicone rubber catheter (for an infant, the internal diameter is 0.025 inch and the outside diameter is 0.047 inch) is passed through the needle. When the needle is withdrawn, the catheter resides in its subcutaneous tract. Before cannulation, the vein is ligated distally and an incision is made between this point and a proximal controlling ligature. If the internal jugular vein has been selected, ligature of the vein can sometimes be avoided by passing the cannula into the vein through an incision made in the center of a pursestring suture. The jugular vein is then cannulated and the tubing is advanced to the region of the right atrium (approximately 5 cm in an infant). Occasionally some manipulation is necessary to obtain entry into the superior vena cava from the external jugular vein. The exact location of the catheter is confirmed radiographically by taking a single x-ray with the catheter filled with radiopaque contrast material.

Antibiotics are administered only when indicated by the child's primary illness, but not specifically to prevent sepsis that might occur from the presence of a central venous line. An antibacterial ointment and a sterile dressing are applied to the exit site on the skin, and, to avoid accidental displacement, a coil of catheter is included in the dressing. Every two days the dressing is removed aseptically, the skin is cleansed with an antiseptic, and a sterile dressing and antibacterial ointment are reapplied. Povidone-iodine (Betadine) ointment is now used routinely because of its effectiveness against both bacteria and fungi. Before the infusion is started, a Millipore filter (0.22μ) is placed in-line to remove particulate matter, microorganisms that may have contaminated the solution, or both. A calibrated buret is placed in the circuit to monitor accurately the volume delivered.

The infusate must be delivered at a slow, uniform rate to ensure proper utilization of the glucose and amino acids. In the small infant this is most readily accomplished by the use of a constant-infusion pump. The entire system is locally referred to as the "lifeline." Figure 2-10 shows such a sys-

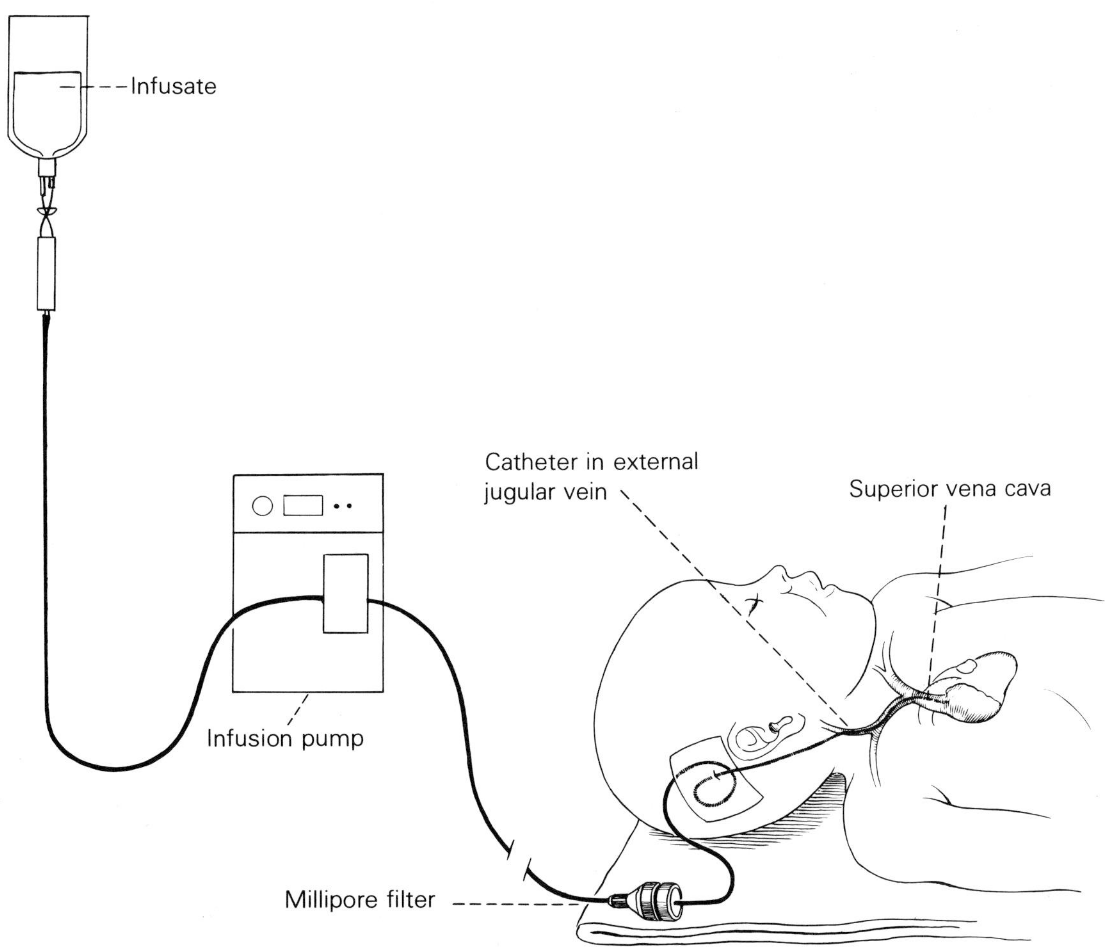

2-10. System for long-term central total parenteral nutrition.

tem for long-term total parenteral nutrition. The amino acid and dextrose infusate flows through a calibrated buret. An infusion pump ensures a uniform hourly flow. The Millipore filter in the circuit will remove any microorganisms that may have contaminated the system. The venous catheter enters the scalp behind the ear. The appropriate position of the catheter in the superior vena cava is confirmed radiographically.

Method for Peripheral Feeding with Fat

In infants a 21- or 23-gauge scalp vein needle (sometimes even a 25-gauge needle) is inserted into a peripheral vein, usually in the scalp, and the intravenous tubing from the bottle containing the amino acids is connected to this needle (Figure 2-11). The tubing from the Intralipid bottle is then inserted into the rubber nipple at the end of the tubing from the first bottle ("piggy-backed"). The tubing from the In-

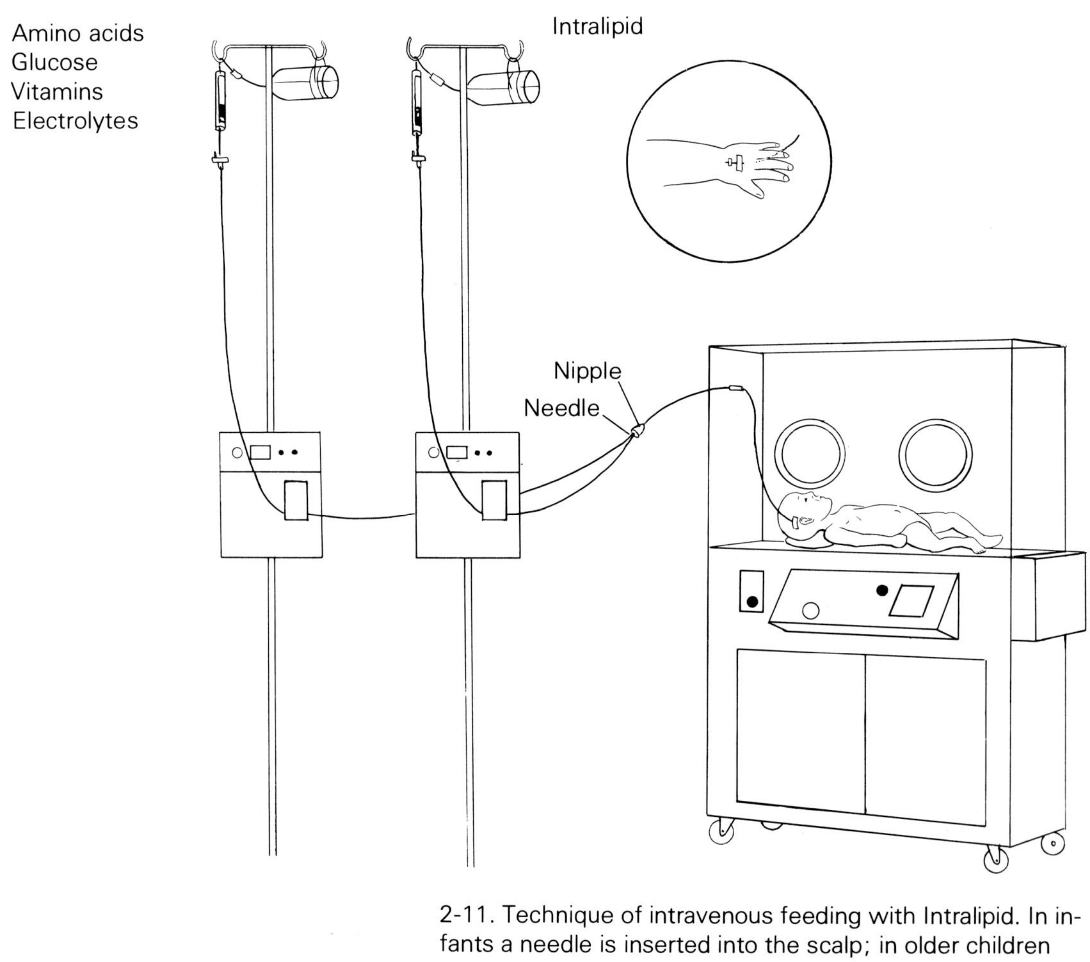

2-11. Technique of intravenous feeding with Intralipid. In infants a needle is inserted into the scalp; in older children the veins on the dorsum of the hand are generally used.

tralipid bottle is secured with tape to the tubing from the amino acid bottle. A calibrated buret is placed in each intravenous line, and both bottles are infused over a 24-hour period using two separate constant-infusion pumps. The 24-hour infusion with two separate pumps is employed to ensure proper utilization of the administered fat, glucose, and amino acids. No filters are used because these would block the infusion of the fat. Because of infiltration, the needle usually must be changed every three to four days.

Method for Peripheral Feeding without Fat

The techniques involved here are no different from those used for routine intravenous infusions. The entire solution is contained in one bottle and is infused into a small needle placed into a peripheral vein in the scalp or an extremity. A Millipore filter (0.22μ) is placed in-line, and the infusion is run over 24 hours, for the various reasons already discussed. The sites for intravenous infusions last 24 to 48 hours and are changed promptly when signs of infiltration or phlebitis are noted. Warm soaks placed over the infiltrated skin reduce the swelling rather quickly. In rare instances a small skin slough results, which heals fairly rapidly with local care.

Metabolic Observations

Clinical measurements that are essential include daily body weight, accurate volume of urine, and other body-fluid losses. The urine sugar content is monitored at each voiding. The important blood tests and the frequency of study in the usual patient are given in Table 2-4. More frequent monitoring of some variables may be necessary in patients with specific metabolic abnormalities, for instance, in patients with renal or hepatic disease.

Precise control of administration of fluids and electrolytes is mandatory. Infusion pumps are useful if they work reliably. A skilled nurse can keep open several intravenous lines with a limit of 5 ml per hour. The volume of fluid used in flushing the monitoring lines must be included as input.

Table 2-4. Blood values monitored routinely during total parenteral nutrition

At Start of Therapy and Weekly	At Start of Therapy and Every 2 Weeks	As Indicated
Na, K, Cl	SGOT, LDH, alkaline phosphatase	Copper
Urea	Bilirubin	Zinc
Glucose	Creatinine	Iron
Magnesium		Ammonia
Calcium, phosphorus		Osmolarity
Total protein		pH
Hemoglobin, hematocrit, white blood count		
Blood culture		
Candida precipitins		
Platelets		

Counseling of Parents

When an infant undergoes major surgery, the parents experience great emotional stress, especially if the child does not survive. Inevitably they experience guilt feelings and they may blame themselves or someone else for the loss. This attitude should be discussed with them. They should be reassured that congenital anomalies are usually random events, out of their control except in certain uncommon genetically inherited conditions. It is not helpful to suggest that earlier action on their part or earlier referral by the family physician might have altered the outcome.

Most parents are also concerned about the possibility that subsequent children might be born with defects. After one child is born with a congenital anomaly, the odds that another child in the family will be so affected are somewhat greater than they are in the general population. This risk is, however, still low enough not to influence the parents' planning unduly. We therefore usually encourage parents to have more children if that is their wish unless we recognize that the family is afflicted by one of the very rare genetically transmitted abnormalities.

Selected References

1. Behrendt, D. M., and Austen, W. G. *Patient Care in Cardiac Surgery.* 2d ed. Boston: Little, Brown and Company, 1976.
2. Filler, R. M., and Coran, A. G. Total parenteral nutrition in infants and children: Central and peripheral approaches. *Surg. Clin. N. Am.* 56:395, 1976.
3. Gregory, G. A., Kitterman, J. A., Phibbs, R. H., Tooley, W. H., and Hamilton, W. Treatment of idiopathic respiratory distress syndrome with continuous positive airway pressure. *N. Engl. J. Med.* 284:1333, 1971.
4. Mustard, W. T., Ravitch, M. M., Snyder, W. H., Jr., et al. (eds.). *Pediatric Surgery.* Chicago: Year Book Medical Publishers, 1969.

3

Tracheostomy

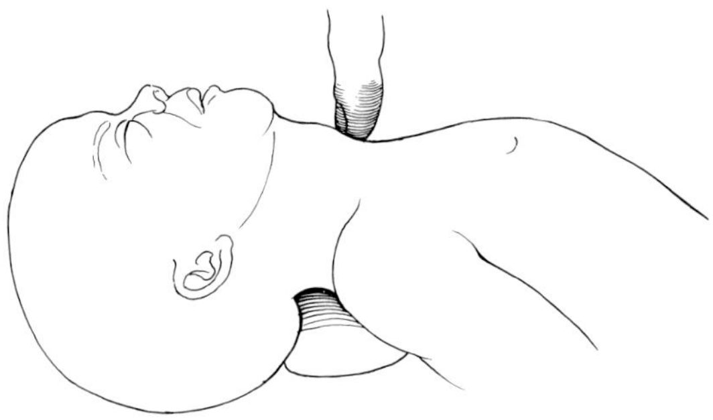

3-1a

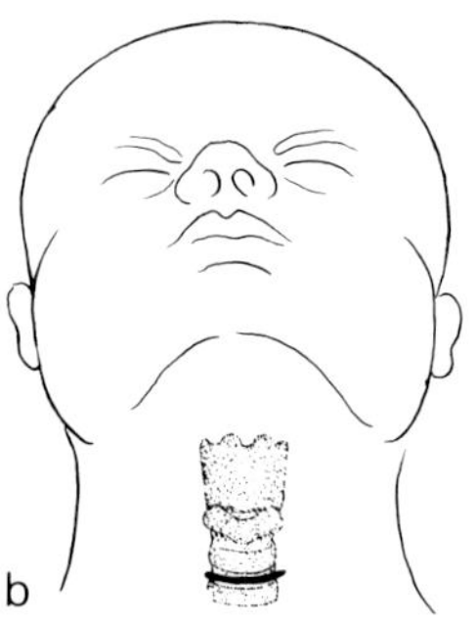

3-1b

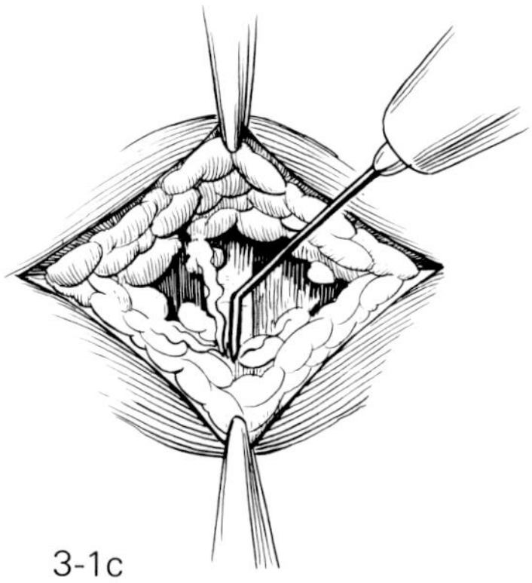

3-1c

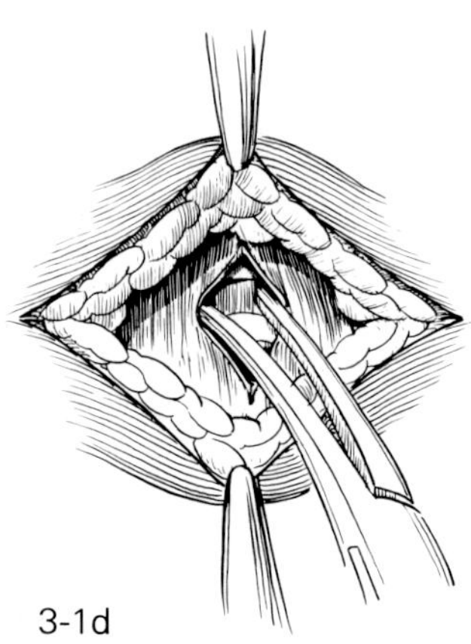

3-1d

Tracheostomy is usually performed in neonates to provide a means of long-term ventilatory support in the postoperative patient, the patient with primary pulmonary insufficiency, the patient with a severe upper airway malformation, or the patient with central nervous system malfunction. The operation is performed less frequently than heretofore because of increased success with prolonged orotracheal and nasotracheal intubation. When ventilatory support is required for more than two weeks, however, we believe tracheostomy is indicated.

Preparation for Operation

No infant should undergo tracheostomy without prior endotracheal intubation, except for the rare infant with mechanical obstruction of the upper airway that precludes intubation. Tracheostomy in the infant should *never* be attempted outside the operating room and it must be performed with general anesthesia, ideal lighting, and proper exposure, suction, and equipment. With these precautions, it is a straightforward, safe procedure.

Operative Technique*

The infant is placed in the supine position with the neck *maximally* extended on an unyielding pack such as a sandbag or rubber wedge, as in Figure 3-1a. This not only serves to provide exposure of the neck but also tenses the trachea and draws its upper portion out of the mediastinum.

The tracheal rings are palpated with the fingernail. It is essential that the cricoid cartilage be identified, because it *must not* be damaged during the procedure.

A transverse skin incision 1 cm long is made over the second tracheal ring; see Figure 3-1b. The infant's skin is very elastic, and this small incision can be readily dilated with a hemostat to allow adequate exposure.

The incision is deepened through the subcutaneous tissues with a needle-point cautery while the skin edges are held apart with fine hemostats (Figure 3-1c). During this and each other step of the operation, *absolute* hemostasis must be obtained.

The strap muscles are teased apart with a fine hemostat, and any blood vessels are cauterized (Figure 3-1d). If necessary, the thyroid isthmus can be divided with the cautery to expose the trachea. Before incising the trachea, the surgeon must be sure that the necessary tracheostomy tubes are at hand and that any adapters necessary to make connection to the anesthesia tubing are available. Small, self-retaining retractors are a great help in obtaining satisfactory exposure.

*Adapted from the techniques developed by Dr. Eoin Aberdeen at the Hospital for Sick Children, Great Ormond Street, London.

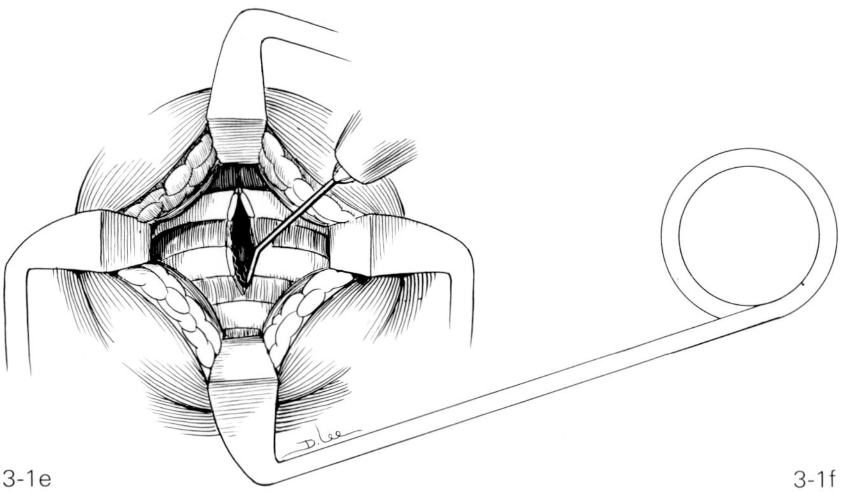

3-1e

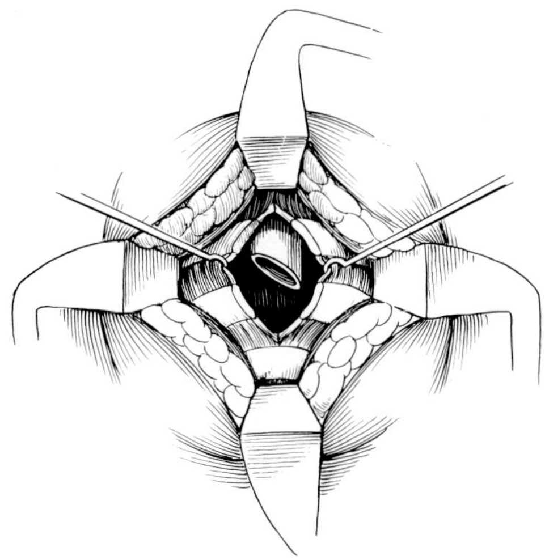

3-1f

(Those illustrated were homemade by attaching blades to a large stainless steel safety pin.) A longitudinal incision through the second and third rings is made with the cautery (Figure 3-1e). The incision must be long enough to allow the trachea to fall open, allowing easy insertion of the tracheostomy tube. Tracheal cartilage is *never* excised in an infant. To do so will lead to loss of tracheal support, with subsequent stricture, and is absolutely unnecessary.

The two cut tracheal edges are held apart with fine skin hooks, and the tracheal incision is enlarged if necessary.

Then under direct vision the anesthetist withdraws the endotracheal tube until its tip is just proximal to the tracheostomy (Figure 3-1f). This tube should *not* be removed until the tracheostomy tube is fixed in position and proved to be satisfactory.

The tracheostomy tube is then inserted into the trachea under direct vision (Figure 3-1g). The tube chosen should be just large enough to fit into the trachea with minimal force. Metal tubes are never used. The flexible plastic tubes manufactured by Shiley, Inc., have proved very satisfactory.

While the retractors and skin hooks are still in place, the anesthetist administers a deep inflation through the tracheostomy tube to determine whether it is airtight. If there is a large air leak, the tube is removed and the next larger size is inserted. (Cuffed tracheostomy tubes are never used in infants.)

Finally, the retractors are removed, and, while *someone holds the tube in place*, the tube is tied securely with tapes encircling the neck (Figure 3-1h). The neck must be flexed to allow the tapes to be tightened sufficiently, and the tapes must be padded to prevent skin damage. Foam rubber with adhesive backing is very satisfactory for this purpose. No one except the surgeon is permitted to loosen these ties until the stoma is well established, in three to five days (Figure 3-1i).

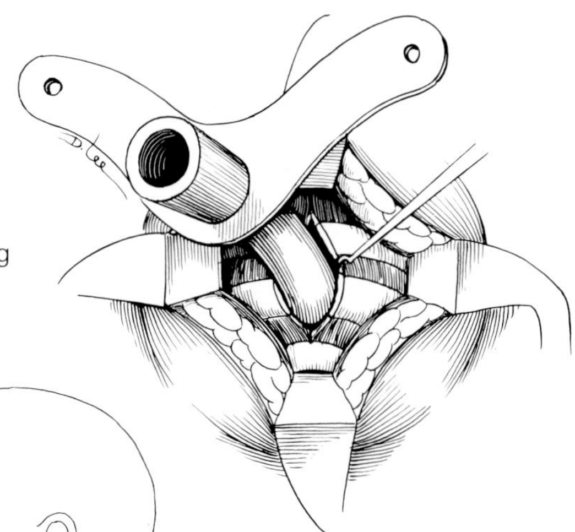

3-1g

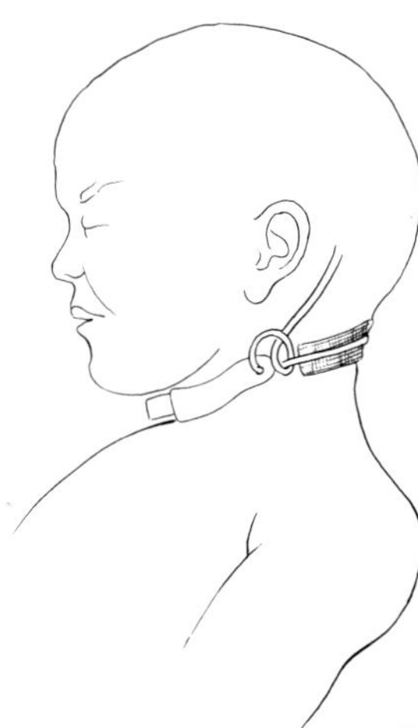

3-1h

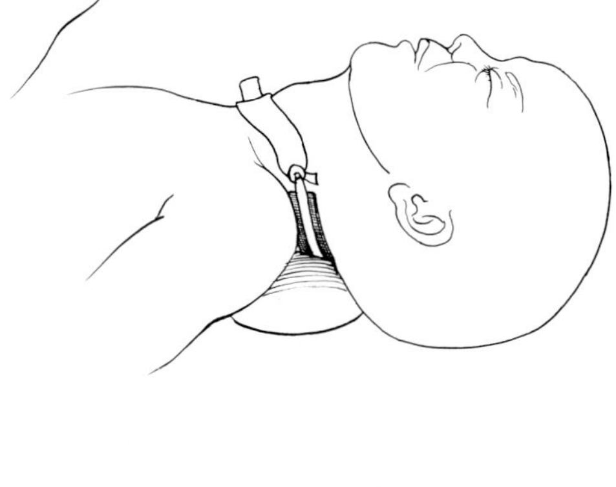

3-1i

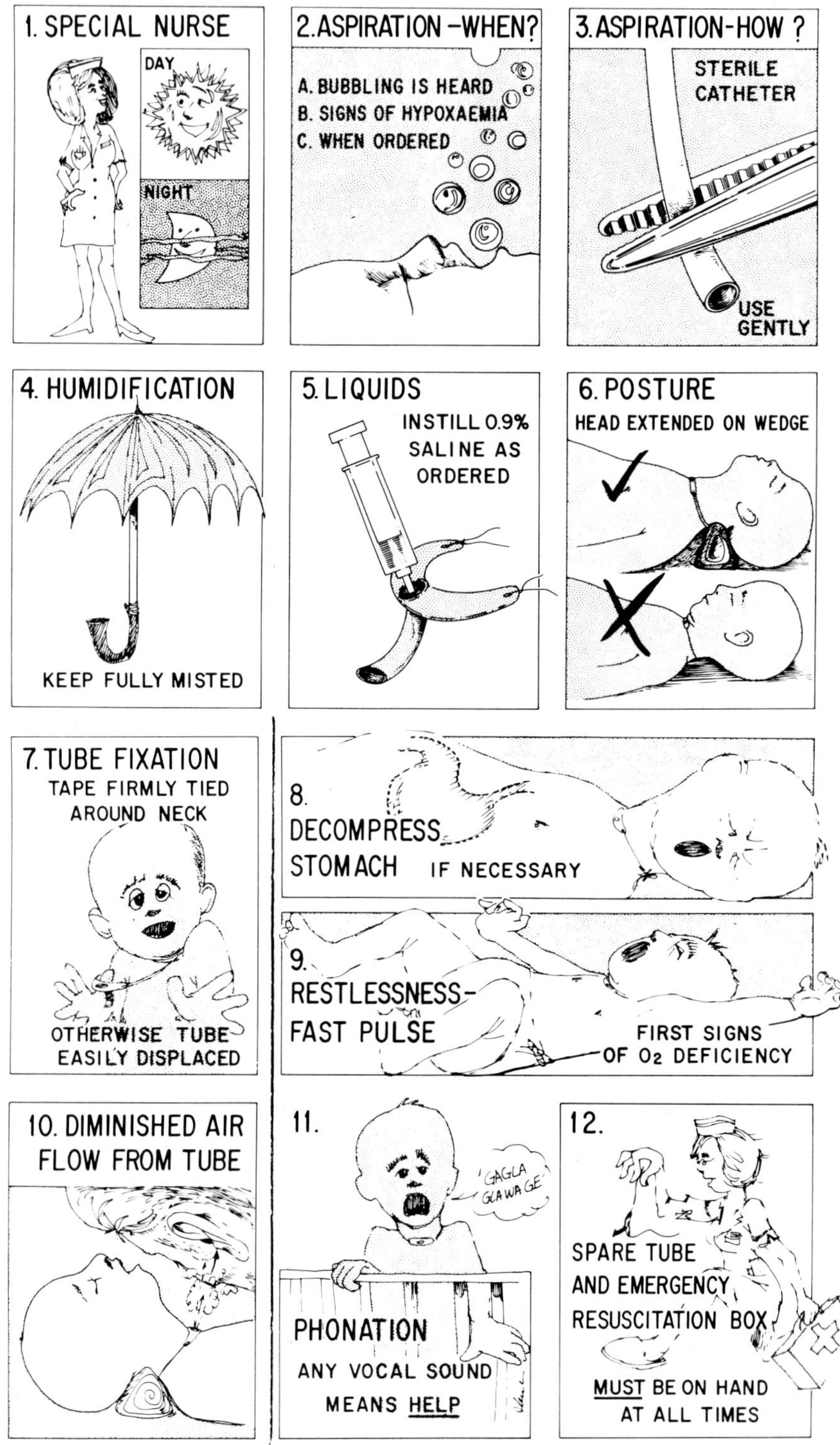

3-2. Tracheostomy nursing care (adapted from educational materials from Hospital for Sick Children, Great Ormond Street, London).

The trachea is then irrigated with 2 ml of saline solution and suctioned. Both sides of the chest are auscultated, and a chest film is obtained to verify the proper position of the tip of the tube *just* above the carina.

In small infants the tip of the tube may extend into the right bronchus. This can be corrected by placing some padding under the flange of the tube to lift it out of the neck slightly. Alternatively, this tube may be cut slightly shorter with scissors, but it must be realized that this increases the risk of inadvertent extubation.

Postoperative Care

Proper nursing care of the infant with a fresh tracheostomy is essential to success. Once the stoma of the tracheostomy has become established, suctioning can be less frequent and humidification less religiously maintained. Occasionally we have successfully managed over a long time infants with tracheostomies who were at home.

We have never failed to extubate an infant because of a complication of the tracheostomy itself, although we have failed when a subglottic stricture had been previously caused by an endotracheal tube.

At the time of extubation the child should be returned to intensive care and placed in a mist tent. His tracheal secretions should be thin and his lungs free of active infection. After the tube has been removed, the stoma should be occluded to be sure that ventilation through the larynx is unobstructed. If there is any hint of stridor, an elective bronchoscopy should be performed. Occasionally a mass of granulation tissue from the stoma protrudes into the trachea, occluding it; the tissue must be removed. Removal is most easily done by revising the stoma from outside rather than endoscopically.

Selected Reference

Aberdeen, E. Tracheostomy in Infants. Page 223 in Rob, C., and Smith, R. *Operative Surgery*. 2d ed. Vol. 1. Philadelphia: J. B. Lippincott Co., 1968.

4

Cystic Hygroma and Other Lesions of the Head and Neck

are removed in five to seven days or when drainage is no longer present. Dressings are not used on the patient because they prevent daily observation of the wound and usually will not stay in place. Because delayed respiratory obstruction may follow this type of surgery, cardiorespiratory monitoring should be maintained, particularly at the time when oral feedings are begun.

Complications

Considerable swelling invariably follows resection of cystic hygromas. Differentiation between recurrence and edema is not possible for weeks or months. Surgery 6 to 12 months later on the residual lesion is frequently curative. The fact that cystic hygroma is almost never encountered in adults implies that many such lesions spontaneously regress.

Trauma to the mandibular branch of the facial nerve should be rare; extreme care should be taken to avoid injury to this structure. If paresis occurs, it is usually the result of edema and is temporary.

Acute infection or hemorrhage of the remaining cystic hygroma should be treated conservatively. Antibiotics are often helpful. Infections are occasionally followed by spontaneous regression. If surgery is necessary, however, a delay of two to three months should make the operative procedure less difficult. Radiation therapy is not indicated in the treatment of cystic hygroma.

Results

Operative mortality for newborns with cystic hygroma should be less than 2 percent. The cosmetic result varies but is almost always satisfactory.

Hemangiomas

Abnormalities of the blood vessels with resultant hemangioma are by no means rare in the head and neck of infants. The lesions are not often noted at birth but, rather, appear seven to ten days later and grow rapidly. The most common type encountered is the mixed capillary and cavernous hemangioma. These lesions grow quickly and often appear grotesque. Spontaneous regression, however, is the rule. Therefore surgery is to be avoided, because it is difficult, bloody, incomplete, and dangerous. If left alone, the hemangioma will disappear, leaving a surprisingly good cosmetic result.

The larger masses can trap platelets, producing a coagulopathy with associated local and systemic hemorrhage. Cortisone and low-dose radiation have been used for this syndrome, with only moderate success. Surgical resection has also been largely unsuccessful except in discrete lesions less than 5 cm in size.

Torticollis (Wry Neck)

The cause of torticollis is unclear; the deformity may result from many different abnormalities. Most instances are diagnosed at two to three weeks of age; birth trauma with a resultant hematoma in the sternocleidomastoid muscle certainly appears to be one cause, since ecchymosis is present over some of these lesions. A rock-hard mass the shape of an olive is felt within the sternocleidomastoid muscle. Treatment in neonates is nonsurgical; stretching exercises are begun by a physiotherapist and are continued on a daily basis by the mother. The mother gently turns the infant's head fully left and right, and touches each ear to its corresponding shoulder. Within several weeks the mass is gone and normal function returns.

Untreated cases progress to fibrosis of the involved muscle and a tendency of the head to stay turned to the other side. In advanced cases the ipsilateral side of the skull and face may flatten out from the pull of the muscles. Exercises, proper positioning of the head (including repositioning of the crib to encourage facing the room light) should be tried. If a satisfactory response is not seen quickly, then surgical division of the fibrosed muscle and underlying fascia colli is effective management.

Midline Cervical Teratoma

A cervical location for a teratoma is exceedingly uncommon, but it must be considered in the newborn who has a large, partly cystic mass in the midline of the neck. Respiratory difficulty may occur with these lesions so that immediate surgical removal is necessary.

A transverse cervical incision is made. The lesion is lobulated and frequently anterior to the strap muscles. It has a pedicle attached to the thyroid and can usually be excised intact with relative ease. The skin may require plastic revision before closure, and the wound should be drained. The final results of this procedure in neonates should be excellent because the lesion is superficial, and no malignant change has been reported in this location in the newborn.

Cleft Lip and Palate

Cleft lips and cleft palates are frequently encountered and are present at the time of birth. Repair of the lip abnormality may be undertaken in the neonatal period, but these procedures are beyond the scope of this book. An excellent description of the operative approach to cleft-lip deformities may be found in *Cleft Lip and Palate: Surgical, Dental, and Speech Aspects,* by Grabb, Rosenstein, and Bzoch [8].

Cleft palates do not require surgical correction early in life but when a cleft palate occurs as part of the Pierre-Robin syndrome the pediatric surgeon is often asked to help care for the child. Children with Pierre-Robin deformity have a

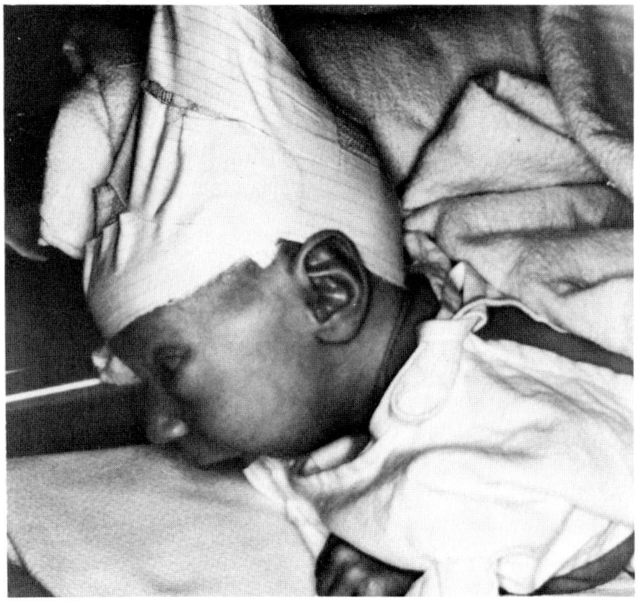

4-4. Child with Pierre-Robin deformity suspended with a stockinette cap.

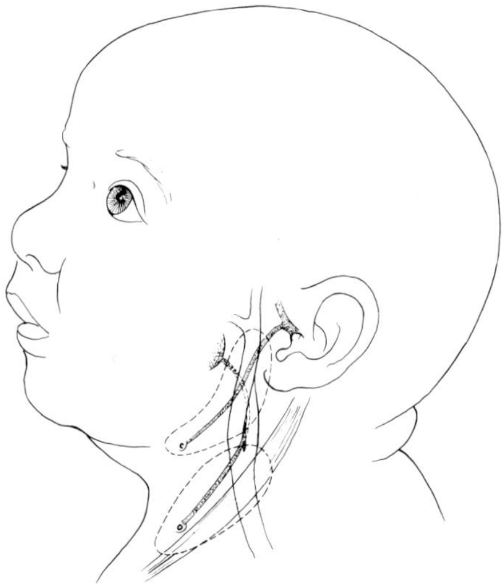

4-5. First branchial cleft is shown as it enters the external auditory canal. The second cleft bisects the carotid bifurcation and enters the tonsillar fossa.

cleft of the soft palate, micrognathia (small chin), and glossoptosis (posterior tongue). This combination of defects forces the airway and pharynx to compete for space. As a result, the child may have considerable difficulty breathing, especially when being fed.

Surgical procedures on the lip, tongue, or mandible do not work and are not advised. Most children with these difficulties do well if placed prone and if fed with a special cleft palate feeder or "lamb's nipple." If this regimen is unsuccessful, the child's neck is hyperextended by a cap apparatus to allow the tongue to fall forward (Figure 4-4). This cap is placed by shaving the head and gluing a stockinette to the scalp with collodion. Almost all the infants with Pierre-Robin syndrome do well after receiving this treatment, but occasionally a gastrostomy is necessary to allow feeding to continue without interfering with respiration. Because these babies spend most of their time on their abdomen, the gastrostomy tube should be brought out more laterally than usual to prevent pressure on its exit site.

Tracheostomy would alleviate almost all the problems seen with the Pierre-Robin syndrome, but the complication rate of tracheostomies in infants is so high that it should be an absolute last resort. A tracheostomy in an infant with the Pierre-Robin syndrome cannot safely be removed for at least a year; during that time the care required by the child is expensive, demanding, and subject to a number of complications.

Branchial Cleft Remnants

Anomalies of the first and second branchial clefts rarely produce symptoms during the neonatal period, but they may be confused with cystic hygromas or torticollis. They can be safely observed for many months before surgical excision is undertaken. An occasional infection can be treated medically (Figure 4-5).

Thyroglossal Duct Cysts

This common condition results from the growth of thyroid-rest tissue left behind when the thyroid migrates from the foramen cecum behind the tongue to the lower anterior neck. The resultant midline cyst is attached to the hyoid bone and moves with the tongue. Surgical excision including a section of the hyoid bone is necessary, but these cysts are rarely encountered in children who are less than a year of age.

Congenital Goiter

Congenital goiter is no longer common. In a newborn with a large collarlike mass in the neck, however, the condition should be suspected, especially if the mother has been on a goitrogenic drug such as iodine for a cough or asthma. Unless severe tracheal compression is present, medical management of the goiter is invariably successful. If acute respiratory obstruction occurs, the goiter should be surgically split in the midline to alleviate the tracheal compression. Tracheostomy may be necessary if tracheomalacia has developed that results in collapse of the trachea with inspiration.

Parotid Gland Lesions

Mixed tumors and malignancies of the parotid glands have been encountered in the newborn, but only rarely. The surgical principles used for parotid exploration in children or adults are applicable in the newborn.

Hemangiomas of the parotid are almost always located near the gland, rather than in it; conservative management is appropriate.

Tongue Tie

Theoretically, a short frenulum between the tip of the tongue and the floor of the mouth should restrict the tongue's movement. This restriction is by and large only theoretical, and surgical release is usually not needed in infants. In older children, a simple incision in the avascular tissue will release the tip of the tongue and solve the problem permanently.

Lymphadenopathy

Enlarged neck nodes are uncommon in small infants and can be safely observed. If the nodes are enlarged secondary to an infectious process in the head and neck area, then appropriate antibiotic coverage should be instituted. If fluctuance occurs, then drainage should be carried out.

Macrostomia

Abnormalities of the mouth, cheeks, and pharynx may make feeding difficult or impossible. A feeding gastrostomy is indicated in infants with these abnormalities until plastic revision of the lesion is undertaken months later.

Choanal Atresia

Infants breathe almost entirely through the nose. If the upper passages are not patent, respiratory difficulty may be encountered. A long airway should be inserted through the mouth to encourage breathing. Because direct surgical repair is not feasible in the young infant, careful airway management is needed until the child learns to breathe through the mouth. A feeding gastrostomy is occasionally needed, but tracheostomy can invariably be avoided.

Selected References

1. Armstrong, D., et al. Torticollis. *Plast. Reconstr. Surg.* 35:14, 1965.
2. Bears, O. H., and Adson, M. A. Surgical anatomy and techniques of parotidectomy. *Am. J. Surg.* 95:885, 1958.
3. Bill, A. H., and Vadheim, J. C. Cysts, sinuses, and fistulas of the neck arising from the first and second branchial clefts. *Ann. Surg.* 142:904, 1955.
4. Brown, P. M., and Judd, E. S. Thyroglossal cysts and sinuses. *Am. J. Surg.* 102:494, 1961.
5. Camishion, R. C., and Templeton, J. Y. Cervicomediastinal cystic hygroma. *Pediatrics* 29:831, 1962.
6. Cherry, J., and Bordley, J. E. Surgical correction of choanal atresia. *Ann. Otol. Rhinol. Laryngol.* 75:911, 1966.
7. Edgerton, M. T. The treatment of hemangiomas. *Ann. Surg.* 183:517–33, 1976.
8. Grabb, W. C., Rosenstein, S. W., and Bzoch, K. R. *Cleft Lip and Palate: Surgical, Dental, and Speech Aspects.* Boston: Little, Brown and Company, 1971.
9. Ninh, T. N., and Ninh, T. X. Cystic hygroma in children. *J. Pediatr. Surg.* 9:191–5, 1974.
10. Rickham, P. P. *Neonatal Surgery: Cervical Teratoma.* P. P. Rickham and J. H. Johnson (eds.). New York: Appleton-Century-Crofts, 1969, pp. 162–6.

5

Esophageal Atresia

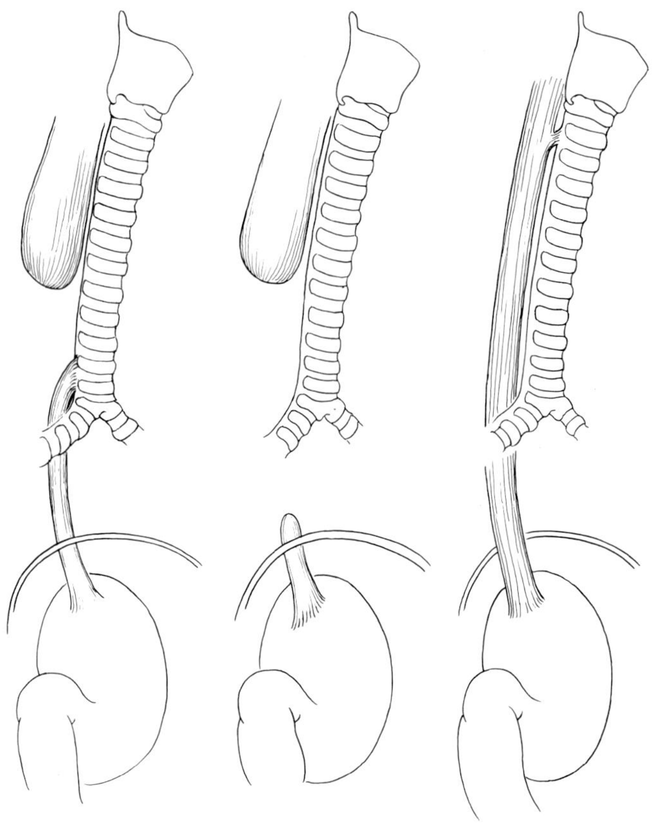

5-1 5-2 5-3

5-1. The most common form of esophageal atresia (85 percent) consists of a dilated proximal esophageal pouch and a connection of the distal esophagus to the carina of the trachea.

5-2. Pure esophageal atresia.

5-3. Fistula of the H type without atresia.

The incidence of congenital atresia of the esophagus with or without tracheoesophageal fistula (TEF) is 1 in every 4,425 live births in Washtenaw County surrounding the University of Michigan. The origin of this anomaly is not well understood, but, in general, esophageal atresia can be divided into four main types to allow a better understanding of the treatment regimens. The largest group includes the cases where the upper pouch ends blindly and the distal esophagus is connected to the trachea in the region of the carina (Figure 5-1). This group accounts for 80 percent to 90 percent of all cases. Pure esophageal atresia without any fistula to the respiratory tract occurs in 5 percent to 8 percent of the cases (Figure 5-2). In infants with pure esophageal atresia, there is a blind dilated upper pouch and a small short distal esophagus. The third group of patients have the so-called H type of fistula between the esophagus and the trachea, but there is no atresia of the esophagus (Figure 5-3). Infants with fistulas of the H type account for only about 2 percent of all cases. The final group, comprising less than 2 percent of all cases, includes all other types of tracheal esophageal fistulas with atresias. These cases are obviously rare and may involve fistulas from the esophagus to the trachea from both the upper and lower pouches. These rare types will not be discussed in this chapter.

Esophageal Atresia with Distal Tracheoesophageal Fistula

This is by far the most common type of TEF encountered. Infants with esophageal atresia and distal tracheoesophageal fistula develop symptoms within the first few hours of life because they have increased salivation, regurgitation of their feedings, or respiratory distress. Attempts to pass a nasogastric tube through the nose or mouth into the stomach are unsuccessful, and a chest x-ray shows that the nasogastric tube is curled up in the proximal esophagus. One to two milliliters of thin barium or 50% Hypaque is placed down the tube under fluoroscopy to delineate the bottom of the blind pouch (Figure 5-4). Because the distal end of the esophagus is almost always attached to the trachea at the level of the carina, it is possible to estimate the approximate distance between the end of the upper pouch and the top of the fistula. In general, a primary anastomosis is possible when there is a distance of two to three vertebral bodies (2 to 4 cm) between the upper and lower pouches on x-ray. The chest x-ray should also be inspected for the presence of aspiration pneumonia or a right-sided aortic arch. Aspiration pneumonia should suggest a delay before primary repair is attempted, whereas a right-sided aortic arch may indicate the need for a left rather than a right thoracotomy for the primary repair.

When the diagnosis of this common type of esophageal atresia with tracheoesophageal fistula is made, the child

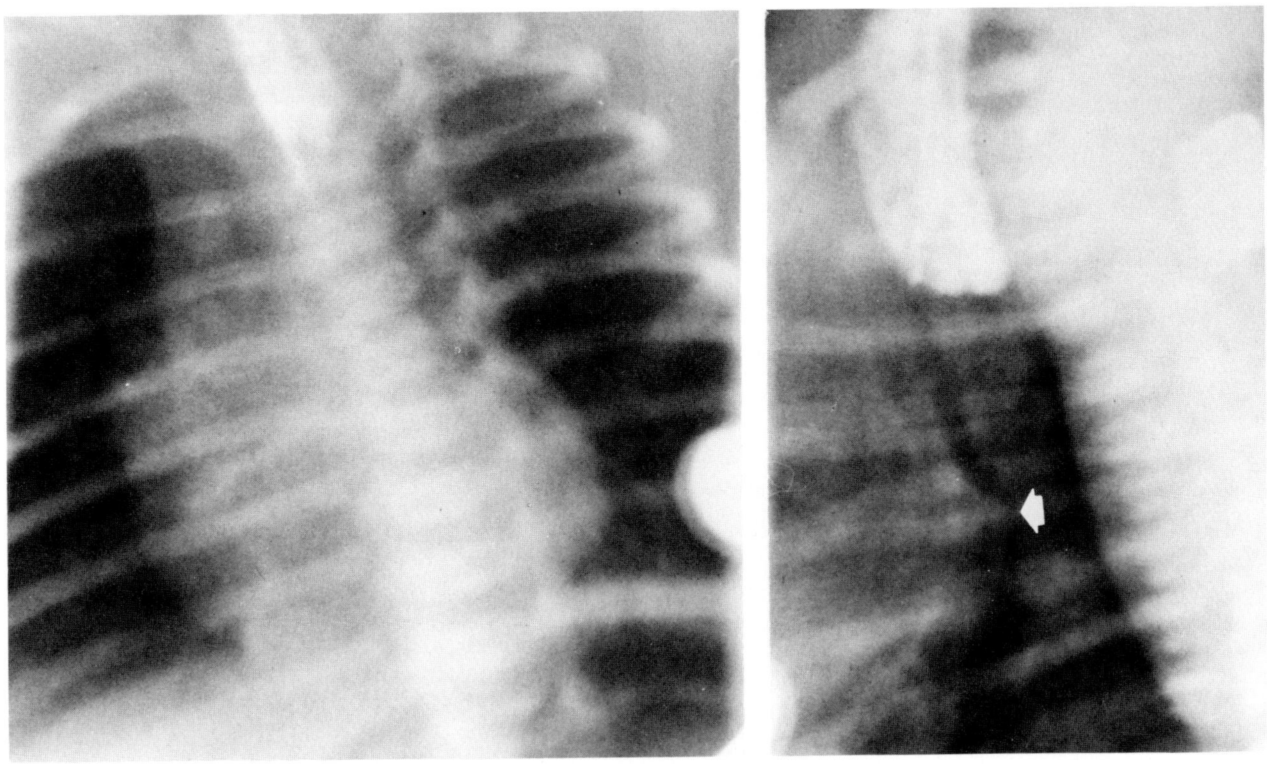

5-4. Enlargement of 70-mm x-ray films of an infant with a common type of esophageal atresia with TEF. Arrow points to junction of esophagus and trachea.

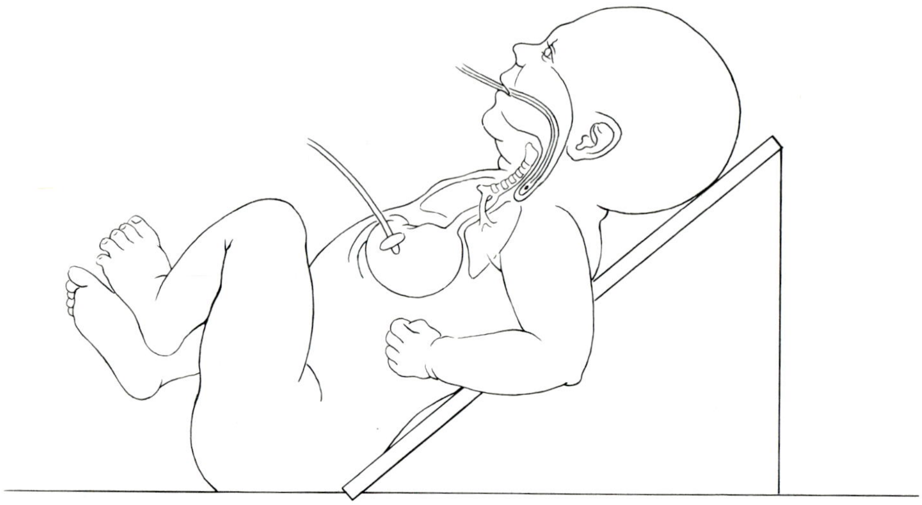

5-5. Proper position of child awaiting primary repair of TEF.

should have a Repolgle sump tube passed through the nose or mouth to the upper pouch; the tube is placed on constant suction to keep saliva from accumulating in the pouch and spilling over into the lungs, with resultant pneumonia. The patient should be placed in an upright position in an infant seat to prevent gastric reflux, and a good intravenous line should be inserted (Figure 5-5). Ampicillin and gentamicin are started, vitamin K is administered, and a type and crossmatch for blood is performed.

It has been our practice to perform an immediate Stamm gastrostomy (see Chapter 12) under local or light general anesthesia and to prepare the child for primary repair sometime during the next 48 hours. On the other hand, there is ample evidence that immediate primary repair can be carried out without a gastrostomy on full-term healthy infants.

Operative Technique

Endotracheal anesthesia is administered and the patient is positioned with the right side directly up. The anesthesiologist will notice an air leak because, with each breath, the gases pass into the trachea and then escape through the fistula into the distal esophagus. A right posterolateral thoracotomy is done with the posterior portion of the incision curved superiorly around the medial aspect of the scapula (Figure 5-6a). This curve in the incision can be helpful for exposure in the retropleural dissection and is preferred to a straight transverse incision. The chest is entered in the fourth intercostal space. The intercostal muscles are slowly and carefully separated until the pleura is seen. Wet cotton-tipped applicators and Kittner sponges are used to dissect

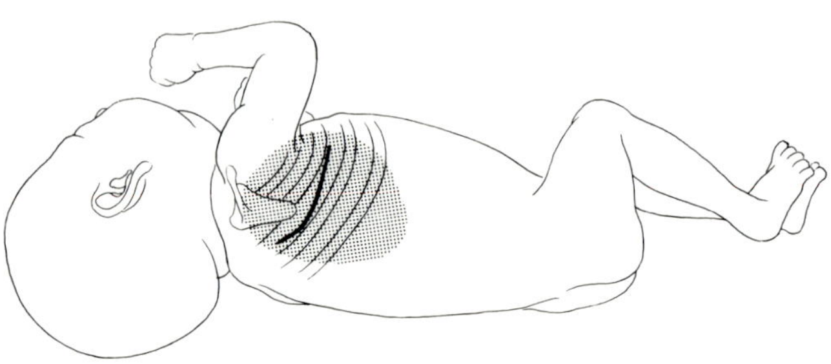

5-6a. Incision for primary repair of TEF. Shaded area denotes extent of extrapleural plane needed.

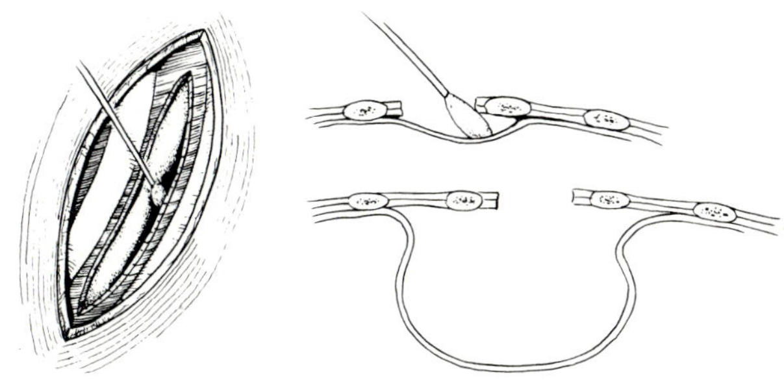

5-6b

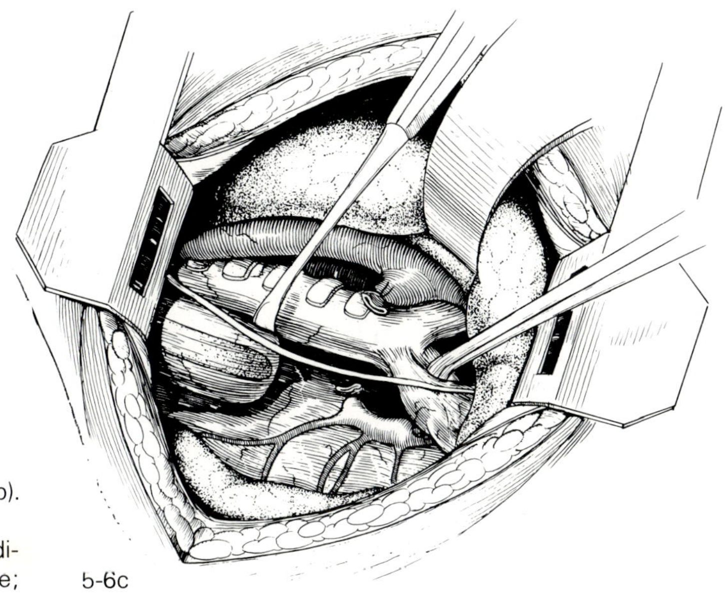

5-6c

the parietal pleura gently off the chest wall (Figure 5-6b). Gentle twisting of the applicators is especially effective.

This technique creates a nice retropleural plane but is tedious, adding as much as 15 minutes to the operative time; however, avoiding entry into the pleural cavity prevents development of an empyema if an esophageal leak should occur. Once the pleura starts to come away from the chest wall, the dissection becomes gradually easier. The dissection is then carried both anteriorly and posteriorly to prevent any area of the pleura from being stuck to the chest wall and tearing during the remainder of the procedure. Posteriorly, as the dissection of the pleura goes past the mediastinum, the surgeon encounters the azygous vein, which is doubly ligated and cut. The orogastric tube aids in the location and dissection of the upper pouch. The distal esophageal fistula is usually directly under the area where the azygous vein has been divided (Figure 5-6c). Usually the fistula can be seen bulging with each breath. It is gently surrounded with a 0 silk for traction (Figure 5-6d). The crotch between the fistula and the trachea is dissected with a right-angle clamp, and a suture of 5-0 or 6-0 cardiovascular silk is placed in the inferior portion of the fistula, which is then partially transected. Two or three more sutures are placed until the fistula has been completely cut across and oversewn (Figure 5-6e). A small rim of esophagus is left on the trachea so that the closure does not compromise the lumen of the trachea. Saline solution is placed over the suture line to check for an air leak. The distal esophagus is then allowed to retract momentarily while attention is directed to the upper pouch. This blind pouch can easily be found by having the anesthesiologist push down on the Repolgle tube. A holding suture of 2-0 silk is then placed in the proximal esophagus to aid in the circumferential dissection. Great care must be taken in dissecting between the upper pouch and the trachea because the trachea can be accidentally entered. The esophagus is dissected free all the way up to the thoracic

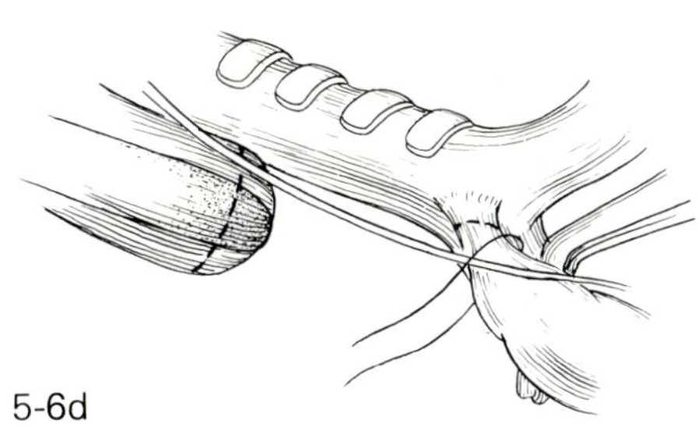

5-6d

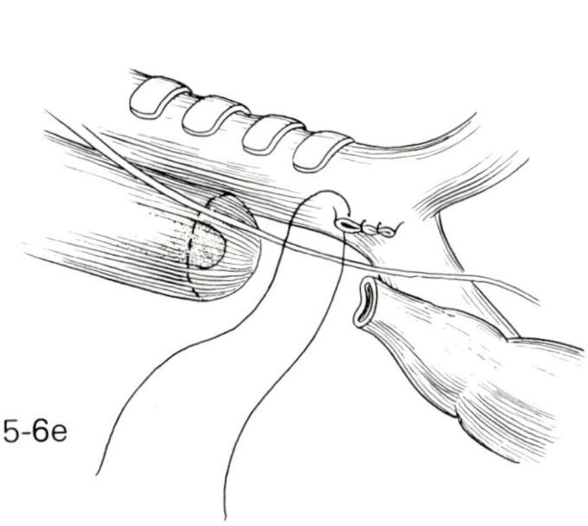

5-6e

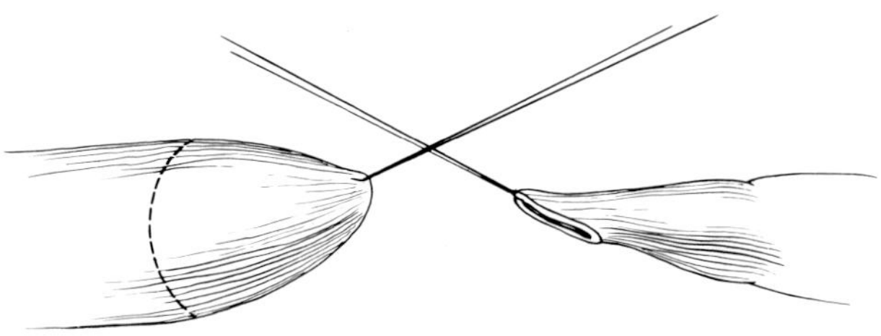

5-6f

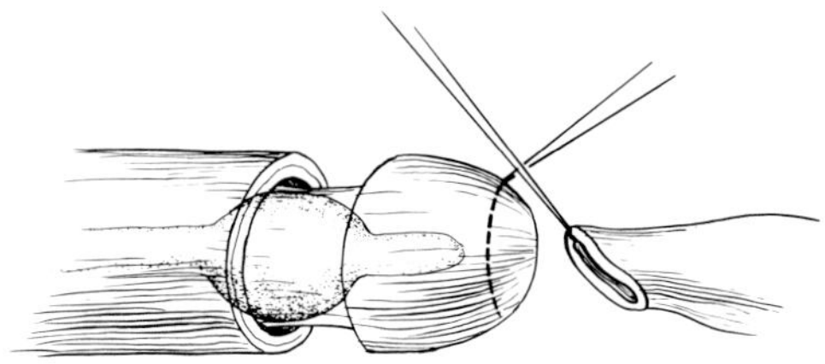

5-6g

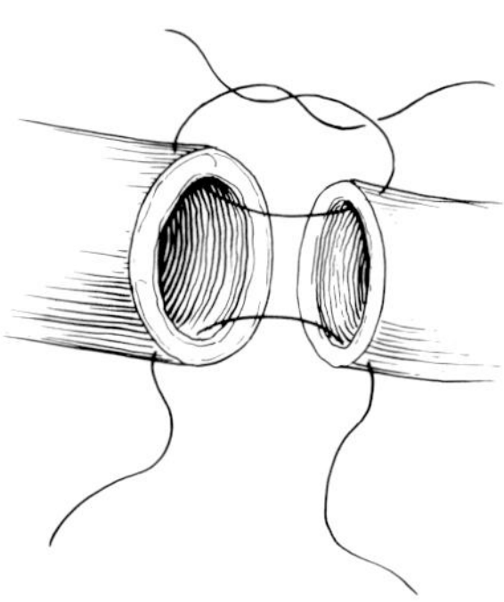

5-6h

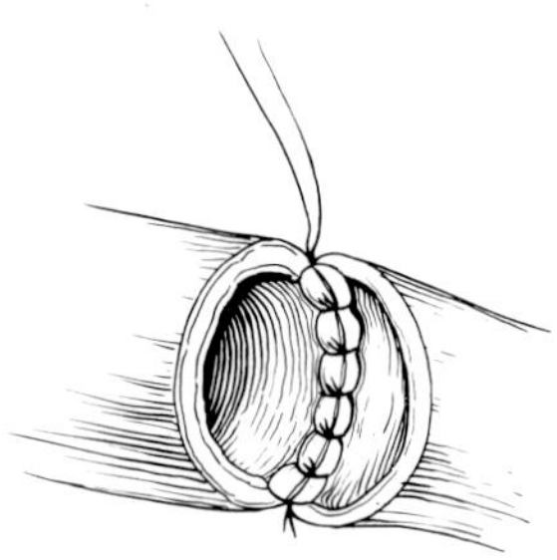

5-6i

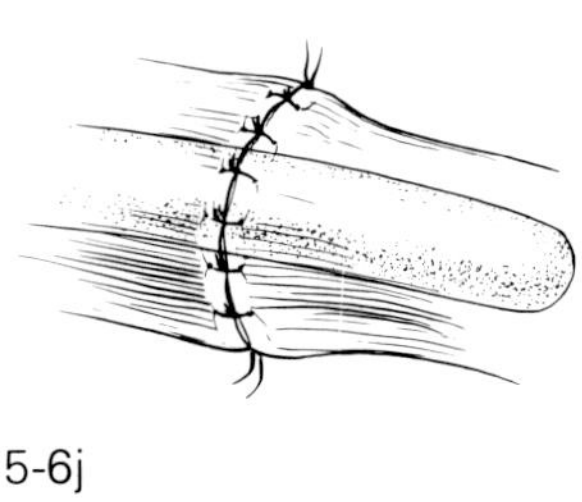

5-6j

inlet. A blunt periosteal elevator makes the dissection easier. At this point the surgeon assesses the feasibility of performing a primary anastomosis. The distal esophageal segment is grasped gently and the distance between the two segments is estimated (Figure 5-6f). Only minimal dissection of the distal esophagus should be carried out because its blood supply is segmental. Dissection of more than 1 to 2 cm distally in order to gain length will increase the risk of necrosis of the distal esophagus and failure of the anastomosis.

Occasionally it will be obvious that primary anastomosis is not possible. In such a situation the surgeon should oversew the distal esophageal segment and tack it as high as possible on the prevertebral fascia. The proximal pouch is not opened, so that in essence the patient has been converted to pure esophageal atresia without fistula. The chest is then closed. Subsequent treatment is similar to that used for patients with pure esophageal atresia except that the repeat thoracotomy is done transpleurally. More recently, circular myotomies performed on the upper pouch 2 cm proximal to the tip have resulted in sufficient extra length to permit primary repair during the initial thoracotomy (Figure 5-6g).

Fortunately, in most cases the segments will reach, and a primary anastomosis with 5-0 or 6-0 silk can be performed. The tip of the dilated proximal segment is transected. Full-thickness bites of both the lower and upper pouches are taken medially and laterally as stay sutures (Figure 5-6h). At this point, the posterior row of silk sutures is placed with both bites being full thickness and the knots tied on the inside (Figure 5-6i). (In patients where there is no tension at all on the two ends of the esophagus, two stay stitches can be tied first and the anastomosis twisted 180 degrees, so that both the anterior and posterior rows can be done under direct vision with the knots on the outside.) In either case, before the anterior row is sutured the anesthesiologist gently passes the Repolgle tube down into the field and the surgeon threads it farther on into the stomach through the distal esophagus. The anterior row is then placed with the knots on the outside (Figure 5-6j). There are usually no more than four or five stitches in either row. When the anastomosis is completed, the Repolgle tube is completely removed by the anesthesiologist.

Many surgeons prefer the Haight anastomosis, which requires a separation of the muscle and mucosa of the upper pouch in order to create a "telescoped" anastomosis (Figure 5-7). In the Haight (two-layer) anastomosis, the inner layer consists superiorly only of mucosa, which is sutured to the full thickness inferiorly. The outer row is taken using muscular bites superiorly to telescope this layer over the transverse muscular bites on the inferior esophageal segment.

A small amount of saline solution is placed in the wound, and the anesthesiologist applies 20 centimeters of constant pressure on the airway to check again for leaks in the tracheal suture line. After it is certain that there is no air leak and that there is no further bleeding, a 14 or 16 French chest tube is paced through a stab wound and fixed in the posterior extrapleural gutter with a plain catgut suture so that it does not lie directly on the anastomosis. The anesthesiologist can then reinflate the lungs, which are still protected by the pleura; 3-0 chromic paracostal sutures are used and the muscle layers are closed with interrupted 3-0 or 4-0 silk or running 3-0 chromic catgut. The skin is closed with a running 5-0 nylon suture. We prefer a collodion dressing because this allows the child to breathe unencumbered by a heavy dressing of gauze and tape.

Postoperative Care

The child is placed erect in an infant seat and a premeasured nasogastric tube is taped near the child's incubator. At the time of surgery the tube is measured from the mouth to the level of the anastomosis. Each time esophageal or tracheal suction is needed, the new catheter is measured against the original standard suction catheter, to prevent any catheter from being placed down to the level of either anastomosis. Antibiotics and intravenous fluids are continued. In children with a gastrostomy, the tube is placed to gravity drainage until the third or fourth postoperative day, when cautious gastrostomy feedings are instituted. Children without a gastrostomy are started on peripheral hyperalimentation the day after surgery. The extrapleural chest tube is placed on underwater seal, and the amount of fluid that comes out is carefully noted. Daily chest films are obtained to determine the presence of mediastinal or pleural fluid. Anastomotic leaks can present with either air or fluid on the chest film as well as with saliva in the extrapleural tube.

Most infants do quite well, and on the tenth postoperative day a Hypaque esophageal swallow is obtained under fluoroscopy. If no leak is seen, the child is begun on a clear liquid diet orally the same afternoon. The following day, if the chest film remains normal and no fluid has been coming from the extrapleural tube, the tube is removed, and the child is started on a progressive oral diet. If a leak is encountered, no oral feedings are given, the gastrostomy feedings are stopped, and alimentation is continued intravenously. Most leaks will heal spontaneously in 7 to 14 days. Before discharge the child undergoes an intravenous pyelogram (IVP) to check for renal anomalies.

Methods for Handling Infants with Associated Problems

Primary repair of esophageal atresia with tracheoesophageal fistula should not be attempted in infants weighing less than 1.5 kilograms, those with severe cardiac anomalies, or those who have significant aspiration pneumonia. Instead, on the day of admission children with these conditions should have

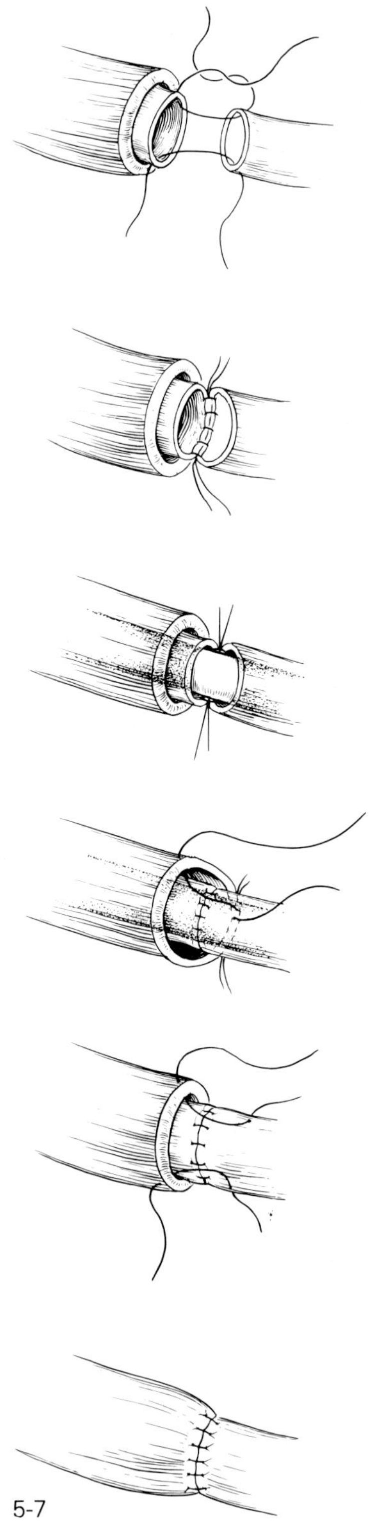

5-7

a gastrostomy performed under local anesthesia. The child is placed erect in an infant seat with a Repolgle tube to suction. Appropriate steps are taken to correct the associated problem; then the primary esophageal repair can be undertaken. If necessary, these infants can be maintained like this for several weeks before definitive repair.

One-third of patients with esophageal atresia have significant associated anomalies, the most common being cardiac and gastrointestinal, especially imperforate anus. Neurologic, genital, urinary, and orthopedic anomalies are also seen, with varying frequency.

The patients with high imperforate anus present a unique combination of diseases, which can be treated in several ways. A gastrostomy and colostomy may be performed on the first day of life through a single transverse abdominal incision, followed by elective thoracotomy several days later. Occasionally a newborn with these two anomalies is extremely vigorous and strong and can tolerate the colostomy, gastrostomy, and primary repair during the same anesthesia.

Complications

Pneumonia, which is frequently encountered in patients with TEF, is treated with gentle thoracic vibration through the use of a battery-operated vibrator in addition to antibiotics given intravenously. With this treatment infants normally recover from their pneumonia rather rapidly.

Leak at the site of the esophageal anastomosis is uncommon but it can occur. The extrapleural thoracotomy eliminates the risk of empyema; saliva and other secretions are removed by the extrapleural chest tube. If oral feedings are stopped and nutrition is provided intravenously, the fistula usually closes spontaneously. Gastrostomy feedings can be continued as long as the patient is propped in an upright position and there is no evidence of leakage of formula into the extrapleural chest tube. One week after clinical evidence of the leak has disappeared, a Hypaque swallow under fluoroscopy is repeated. This usually demonstrates closure of the leak. Oral feedings are then started. Even with disruption of as much as half of the anastomotic suture line, it is possible to salvage a functioning esophagus using this conservative program followed by esophageal dilatation.

Recurrent fistulas between the trachea and the esophagus do occur and are best treated with a gastrostomy, long-term hyperalimentation, and subsequent transthoracic reoperation for division of the fistula.

By far, the most common late complication is anastomotic stricture. Three weeks after repair the esophagus should be of sufficient size to accept a size 24 French catheter passed through the mouth into the stomach. Approximately half the patients who have undergone TEF repairs require no dilatations, while the other 50 percent require from one to several dozen dilatations over the following weeks, months, or years until such time as the anastomosis is sufficiently wide to provide a good conduit for swallowed food. After the infant has been discharged from the hospital, any attack of gagging or coughing should be reported by the parent to the surgeon. Almost always such an attack is an indication for esophagoscopy and careful dilatation.

Recent reports have pointed out the increased incidence of gastroesophageal reflux (GER) with or without hiatus hernia in infants following repair of esophageal atresia. If a postoperative esophagram demonstrates significant GER, serious consideration for transabdominal fundoplication should be entertained.

Fortunately it is uncommon for the tracheal suture line to cause any significant problem except for the rather raspy cough that these children typically develop. Tracheal stenosis and granulomas are uncommon.

Children who have had these repairs appear to grow and develop normally. Cine-esophagrams reveal, however, that the esophagus does not develop a normal propulsive motion in the area of the anastomosis, and the x-ray findings may stay abnormal for many years despite the obvious normal swallowing function of the esophagus.

Esophageal Atresia without Tracheoesophageal Fistula

Patients with pure esophageal atresia develop symptoms in the first few hours of life that are essentially identical to those seen in patients who have esophageal atresia with an accompanying tracheoesophageal fistula. There is increased salivation, respiratory difficulty, and intolerance to feeding. An attempt to pass a tube into the stomach is unsuccessful, and contrast studies reveal a blind upper esophageal pouch. One striking difference between these children and those who have an associated fistula is the total absence of intestinal or gastric gas on x-ray film, because there is no connection between the gastrointestinal tract and the pharynx (Figure 5-8). Initial management of these patients is the same as that described for patients with a fistula.

Unlike the patients discussed in the previous section who have an associated distal fistula, babies with pure esophageal atresia do not ordinarily have sufficient length in the lower esophageal segment to allow primary anastomosis initially. Therefore immediate thoracotomy is inadvisable in these infants. Instead, a gastrostomy under local or general anesthesia is performed. The stomach and intestines are usually small in these infants, and the gastrostomy must be made with great care. Because gastric tube interposition is frequently used for esophageal replacement at a later date, the gastrostomy should be placed away from the greater curvature of the stomach, to make future surgery less difficult.

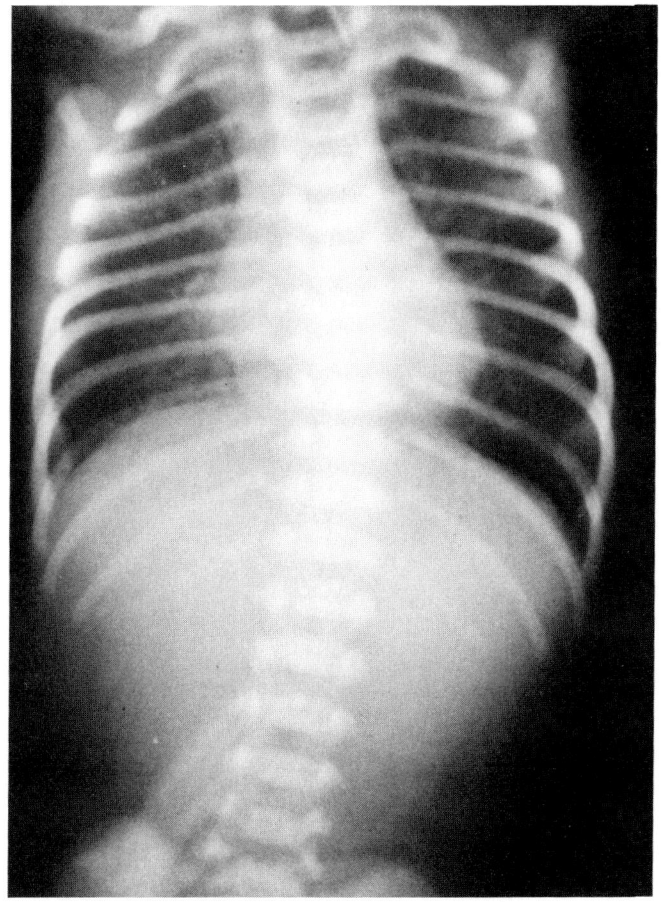

5-8. X-ray film of child with pure esophageal atresia demonstrates the absence of abdominal gas.

There is considerable disagreement as to the next step in the care of these children. Cervical esophagostomy performed at the same time as the gastrostomy has been done for many years and is a safe procedure that, when followed at one year of age by esophageal replacement, can give satisfactory long-term results. On the other hand, it is possible to dilate and stretch the upper pouch over several weeks in an attempt to create a situation amenable to primary anastomosis, thereby avoiding the problems of esophageal replacement.

We believe that cervical esophagostomy should not be performed except in those infants with significant associated problems in whom esophageal stretching and subsequent thoracotomy would be hazardous. Instead, after the gastrostomy, the child is returned to the intensive care ward with the Repolgle tube on constant suction and the infant propped in an infant seat. Each day the surgeon takes a 32 French bougie and gently stretches the upper esophageal pouch in an effort to elongate it. Once each week the patient is stretched under fluoroscopy to measure the downward progression of the upper esophageal pouch. In approximately three to five weeks, the upper esophageal pouch will have stretched to a level of the third or fourth thoracic vertebra, and a primary repair can be undertaken. The operative procedure is done extrapleurally in a manner similar to that described in the previous section except for the fact that there is no fistula that requires division. The anastomosis is usually made under slightly more tension than is necessary with the more common TEFs; even with a partial disruption of the anastomosis, however, the patient's own esophagus can usually be salvaged with conservative treatment and repeated dilatations. At the time of thoracotomy, if the distance between the two segments is still wide, a circular myotomy of the upper pouch should be attempted in order to obtain further length. Cervical esophagostomy is used only in extreme cases.

Cervical Esophagostomy

The cervical esophagostomy is done on the left side because most forms of esophageal replacement are brought through the left chest or under the sternum. The patient is placed with the head facing toward the right and a 1.5- to 2-cm transverse incision is made 1 cm above the clavicle over the left sternocleidomastoid muscle. With both sharp and blunt dissection, the tip of the Repolgle tube is palpated, and the esophagus is located. The strap muscles are retracted anteriorly, and the sternocleidomastoid and omohyoid muscles and the carotid sheath are moved posteriorly. By using the catheter as a guide, the end of the blind pouch of the esophagus is freed and brought out through the incision. Interrupted sutures of 4-0 silk are used to anchor the side of the esophagus to the subcutaneous tissue and sternocleidomastoid muscle. The tip of the esophagus is then opened, and interrupted 4-0 Dexon sutures are used to sew the full thickness of the esophagus to the skin (Figure 5-9). A sponge left on the left shoulder will absorb the saliva.

These children need to associate the act of eating with fullness in the stomach. With this in mind, at the time of each gastrostomy feeding the child is fed a small amount of sugar water or given a pacifier in the mouth to create this sensation. At one year of age, when the child weighs more than 20 pounds, esophageal replacement can be undertaken.

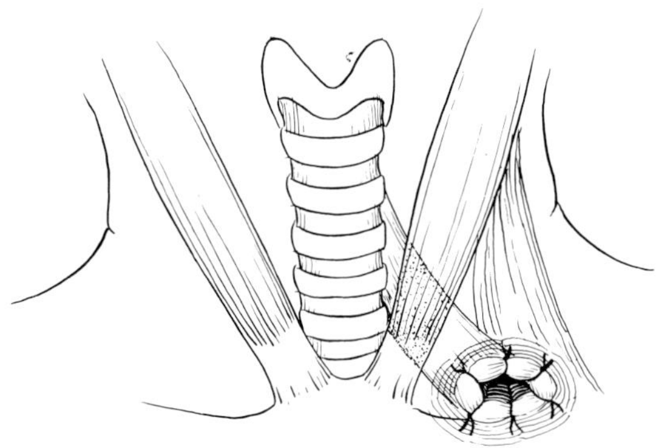

5-9

Complications

Most of the complications described in the section under Esophageal Atresia with Distal Tracheoesophageal Fistula are seen in patients with pure esophageal atresia. One additional complication is temporary closure of the esophagostomy caused by postoperative edema. The surgeon should be alert to this possibility and should be certain that the child has adequate oral suctioning during this phase to prevent aspiration. Sham feedings must be continued throughout the first year of life to make certain the child does not lose the suck reflex.

Tracheoesophageal Fistula without Esophageal Atresia (H Type)

The H type of TEF is rare, although it is frequently considered in the work-up of infants. The diagnosis is suspected in children who cough when eating, in infants with coughing spells or cyanosis, and in babies with recurrent unexplained attacks of pneumonia. The diagnosis is difficult to make because there is no completely reliable diagnostic test. Children with TEFs of the H type range in age from two days to several years, but about two-thirds develop symptoms in the first month of life. A cine-esophagram with barium is frequently helpful and should be tried first. On lateral view the fistula is seen running up from the esophagus toward the trachea. In patients with a good history, several repeat studies may be needed to delineate the fistula (Figure 5-10).

Bronchoscopy and esophagoscopy using the Storz pediatric telescope has greatly aided the early diagnosis of H-fistulas. If none is seen, a Cole endotracheal tube is placed in the trachea and the esophagoscope is then inserted. One-half milliliter of methylene blue dye is placed down the endotracheal tube, the lungs are hyperinflated, and the esophagus is then inspected for leakage of the blue dye through the fistulous opening. It is important to realize that H-fistulas are much more cephalad than are fistulas associated with esophageal atresia and that the H-fistula enters the trachea at a higher level than its connection with the esophagus.

If no fistula is discovered by using these techniques, the diagnosis should be temporarily abandoned. Repeat studies

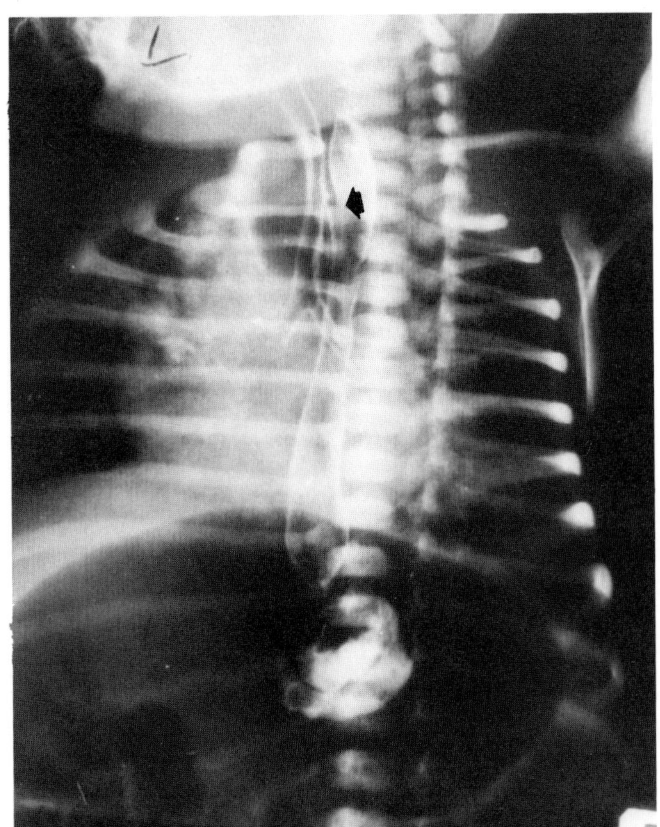

5-10. X-ray film of H-type fistula.

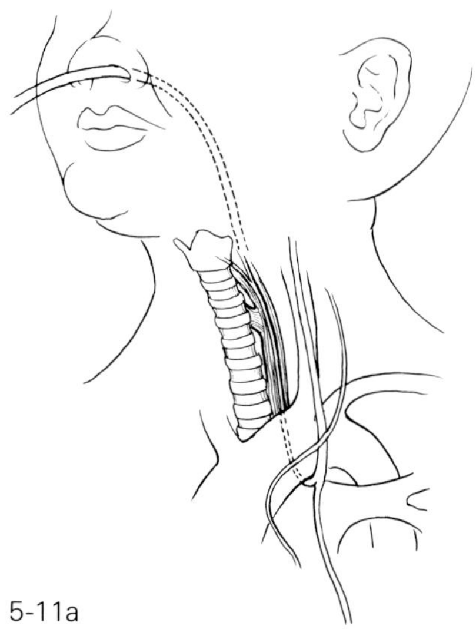

5-11a

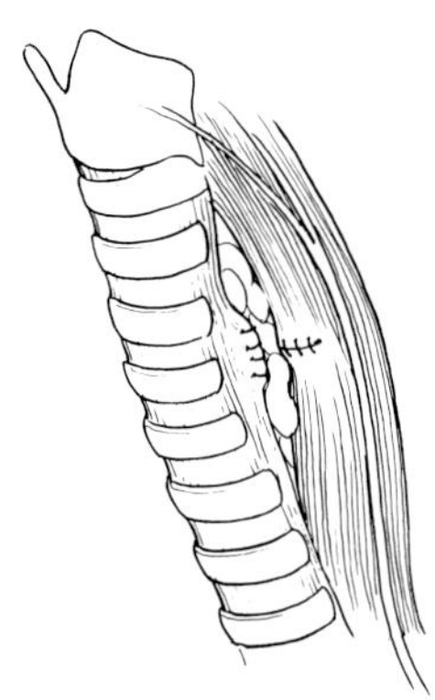

5-11b

may be indicated if symptoms persist, but blind surgical exploration should *not* be undertaken.

Operative Technique

The procedure is carried out under general anesthesia with the patient's head turned toward the right. A 3-cm transverse incision is made 1 to 2 cm above the clavicle over the left sternocleidomastoid muscle. A nasogastric tube in the esophagus aids identification. The sternocleidomastoid and omohyoid muscles are retracted laterally and posteriorly. The strap muscles are usually moved anteriorly but can also be moved out laterally if appropriate. The inferior thyroid vessels are ligated and divided. The middle thyroid vessels are exposed and the recurrent laryngeal nerve is identified and preserved before dividing these vessels (Figure 5-11a). The esophagus and thyroid are retracted to expose the fistula. The recurrent nerve, the vagus, and the phrenic course through the field. Occasionally, at the beginning of the procedure, to make identification easier, it is possible to place a Fogarty catheter through the fistula during endoscopy. When the fistula has been dissected completely free, it is transected close to the esophageal side. This allows a careful closure of the trachea with 4-0 or 5-0 silk without the danger of stenosis. The esophagus is closed with one or two layers of 4-0 silk; usually this can be done in a transverse direction to prevent esophageal stenosis. A pedicle of mediastinal fat or connective tissue is interposed between the two suture lines (Figure 5-11b) and a small Penrose drain is left near but not on the suture line before the platysma and skin are closed.

Postoperative Care and Complications

Oral feedings should be withheld for three to five days. The patient is given intravenous feedings and antibiotics during the healing phase. If the infant is swallowing saliva well, a Hypaque swallow on the fifth postoperative day is checked before clear liquids are started cautiously.

Early postoperative tracheal obstruction must be guarded against. Intravenous steroids, mist, and even tracheostomy may be necessary. Recurrent nerve injury is almost always temporary, so that conservative observation is indicated.

Esophageal cutaneous fistulas are uncommon and should be treated with hyperalimentation. Recurrent tracheoesophageal fistulas require proper nutritional support and reexploration.

Selected References

1. Bedard, P., Girvan, D. P., and Shandling, B. Congenital H-type TEF. *J. Pediatr. Surg.* 9:373, 1974.
2. Ein, S. A further look at the gastric tube as an esophageal replacement in infants and children. *J. Pediatr. Surg.* 8:859, 1973.

3. Eraklis, A. J., Rossello, P. J., and Ballantine, T. V. N. Circular esophagomyotomy of the upper pouch in primary repair of long segment esophageal atresia. *J. Pediatr. Surg.* To be published.
4. Haight, C. The esophagus. In W. T. Mustard, M. M. Ravitch, W. H. Snyder, Jr., et al. (eds.). *Pediatric Surgery.* Chicago: Year Book Medical Publishers, 1969, pp. 357–82.
5. Holder, T. M. Esophageal atresia and tracheoesophageal fistula: A survey of its members by surgical section of the American Academy of Pediatrics. *Pediatrics* 34:542–9, October 1964.
6. Holder, T. M. Esophageal atresia and tracheoesophageal fistula. *Curr. Probl. Surg.* 1–68, August 1966.
7. Killen, D. A., and Greenlee, H. B. Transcervical repair of H-type congenital TEF. *Ann. Surg.* 162:145, 1965.
8. Mahour, G. H., Woolley, M. M., and Gwinn, J. L. Elongation of the upper pouch and delayed anatomic reconstruction in esophageal atresia. *J. Pediatr. Surg.* 9:373, 1974.

6

Pulmonary Anomalies

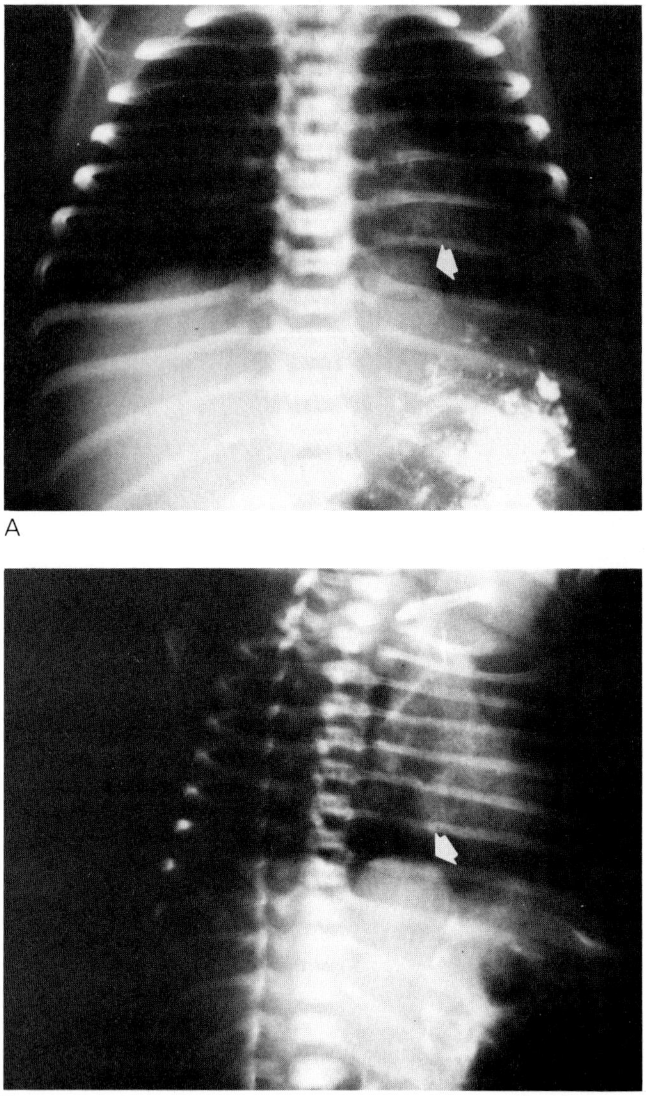

A

B

6-1. (A) Posteroanterior x-ray film of chest shows a mass lying over the costophrenic angle of the diaphragm. The mass has a rounded, smooth contour. This is a typical radiographic picture of an extralobar sequestration. (B) Oblique view shows the same mass more clearly.

Malformations of the lungs in neonates and infants are rare and usually do not cause serious symptoms that require emergency surgery. Three conditions are encountered in the neonate and infant: congenital lobar emphysema, cystic adenomatoid malformation, and extralobar sequestration. The first two can cause acute respiratory distress in the newborn and may require immediate surgery. Extralobar sequestration is almost always an asymptomatic condition that is discovered incidentally on a routine chest roentgenogram.

An *extralobar pulmonary sequestration* (Figure 6-1) is a rounded, smooth, soft mass lying between the top of the diaphragm and the inferior surface of the lung, almost always on the left. The accessory lobe is not attached to the lung and is covered by smooth, glistening visceral pleura. These masses do not contain air. They are usually attached to a pedicle containing an artery that has pierced the left diaphragm, having arisen from the abdominal aorta. Surgery for this condition is usually not difficult: It merely involves excision of the accessory lobe, with care taken to divide the arterial pedicle properly. Thus no further details of this entity will be presented.

Congenital lobar emphysema is the overdistention of one or more lobes of the lung. Shortly after birth this condition may progress rapidly, causing compression of the other pulmonary lobes and gross displacement of the mediastinum. Rapidly increasing dyspnea and cyanosis result. Commonly the emphysema is gradual in onset, and symptoms do not occur until later in life. The affected lobe cannot deflate normally, perhaps because of a deficiency of cartilage in the bronchus that supplies the lobe. This condition is frequently associated with congenital malformations of the heart and great vessels. On examination of the chest the signs most frequently encountered are absent or diminished breath sounds over the affected side, hyperresonance on percussion, and displacement of the mediastinum. The chest roentgenogram is characteristic (Figure 6-2). There is increased translucency of the affected side of the chest, almost always involving the upper or middle lobes. Rarely is a lower lobe involved. If the infant is in severe respiratory distress, no further diagnostic studies should be carried out, and the surgeon should proceed immediately with an operation.

Cystic adenomatoid malformation of the lung is an adenomatous epithelial hyperplasia of the pulmonary tissue. Cysts lined by proliferating bronchial epithelium lie between normal portions of the lung. Cartilage is almost always absent from the walls of the cysts. Although this condition is rare, it is being recognized preoperatively more often by radiologists and pediatric surgeons. In fact, today this condition is more common than congenital lobar emphysema and pulmonary sequestration. In the neonatal period these infants often have acute respiratory distress associated with

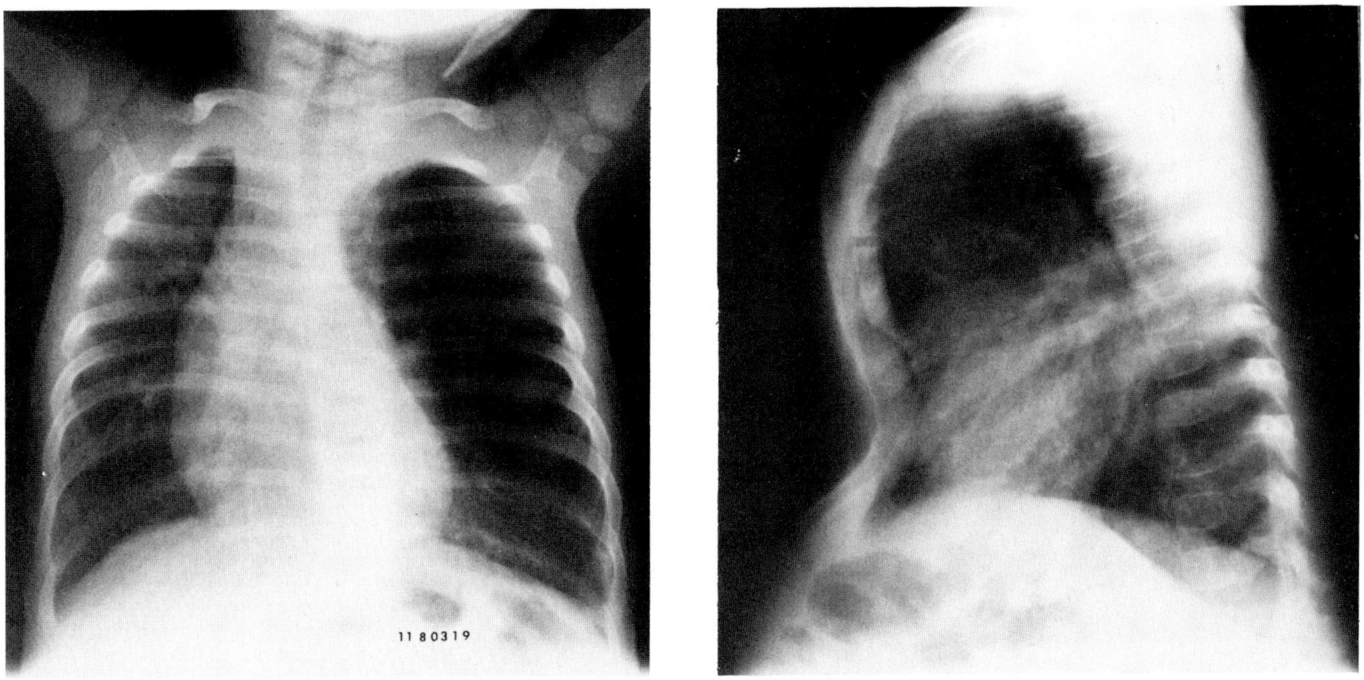

A B

6-2. (A) Posteroanterior x-ray film of chest showing congenital lobar emphysema of the left upper lobe. Note the overexpansion of the left upper lobe and compression of the left lower lobe with a shift of the mediastinum to the right side. (B) A lateral x-ray film shows overexpansion of the left upper lobe. Retraction of the sternum is secondary to respiratory distress in this infant.

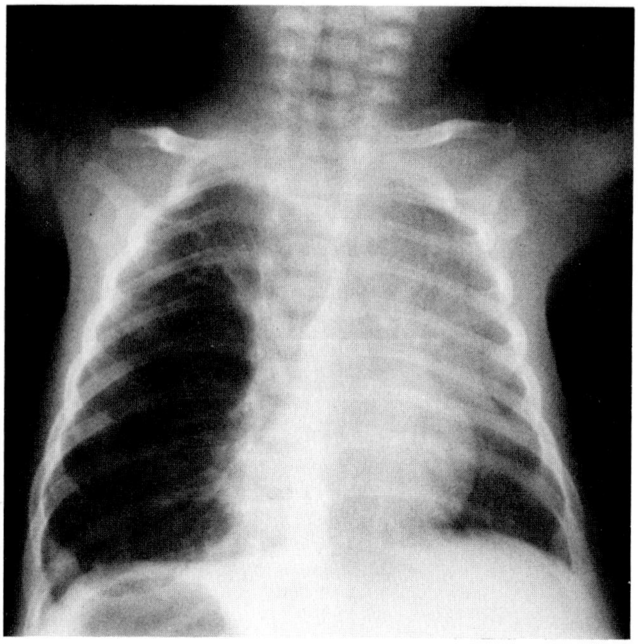

A

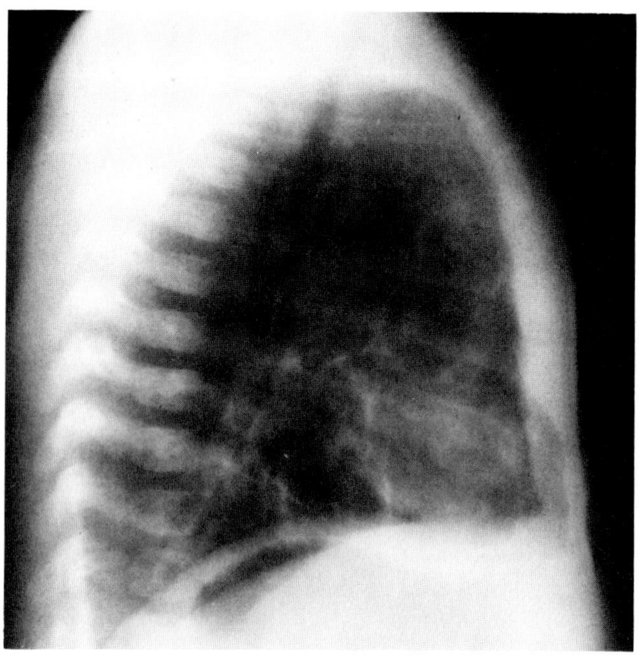

B

6-3. (A) Posteroanterior x-ray film of chest of an infant with cystic adenomatoid malformation of the left lung. Note the overexpansion of the left lung, several cystic areas of the midleft lung field, and a marked mediastinal shift to the right side. (B) The lateral film shows cystic spaces in the lung.

severe dyspnea and cyanosis. The affected lobe is often considerably expanded, compressing the remainder of the ipsilateral lung and shifting the mediastinum to the opposite side. The radiologic picture is variable, depending on the extent and location of the lesion. There may be a large cystic space on one side with marked displacement of the mediastinum (Figure 6-3) or a persistent area of opacity in one of the lobes. On x-ray film multiple cysts are found to be far more common than a single cyst. These can easily be confused with a congenital diaphragmatic hernia. Location of the stomach bubble on the radiograph will help to differentiate these two conditions. As in the case of lobar emphysema, immediate thoracotomy should be carried out when there is severe respiratory distress. Preoperative preparation in the neonate consists simply of administration of broad-spectrum antibiotics and vitamin K intramuscularly.

Operative Technique

After the infant has been anesthetized and an endotracheal tube and a reliable intravenous line have been placed, he is positioned in a lateral thoracotomy position with the affected side up. A towel is placed between the knees, and the patient is secured to the operating table with a large piece of adhesive tape placed over the iliac crest (Figure 6-4a). An axillary pad is unnecessary in infants. For an extralobar sequestration and for a lower lobectomy, the fifth intercostal space is entered; the fourth intercostal space is used for an upper lobectomy. In infants a straight transverse incision is employed starting at the anterior axillary line. The muscles of the chest wall (latissimus dorsi and serratus anterior) are cut with cautery and the proper intercostal space is identified. In infants it is easy to find the correct intercostal space by counting down from the first rib, which is easy to palpate under the scapula (Figure 6-4b). The fifth intercostal space is opened, and the ribs are spread with an infant Finochietto rib spreader. Even though the skin incision may be more limited than in adults, the intercostal space must be opened to its full extent. In the case of congenital lobar emphysema, the affected lobe often herniates through the incision once the pleural space is entered, promptly relieving the respiratory distress. Once the abnormality has been located, the surgeon can proceed with the appropriate lobectomy. For the purposes of this discussion, we shall describe only the technique of a left lower lobectomy in an infant.

The major fissure of the lung is opened by retracting the upper lobe superiorly; the mediastinal pleura is incised, and the left pulmonary artery is exposed. The individual branches of the pulmonary artery to the left lower lobe are identified, dissected free, and individually ligated. Each branch is doubly ligated proximally with 3-0 and 4-0 silk; suture ligatures are not used (Figure 6-4c). Once all the arterial branches are

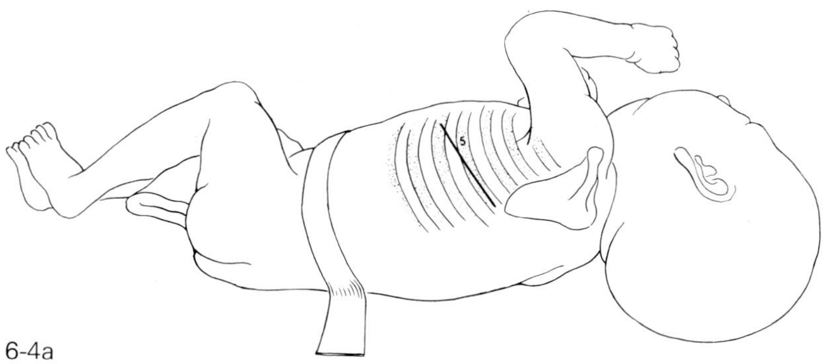

6-4a

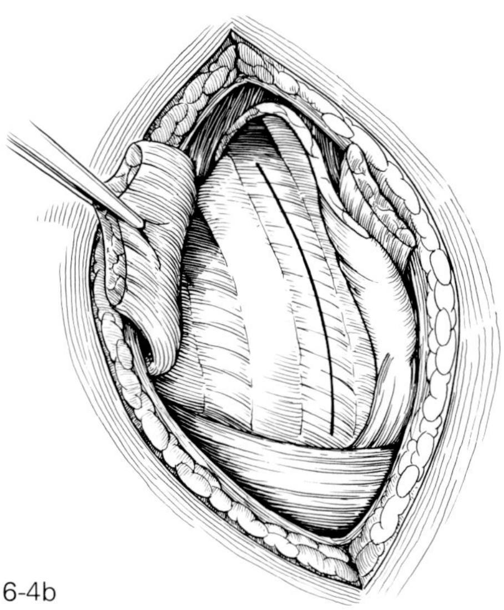

6-4b

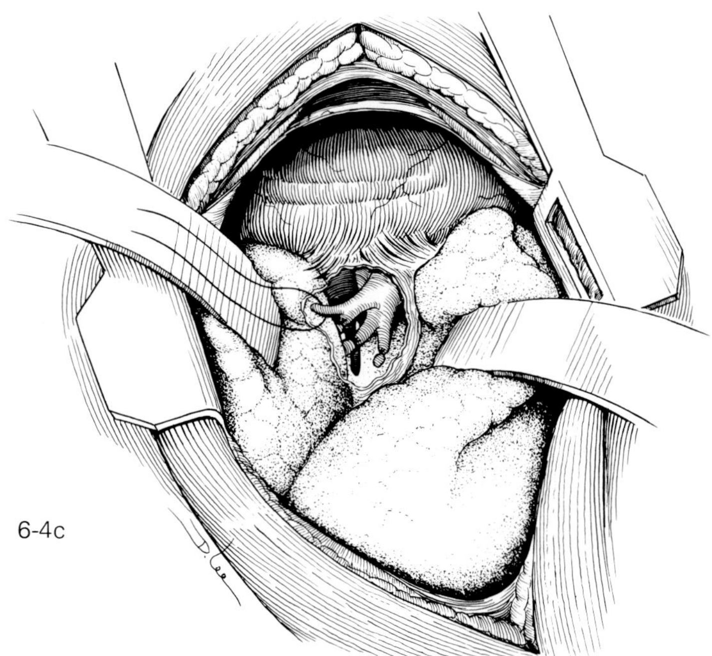

6-4c

divided, the inferior pulmonary vein is identified and dissected free. This vein is exposed by retracting the lung anteriorly to expose the posterior hilum and the inferior pulmonary ligament. The ligament is divided, and the vein is exposed. The vein and its three branches are dissected free, and each branch is individually ligated with 3-0 silk. The main trunk is then doubly ligated with two 3-0 silk ligatures and the vein is divided (Figure 6-4d).

The upper lobe is then retracted anteriorly and the lower lobe bronchus is isolated. Two stay sutures of 4-0 Tefdek are placed on either side of the bronchus, and the bronchus is cut across and sutured in segments. The bronchial closure is performed with interrupted sutures of 4-0 Tefdek placed through the full thickness of the bronchial wall. Once the bronchus is completely cut across, the lobe is removed from

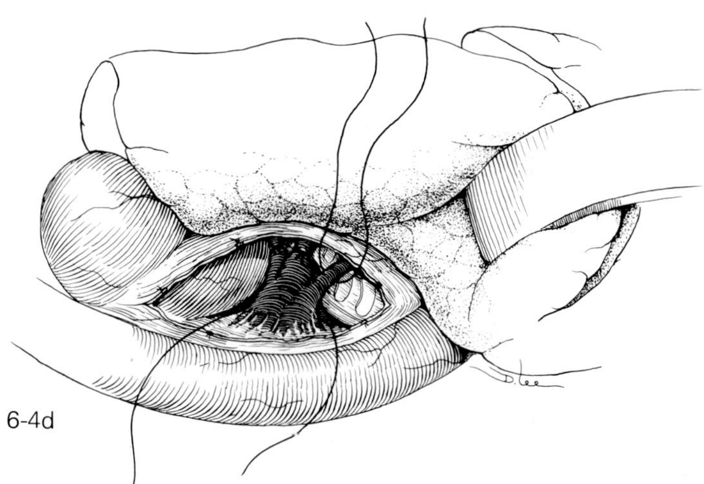

6-4d

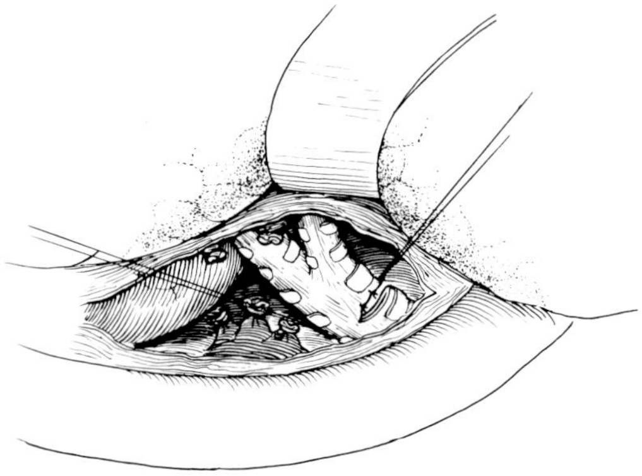

6-4e

the operative field (Figure 6-4e). The pleural cavity is filled with warm saline solution, and gentle positive pressure is applied to the lungs to be sure there is no air leak from the bronchial suture line. A number 20 French chest tube is inserted into the pleural cavity through a separate stab incision below the main incision. The ribs are reapproximated with several interrupted paracostal sutures of 3-0 chromic catgut. The muscles of the chest wall are closed individually with running sutures of 3-0 chromic catgut, and the skin is closed with either a running 5-0 nylon or a running 5-0 subcuticular Dexon suture. The wound is dressed with collodion.

Postoperative Care

The infant is maintained in an intensive care unit until the chest tube is removed. The chest tube is maintained on underwater seal or suction with a negative pressure no greater than 5 cm of water. Any greater negative pressure may cause a mediastinal shift in an infant, which can lead to emphysema of the contralateral lung. The chest tube is left in place for three to five days or longer if full expansion of the remaining lobe on the affected side is delayed or if there is an air leak. Before removal, the chest tube is clamped for a period of 12 hours, and a roentgenogram is obtained to determine if there is significant air accumulation in that pleural cavity. If no pneumothorax has developed, the chest tube is removed. The stab wound should be closed by a suture to prevent pneumothorax. The morning following surgery the infant is started on regular feedings, which he usually tolerates well. One must be careful that no significant gastric dilatation occurs during the first 12 to 24 hours after surgery by carefully observing the stomach bubble on the postoperative chest roentgenogram. If gastric dilatation does occur, a nasogastric tube should be passed and the air removed. Antibiotics are continued for five days postoperatively, or until the chest tube has been removed. The infants are usually ready for discharge from seven to ten days after the operative procedure. They are seen in the office one to two weeks after discharge.

Results

These patients do quite well following pulmonary surgery and usually have no further problems. Major complications such as bronchopleural fistulas or emphysema are rare among infants. Pulmonary function almost always returns to normal.

Selected References

1. Buntain, W. L., Isaacs, H., Jr., Payne, V. C., Jr., et al. Lobar emphysema, cystic adenomatoid malformation, pulmonary sequestration, and bronchogenic cyst in infancy and childhood: A clinical group. *J. Pediatr. Surg.* 9:85, 1974.
2. Gibbon, J. H., Jr., Sabiston, D. T., Jr., and Spencer, F. C. *Surgery of the Chest.* Philadelphia: W. B. Saunders Co., 1969.
3. Mustard, W. T., Ravitch, M. M., Snyder, W. H., Jr., et al. (eds.). *Pediatric Surgery.* Chicago: Year Book Medical Publishers, 1969.
4. Rickham, P. P., and Johnston, J. H. *Neonatal Surgery.* New York: Appleton-Century-Crofts, 1969.

7

Palliative Cardiac Operations

Systemic-to-Pulmonary Shunts

In a number of congenital cardiac defects, obstruction to the flow of blood out of the right ventricle is so severe that blood is preferentially shunted right to left within the heart to the systemic circulation. When the resulting cyanosis is profound (Po_2 below 40 mm Hg), operation is indicated.

Tetralogy of Fallot (Figure 7-1) is the most typical of the congenital cardiac anomalies characterized by diminished pulmonary blood flow. The obstruction to pulmonary blood flow is caused by severe pulmonary valvular, subvalvular, or supravalvular stenosis. Right-to-left shunting occurs proximal to this obstruction across a large ventricular septal defect. When the pulmonary obstruction is caused by hypertrophy of infundibular muscle, the degree of right-to-left shunting may vary according to the degree of spasm of this musculature. In infants with tetralogy of Fallot, severe cyanosis tends to occur in spells rather than continually. Infants with severe pulmonary stenosis or pulmonary valve atresia with an intact ventricular septum also have right-to-left shunting, in this instance through a patent foramen ovale, as discussed later in this chapter.

In patients with *tricuspid atresia* (Figure 7-2) there is obligatory right-to-left shunting across the atrial septum, because there is no other way for blood to leave the right atrium. Pulmonary flow in tricuspid atresia depends upon the mixed saturated and unsaturated blood from the left ventricle being able to traverse a ventricular septal defect into the right ventricle and pulmonary artery. This flow is usually limited by associated pulmonary valve stenosis, hypoplasia of the entire right ventricle, a ventricular septal defect that is small enough to restrict flow, or a combination of these conditions.

All these anomalies, and some others, such as complex transposition with pulmonary stenosis and truncus type IV, share two basic physiologic problems, both of which lead to severe cyanosis:

1. Pulmonary blood flow is markedly reduced, because blood is shunted away from the lungs. Often blood is supplied entirely through bronchial collaterals or a patent ductus.
2. There is mixing of saturated and unsaturated blood within the heart.

Diagnostic Studies Prior to Shunt Operations

Infants with obstruction to blood flow out of the right ventricle have obvious cyanosis, the severity depending on the amount by which pulmonary blood flow is deficient. Pulmonary vascular markings are reduced on the roentgenogram. Electrocardiogram and physical examination may provide clues to the exact diagnosis, but surgical therapy depends on accurate definition of the intracardiac anatomy by cardiac

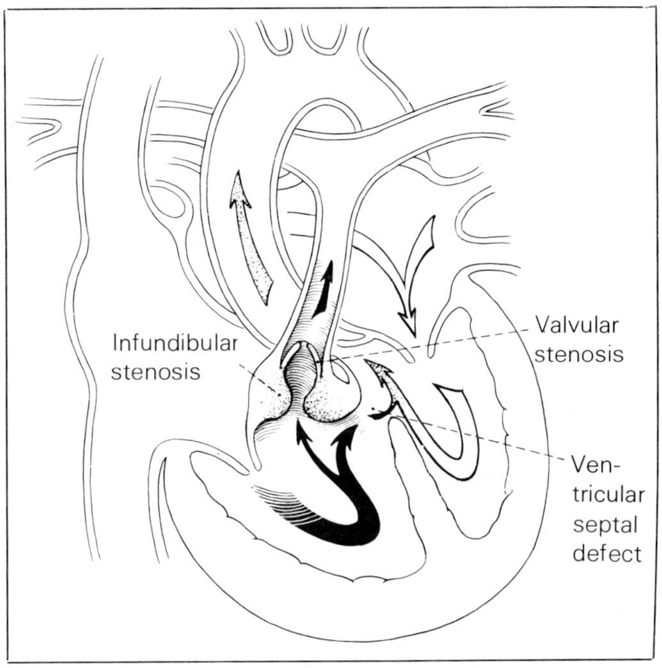

A

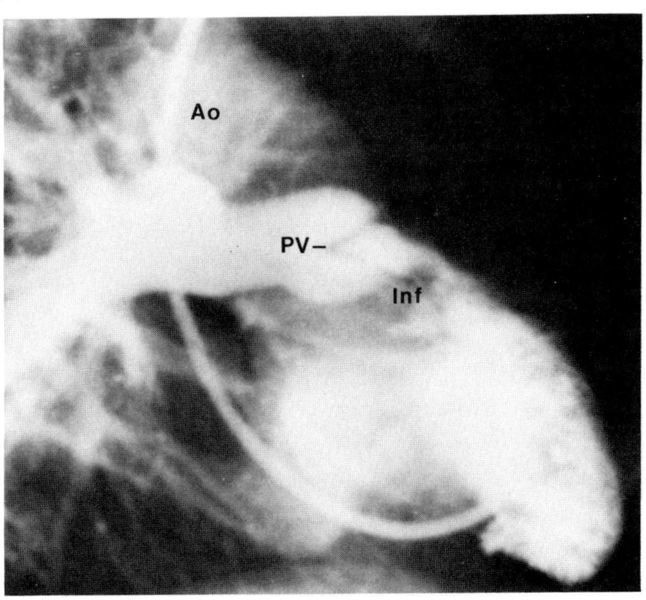

B

7-1. (A) Diagram of anatomy of tetralogy of Fallot illustrating valvular and infundibular pulmonary stenosis, a large ventricular septal defect, and right ventricular hypertrophy. (B) Lateral angiocardiogram in tetralogy of Fallot. Injection of contrast into the right ventricle reveals severe infundibular stenosis (Inf) and a thickened stenotic pulmonary valve (PV). Contrast appears early in aorta (Ao) from right-to-left shunting across the ventricular septal defect.

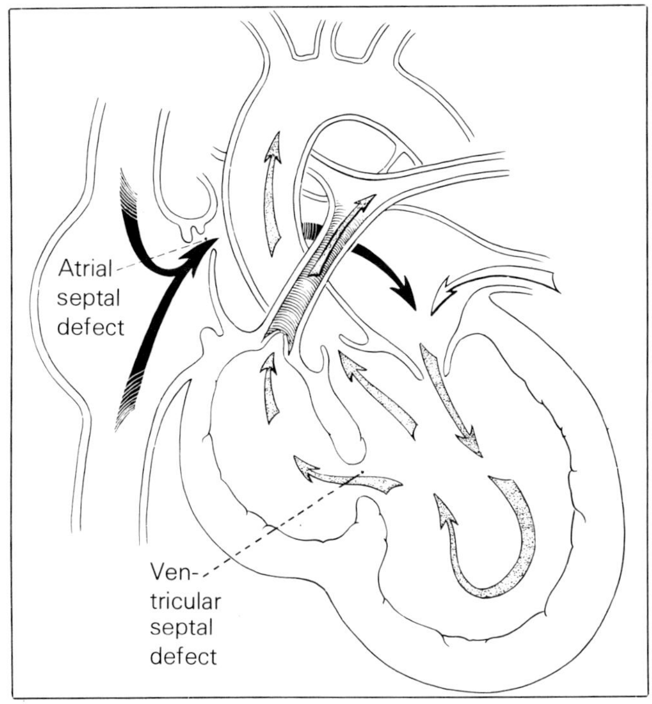

A

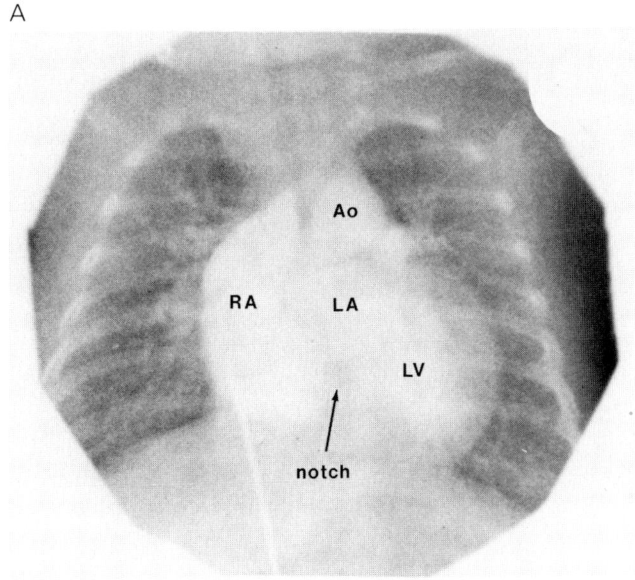

B

7-2. (A) Diagram of typical anatomy in tricuspid atresia illustrating the atrial septal defect (ASD), ventricular septal defect (VSD), and hypoplastic right ventricle and pulmonary artery. (B) Frontal angiocardiogram in tricuspid atresia. Contrast injected into right atrium (RA) crosses an atrial septal defect (ASD) into the left atrium (LA), left ventricle (LV), and aorta (Ao). A characteristic notch is seen in the space usually occupied by the right ventricle.

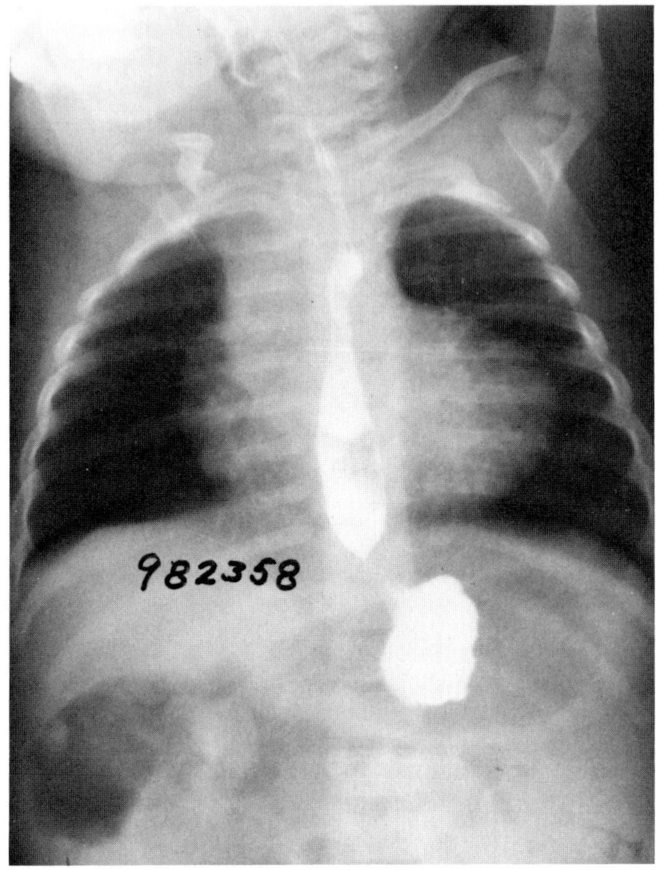

7-3. Typical chest roentgenogram in tetralogy of Fallot showing reduced pulmonary blood flow.

catheterization, angiography, or both. Specifically, these studies must delineate, if possible:

1. The site of intracardiac shunting.
2. The nature of the obstruction to pulmonary blood flow.
3. The source of pulmonary collateral flow, that is, whether there are large bronchial arteries or a patent ductus.
4. The configuration of the aortic arch vessels that might be utilized in creating an artificial shunt.
5. The size of the right and left pulmonary arteries, to allow selection of one suitable for operation. (Failure of visualization of a pulmonary artery does not contraindicate operation. Often an adequate pulmonary artery is present, but it simply fails to opacify on the angiogram because of inadequate blood flow.)

Choice of Shunt Procedure

Palliation can be achieved by creating a systemic–pulmonary artery shunt to increase pulmonary blood flow. Of course there will still be cyanosis because of the intracardiac mixing, but arterial saturation is usually improved sufficiently (to the 70% to 80% range) so that there is marked clinical improvement.

In the past we performed Waterston shunts between the ascending aorta and the right pulmonary artery in the belief that this was the easiest and quickest anastomosis in small babies. Recently it has become apparent that a high incidence of thrombosed or kinked pulmonary arteries follows Waterston shunts (Figure 7-4), which complicates subsequent total repair. Therefore we now perform Blalock-Taussig shunts by preference in almost all patients, regardless of size, and we have found them to be very satisfactory. Potts shunts are rarely performed, because of difficulties in regulating their size and in taking them down at the time of total repair. We have no experience with Glenn shunts.

Primary total correction of tetralogy of Fallot has become a realistic consideration in centers with a large neonatal cardiac experience (see Chapter 9). Total correction of the other anomalies in this group, such as pulmonary atresia with intact ventricular septum, tricuspid atresia, and truncus type IV, at present is delayed until later childhood.

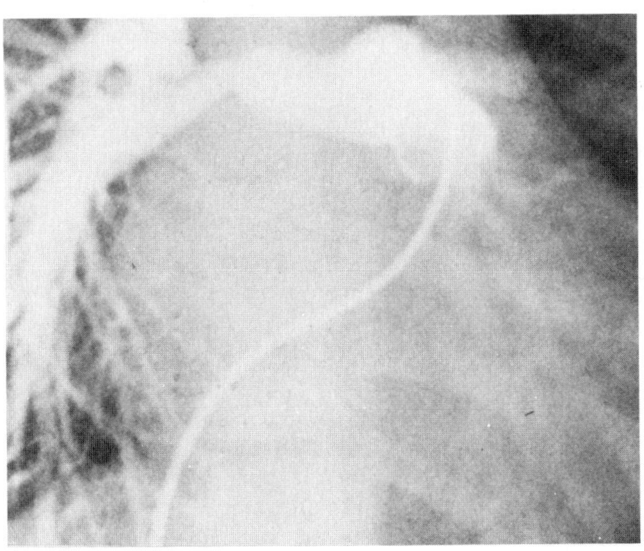

7-4. Stenosis of right pulmonary artery following Waterston shunt.

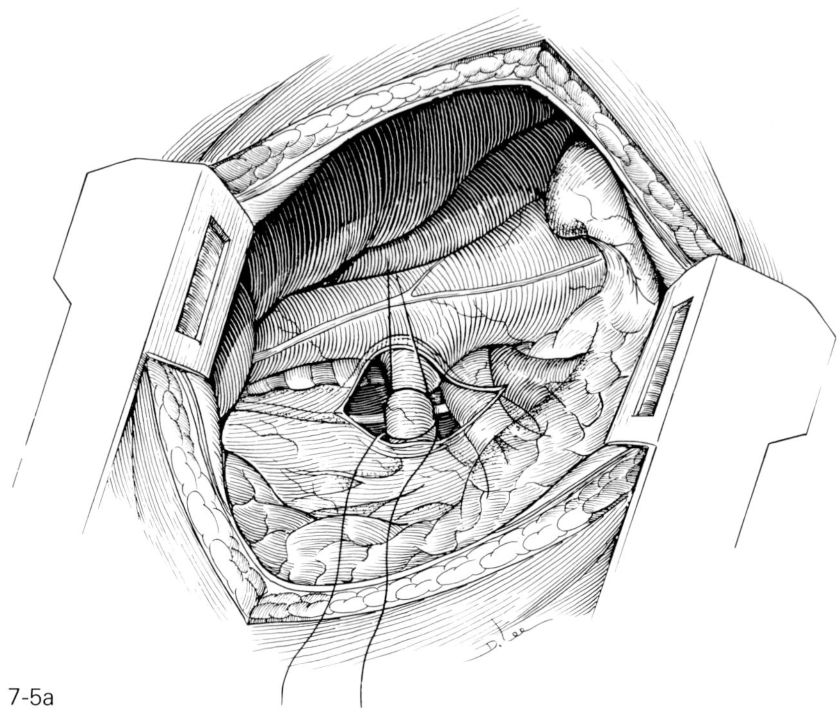

7-5a

Preoperative Preparation for Systemic–Pulmonary Shunt

One unit of blood and 250 ml of plasma are prepared. If the hematocrit is elevated, plasma is used to replace intraoperative blood loss, which should be minimal in any case. No special laboratory studies are necessary. Acidosis, if present, is corrected by administration of sodium bicarbonate or, in urgent situations, by mechanical ventilation as appropriate.

Technique of Waterston Shunt

Intravenous and intraarterial catheters are inserted. The infant is placed in the left lateral decubitus position, and the hemithorax is entered through the fourth intercostal space (see Chapter 6).

The mediastinal pleura is incised, and the azygous vein is divided (Figure 7-5a). A series of stay sutures is used to retract the vena cava medially and anteriorly.

The pulmonary artery is mobilized, and its branches are circumscribed with heavy silk loops (Figure 7-5b). As the pulmonary artery is dissected medially, the pericardium is entered and the ascending aorta is identified.

A partial occlusion clamp is placed with one jaw posterior to the right pulmonary artery and one jaw anterior to the aorta. The handle should face the patient's head if the surgeon is right-handed. When the jaws are approximated, a generous portion of the aorta is juxtaposed to the pulmonary artery.

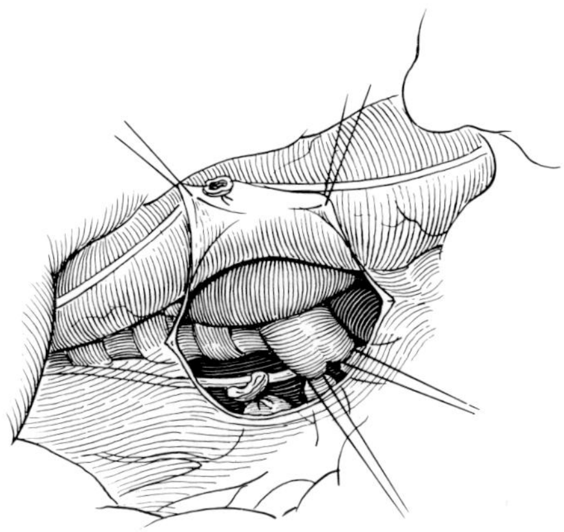

7-5b

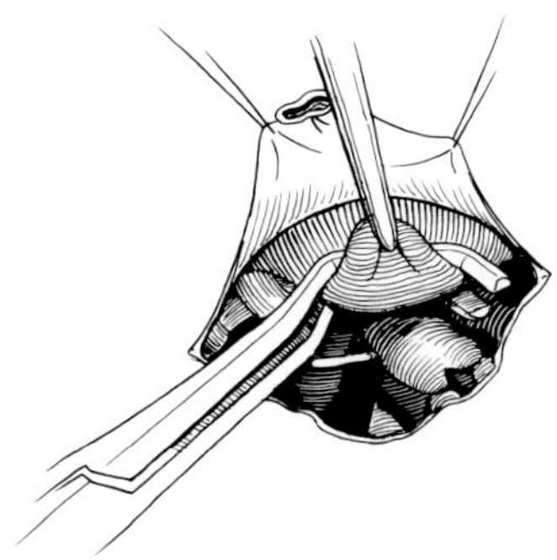

7-5c

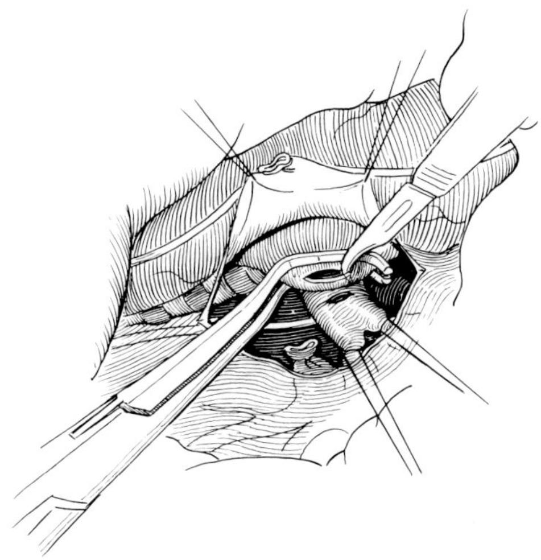

7-5d

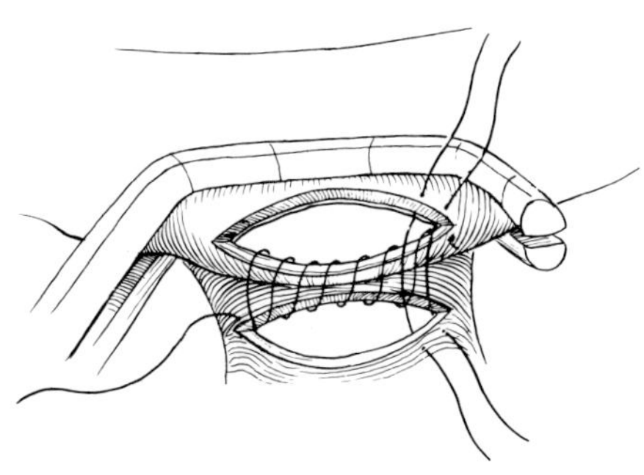

7-5e

It is essential that the incision in the aorta be made as far posterior as possible. Therefore, as the clamp is closed, the posterior surface of the aorta is grasped with atraumatic forceps and rotated anteriorly into the clamp (Figure 7-5c).

An aortotomy is made with a number 12 scalpel blade. This should be 3.0 mm long in the neonate. If this aortotomy is too large, pulmonary edema will result.

A parallel incision is made in the pulmonary artery, care being taken to leave a sufficiently long lip medially to allow suturing (Figure 7-5d). In general, it is best to make this incision smaller than the aortotomy because it enlarges as suturing progresses.

The back row of the anastomosis is performed with a 6-0 nonabsorbable running suture (Figure 7-5e). The anterior row is completed with interrupted sutures, to minimize the chance of pursestringing the anastomosis.

The snares and then the partial occlusion clamp are released. If bleeding is not severe, the anastomosis is packed with Oxycel for five minutes. Persistent bleeding is controlled by placement of extra sutures.

A thrill should be evident in the pulmonary artery upon removal of the clamp, and there may be a noticeable widening of the arterial pulse pressure and a fall in the mean arterial pressure. In our experience, the absence of a thrill generally signifies a technical error or too small a shunt. The clamp should be reapplied and the shunt remade.

Daicoff [2] has suggested that if the mean arterial pressure falls more than 20 percent when the shunt is opened, the anastomosis is too large, and postoperative pulmonary edema is likely. In this event, the anastomosis can be narrowed by an additional suture in one corner of the aortic incision. One can measure the pulmonary artery pressure if the shunt is suspected of being excessive. If the systolic pressure is above 40 percent of systemic, the shunt should be narrowed. For these tests to be valid, the patient cannot be acidotic or in a state of low cardiac output.

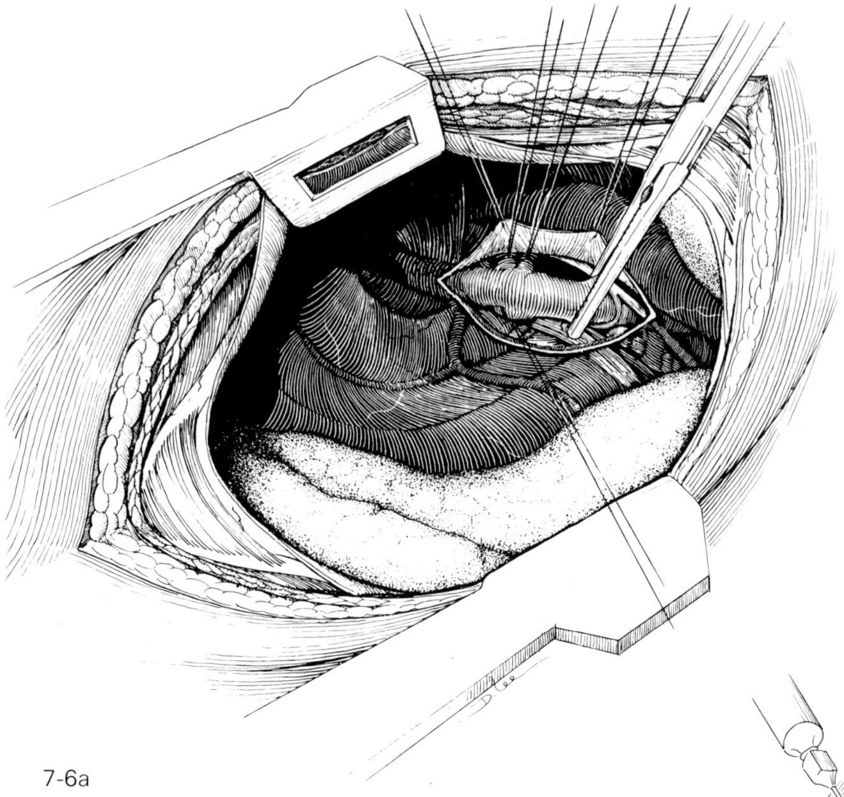

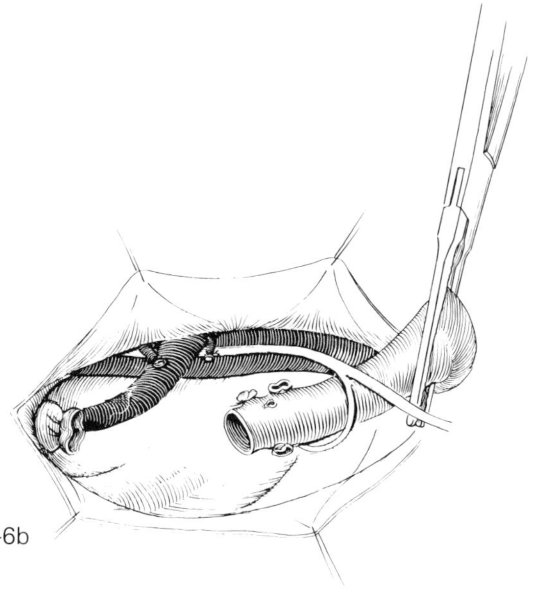

7-6b

7-6a

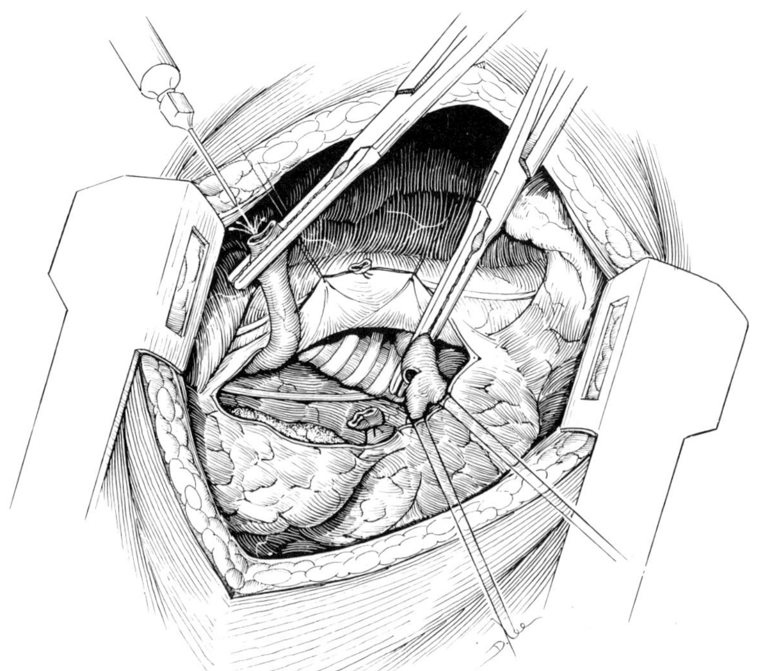

7-6c

Technique of Blalock-Taussig Shunt

The Blalock-Taussig operation is preferentially performed on the side opposite the aortic arch, because the subclavian artery is less likely to kink if it branches from the innominate artery than if it branches directly from the aorta.

A posterolateral incision is performed, and the thorax is entered through the third intercostal space (see Chapter 6). The azygous vein is divided, and the mediastinal pleura is incised from the lung hilum to the apex of the chest. A trough is created by dividing the areolar and lymphatic tissues between the phrenic and vagus nerves. The subclavian artery is isolated, and its branches are divided. There are usually four branches (Figure 7-6a).

The pulmonary artery is mobilized and its branches are circumscribed with heavy silk loops. The pericardium is entered so that the shunt can be created as far medially as possible.

In neonates we then administer 100 IU heparin per kg of body weight. The subclavian artery is next double-ligated as far distally as possible and divided just proximal to its branches. It is drawn through the sling created by the recurrent nerve (Figure 7-6b). The adventitia is removed. It is helpful to lift the adventitia up by forceful irrigation with heparinized saline solution through a 22-gauge needle (Figure 7-6c).

In order to obtain sufficient length to allow anastomosis without tension, the innominate and common carotid arteries must be dissected entirely free of attachments right up to the apex of the chest (Figure 7-6d). Because there are no branches of the carotid in this area, this can safely be done by blunt dissection.

The pulmonary artery is then occluded proximally and distally, and a transverse incision is made, slightly less than the diameter of the subclavian orifice. It will enlarge as suturing proceeds.

During the anastomosis it is essential that the assistant hold the two vessels in precise alignment, so that no tension is placed on the anastomosis while it is only partially completed. Use of straight, atraumatic clamps instead of Cooley- or Blalock-type clamps allows the most room. The back wall is completed first, starting halfway up the pulmonary artery incision toward the surgeon with a 7-0 suture that is tied on the outside, then brought inside and run as a simple over-and-over stitch away from the operator (Figure 7-6e). We prefer to end this suture halfway around and to complete the anterior portion with interrupted 7-0 sutures, all of which are placed before tying (Figure 7-6f). This permits precise alignment and prevents inadvertently suturing the back wall to the front.

The clamps and ligatures are removed, distal pulmonary artery first. Rarely is it necessary to place another suture for hemostasis. The heparin is not reversed (Figure 7-6g).

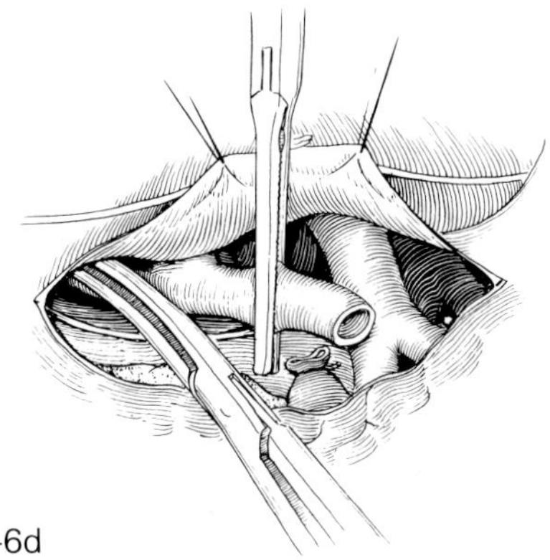

7-6d

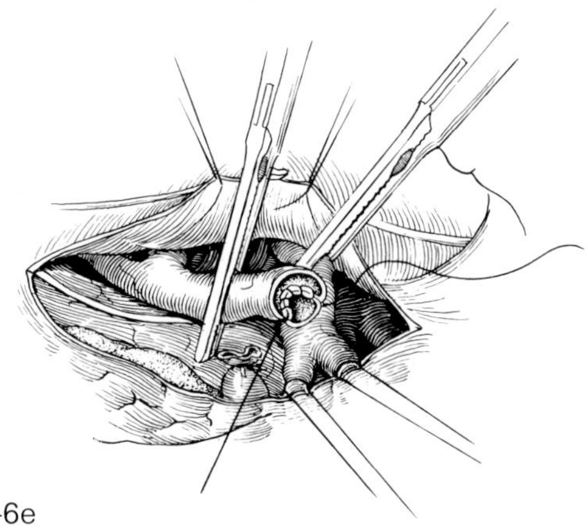

7-6e

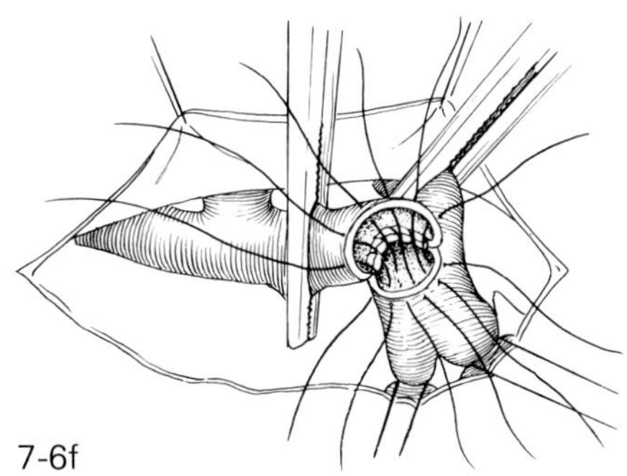

7-6f

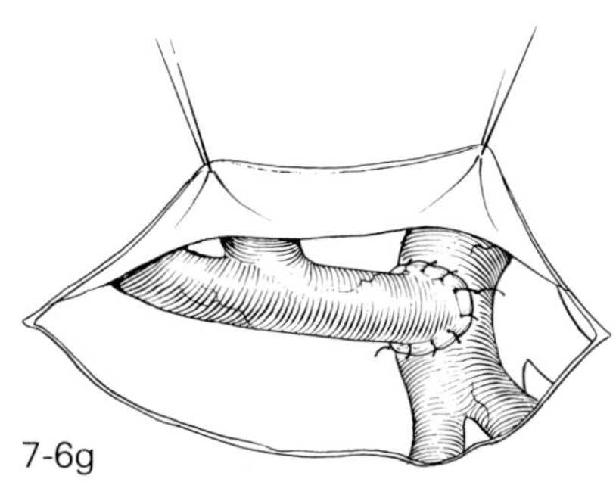

7-6g

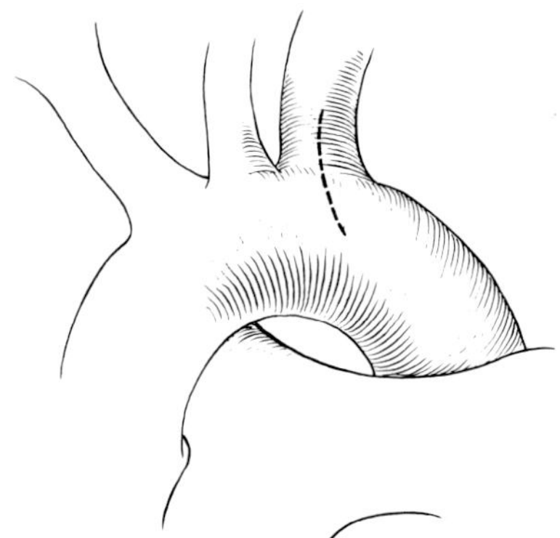

7-7a

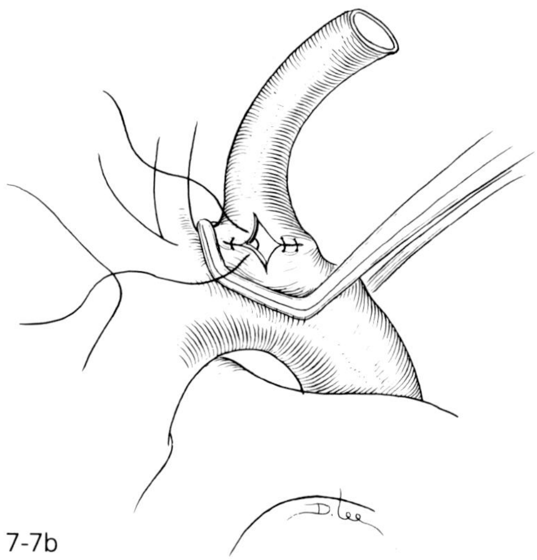

7-7b

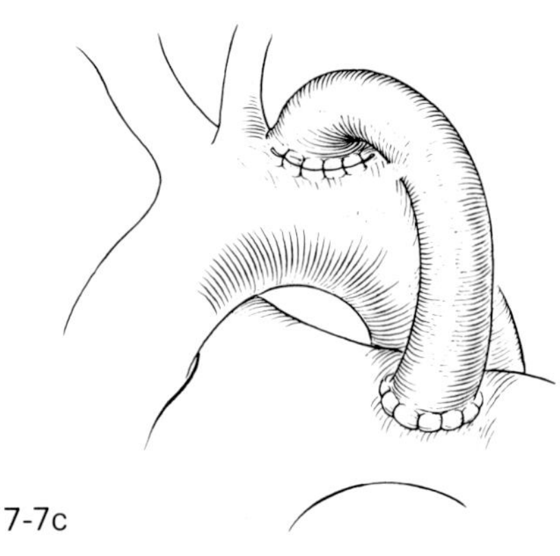

7-7c

Sometimes it may be necessary to construct a Blalock shunt on the side of the aortic arch, which often results in kinking of the subclavian artery where it arises from the aorta. Laks and Castaneda [3] have described a technique for relieving this by subclavian arterioplasty, which we have found very helpful. A longitudinal incision is made across the junction of the subclavian artery and aorta. This incision is sutured transversely to enlarge and reposition the subclavian orifice (Figure 7-7).

Postoperative Care Following Shunts

Most patients can be promptly extubated after operation unless preoperatively they have been extremely hypoxic and acidotic. It is not unusual for the shunt murmur to be inaudible for several days postoperatively, and sometimes there is concern about its patency. During this time the patient's oxygenation provides the most helpful measure of the adequacy of the shunt. For this reason we prefer to leave in an arterial catheter as a means of easily measuring the arterial blood gases. It must be remembered that all these patients continue to have right-to-left intracardiac shunting; therefore, the arterial Po_2 is usually not more than 30 to 50 mm Hg, with a resulting arterial oxygen saturation of 70% to 80% even with a good shunt.

Most of the flow through a shunt is directed to the ipsilateral lung. If this flow is excessive, unilateral pulmonary edema may result. Chest films taken during the 48 hours following operation should be inspected for signs of excessive flow to the ipsilateral lung. When pulmonary edema occurs (and this is rare), it can usually be managed by diuresis and, if necessary, positive-pressure ventilation for a few days. When these measures fail, one must occasionally reoperate and reduce the size of the shunt.

Another postoperative hazard is shunt thrombosis, which is promoted by hypotension, dehydration, and polycythemia. We therefore give these patients fluid liberally (two-thirds normal maintenance), we use plasma to replace any blood loss, and we carefully monitor the hematocrit reading and arterial pressure.

These patients, as all cyanotic neonates, tend to become hypoglycemic, hypercalcemic, or both. Levels of blood sugar and calcium should be monitored and abnormalities treated appropriately.

Results

A substantial operative mortality has attended shunting procedures for cyanotic heart disease in infants. Furthermore, every study has shown that mortality is directly related to age at operation, with mortality for neonates being much higher even than that illustrated in Table 7-1.

Table 7-1. Mortality following shunts in infants

Reports	Tetralogy	Tricuspid Atresia
Waldhausen 1968	0%	25%
Mustard 1970	23%	15%
Bernhard 1971	21%[a]	36%[a]
Waterston 1972	31%	15%
Truconne 1974	16%	42%
Reitman 1974	41%	0%[a]
Daicoff 1974	40%	53%

[a]Includes late deaths.

Our operative mortality for shunts in neonates in the past five years has been 25 percent, although there has been some recent improvement.

Additional complications can occur in the survivors: Shunts can fail after initially appearing to be satisfactory. When later failure occurs, the pulmonary artery itself may thrombose; the pulmonary artery may become kinked and narrowed at the site of the shunt (see Figure 7-4), especially in a Waterston shunt; and the infundibular stenosis in tetralogy can progress to complete occlusion. Thus these patients must be carefully followed postoperatively and they must be thoroughly restudied by cardiac catheterization and angiography before subsequent total correction.

Atrial Septectomy

In transposition of the great arteries, tricuspid atresia, and pulmonary atresia with intact ventricular septum, survival depends upon there being a large atrial patency. In 1950 Blalock and Hanlon [1] devised a procedure to create such a patency by a closed operative technique. This was the first really effective means of treating transposition.

Transposition of the Great Arteries

Transposition of the great arteries (TGA) comprises only about 5 percent of all congenital cardiac anomalies. However, among the cyanotic conditions of the newborn it is the most common cause of morbidity and mortality. The reason for this is that in uncomplicated TGA the pulmonary and systemic circulations are entirely separate, that is, in parallel, which allows no exchange of oxygenated and unoxygenated blood between the lungs and peripheral tissues (Figure 7-8). Usually the foramen ovale is patent, which permits some interatrial mixing, but it is rarely sufficient to allow more than a brief period of survival. In these patients improved mixing of red and blue blood is urgently required.

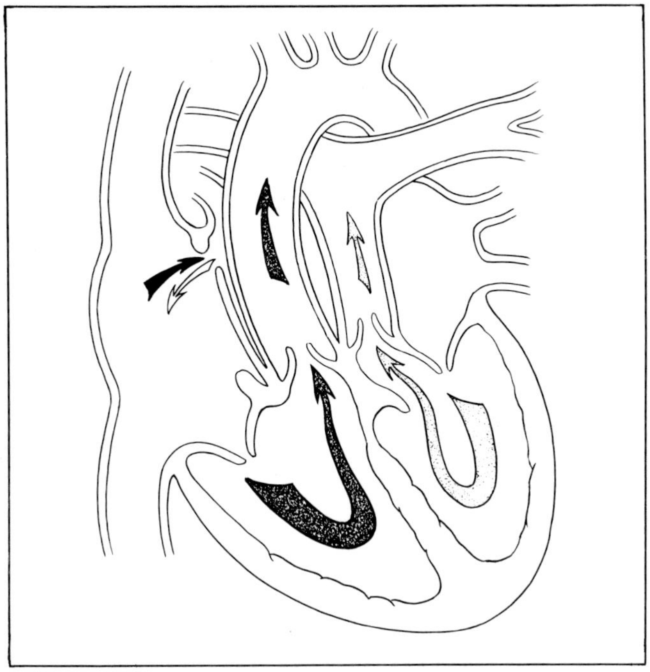

A

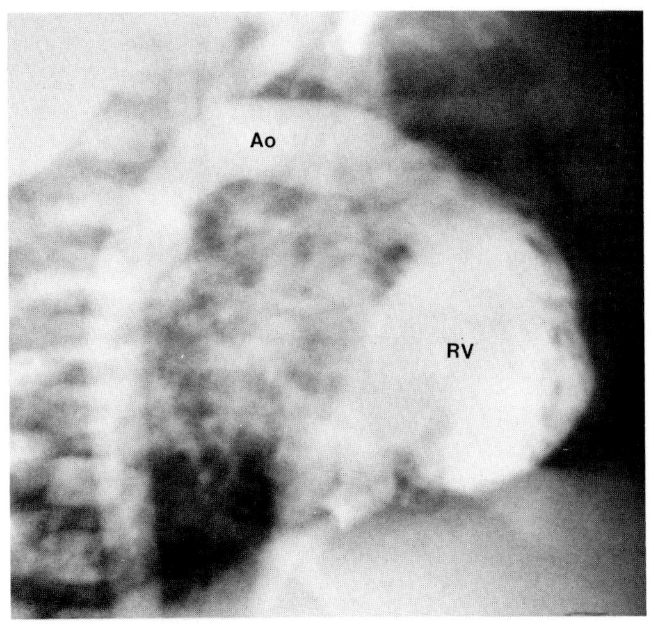

B

7-8. (A) Diagram of usual anatomy in transposition of great arteries. The atria and ventricles are normally situated, but the great arteries are transposed. (B) Lateral angiocardiogram in TGA. The aorta (Ao) arises anteriorly from the right ventricle (RV).

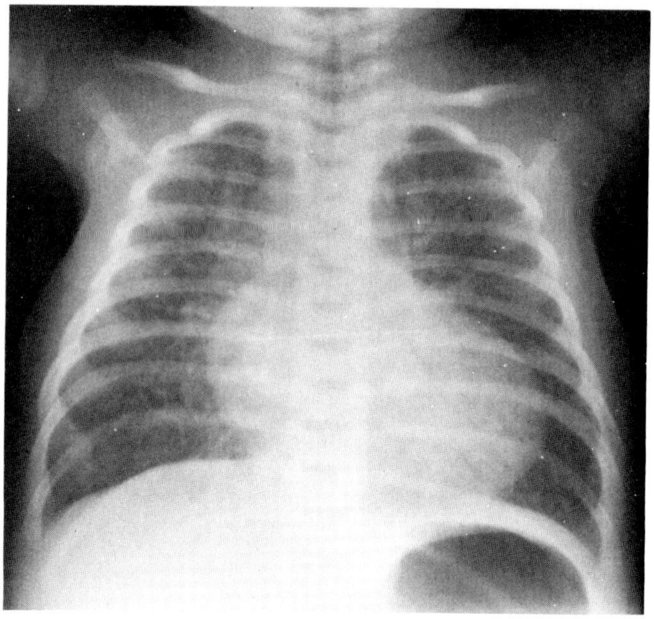

7-9. Typical chest roentgenogram in transposition of the great arteries without associated anomalies.

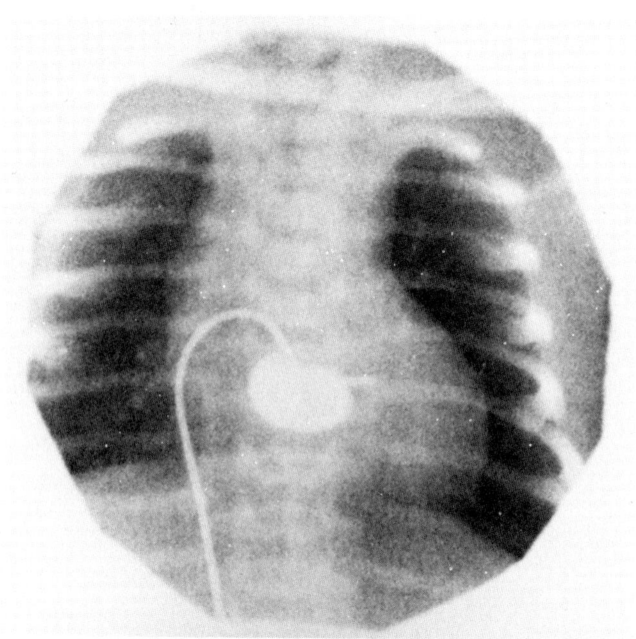

7-10. The Rashkind procedure. A balloon-tipped catheter, inflated with radiopaque contrast material, has been forcibly pulled through the foramen ovale from left atrium into right atrium.

Diagnosis

The diagnosis of TGA should be suspected in any severely cyanotic infant who has increased pulmonary vascular markings on chest film (Figure 7-9). Usually there is no cardiac murmur unless an associated anomaly is present. The diagnosis can be confirmed and associated defects delineated only by cardiac catheterization and angiography, which demonstrate the essential features of the condition in its usual form:

1. The aorta arises from the anterior ventricle, which is morphologically a right ventricle.
2. Interatrial mixing occurs through a patent foramen ovale.
3. A ventricular septal defect (VSD) may be present (in one-third to one-half of the cases).
4. Subvalvular (or valvular) pulmonary stenosis (PS) may be present (in 9 percent of cases).

Measurement of pressures and oxygen saturations allows pulmonary and systemic vascular flows and resistances to be calculated.

Selection of Operation

Once the intracardiac anatomy is known, the proper operation(s) can be selected for that patient's problem, that is, (1) to increase intracardiac mixing, the usual problem; (2) to decrease pulmonary blood flow in patients with TGA and a large VSD; or (3) to increase pulmonary blood flow in patients with TGA and severe PS.

Intracardiac mixing can be increased either by (1) enlargement of the foramen ovale by balloon catheter rupture, the Rashkind procedure (Figure 7-10), or by (2) surgical atrial septectomy by the Blalock-Hanlon or some other technique. Although the Rashkind septostomy is usually satisfactory [5], there is a substantial mortality and failure rate in some hands, and the palliation afforded may be short-lived. Thus some have preferred primary surgical septectomy. Surgical septectomy is sometimes necessary also as a secondary procedure following a Rashkind septostomy that has failed.

Pulmonary blood flow may be decreased by pulmonary artery banding (described later in this chapter). This should be done early in infancy because of the marked propensity for patients with TGA and VSD to develop pulmonary vascular disease. Banding is particularly hazardous in the presence of TGA because, as the band is tightened, cyanosis may increase, which of course does not occur when the great arteries arise normally. Thus the degree of tightness of the band must be judged not only by the fall in distal pulmonary artery pressure but also by the fall in atrial oxygen saturation. At present, our objective is to repair TGA and VSD primarily in infancy, because we have found the additional risks imposed by banding and later debanding to be unacceptable.

Patients with severe pulmonary stenosis (usually in addition to VSD) may have their pulmonary blood flow increased if necessary by means of a systemic-to-pulmonary shunt, discussed at the opening of this chapter. An atrial septectomy may also be required to allow the newly augmented pulmonary blood flow to enter the systemic circulation, permitting the patient to reach a size (five to ten years of age) where a definitive repair can be carried out by the Rastelli technique.

Tricuspid Atresia

In all cases of tricuspid valve atresia (see Figure 7-2), an atrial septal defect provides the only way for blood to leave the right atrium. The systemic and pulmonary venous blood then mixes in the left atrium and ventricle before some of it is pumped into the aorta and the pulmonary artery. Four variations can be identified according to whether or not there is obstruction in the right ventricular outflow and whether the great vessels are transposed or normally related. The right ventricle is invariably hypoplastic to some degree. Without effective palliation, half the infants with this anomaly die before the age of six months and two-thirds die before the age of one year.

Diagnosis

Atresia of the tricuspid valve is suspected in cyanotic infants when the electrocardiogram shows a normal or left axis and preponderance of left ventricular forces. Other cyanotic conditions generally show right ventricular preponderance on the electrocardiogram. The pulmonary blood flow is reduced on the chest roentgenogram in the usual case, where there is obstruction of right ventricular outflow.

The diagnosis is confirmed by cardiac catheterization and angiography, which also serve to delineate (1) the adequacy of the atrial septal defect, (2) the adequacy of pulmonary flow, (3) the size of the right ventricle, and (4) the relationship of the great vessels.

Selection of Operation

In the typical case of tricuspid atresia, pulmonary blood flow is so reduced that a systemic-to-pulmonary shunt is indicated (see the first portion of this chapter). Rarely, when there is a large VSD and normal pulmonary valve, pulmonary blood flow may be excessive, and pulmonary artery banding is required (see the last section of this chapter). In the 20 percent of cases in which the atrial septal patency is small enough to obstruct the free flow of blood from the right atrium to the left atrium, the atrial septum must be enlarged by surgical atrial septectomy or balloon atrial septostomy.

Pulmonary Atresia with Intact Ventricular Septum

In many patients with atresia (or even severe stenosis) of the pulmonary valve, right atrial blood is preferentially shunted across the foramen ovale, which causes cyanosis. It would seem that relief might be afforded simply by opening up the right ventricular outflow. Often, however, the right ventricle is so underdeveloped or the tricuspid valve so incompetent that an adequate stroke volume cannot be attained after pulmonary valvotomy. In this case it may be preferable to approach the problem in stages, by:

1. Bypassing the right ventricle by creating a large atrial septal patency (if one does not exist naturally) and performing a systemic-to-pulmonary shunt.
2. Subsequently performing a pulmonary valvotomy to allow right ventricular and pulmonary artery development.
3. Considering definitive reconstruction of right ventricular outflow at a later date.

In the unusual patient with a well-developed right ventricle and a competent tricuspid valve, primary definitive repair may be performed, as described in Chapter 9.

Preparation for Operation

Because of the severity of hypoxia in most infants with this anomaly, preparation for operation must sometimes be carried out in parallel with diagnostic procedures. Oxygen is, of course, administered, although it is unlikely to raise the Po_2 much above the range of 20 to 30 mm Hg because the fully saturated pulmonary venous blood simply is unable to reach the systemic circulation. Arterial pH and Pco_2 are monitored closely. Sodium bicarbonate is administered as necessary to correct metabolic acidosis, which may be profound. The patient is intubated and ventilated to correct respiratory acidosis if necessary. One unit of blood is crossmatched.

If the patient is in critical condition, the catheter used for diagnostic catheterization is left in place as an intravenous route, and the patient is taken directly to the previously prepared operating room. An arterial line is inserted if time allows.

In the older neonate who has been on digitalis or diuretics, serum electrolytes should be measured. This is unnecessary in the newborn. Preoperative coagulation studies are unnecessary.

Technique of the Blalock-Hanlon Operation

The chest is entered through the right fifth intercostal space (see Chapter 6). The pericardium is incised posterior to the phrenic nerve, which is reflected anteriorly if necessary. Heavy silk sutures are looped about the pulmonary artery and veins, and the sutures are tightened to occlude blood flow (Figure 7-11a). It is essential that the pulmonary artery be occluded first and released last, to prevent the lungs from being engorged with blood while the pulmonary veins are occluded.

A curved vascular clamp is positioned with one blade anterior on the right atrium and the other blade posterior to the right pulmonary veins. The clamp should be placed with the handle pointing cranially if the surgeon is right-handed, or it will interfere with his suturing.

Sutures are placed at each end of the proposed incision and tied. These will be used subsequently to close the incision, when time is of the essence. As the clamp is closed, the arterial pressure is observed. Often the clamp must be replaced to achieve a position that will be tolerated. Never proceed hurriedly until a stable position is found! It is essential that a generous amount of atrium be included in the clamp.

A 2-cm incision is made in the right atrium until the endocardium is *clearly* identified. A fine suction tip is necessary for this (Figure 7-11b). The anterior lip of the incision can be grasped with a straight hemostat. Then a parallel incision is made in the confluence of the right pulmonary veins.

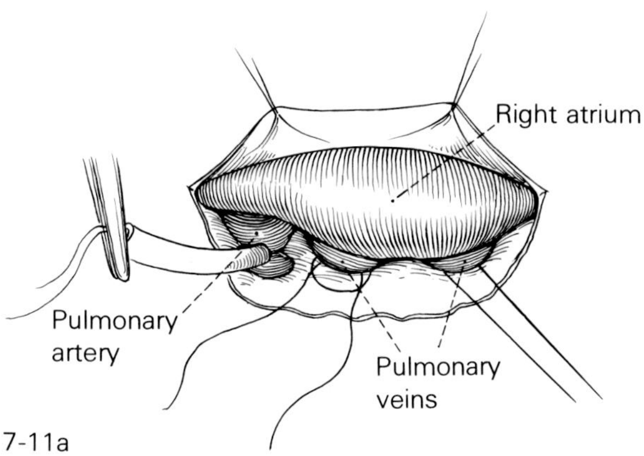

7-11a

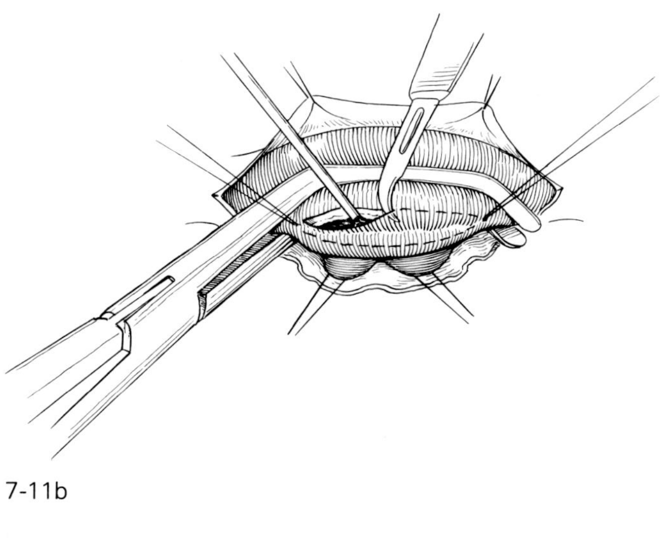

7-11b

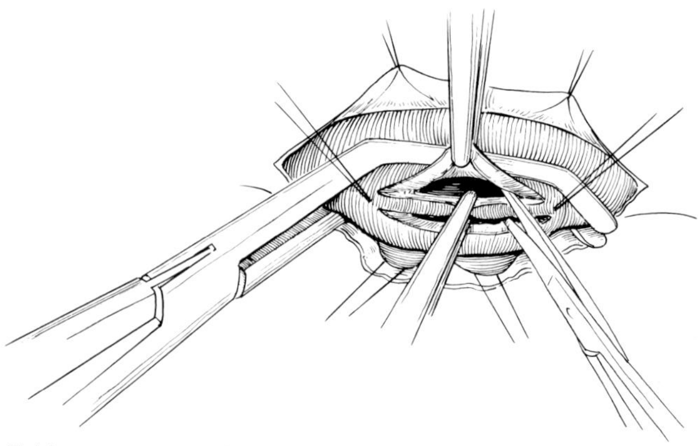

7-11c

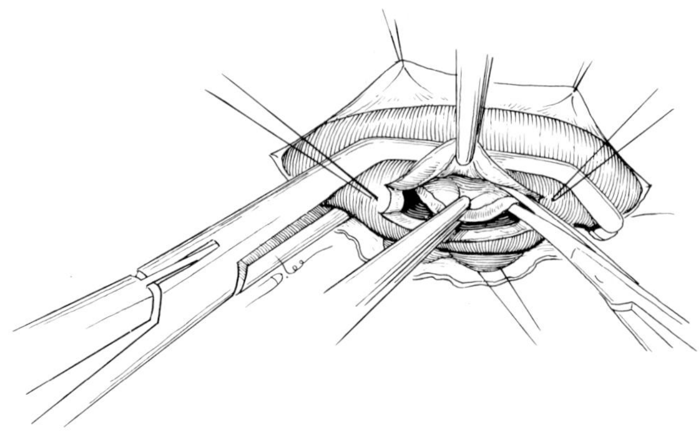

7-11d

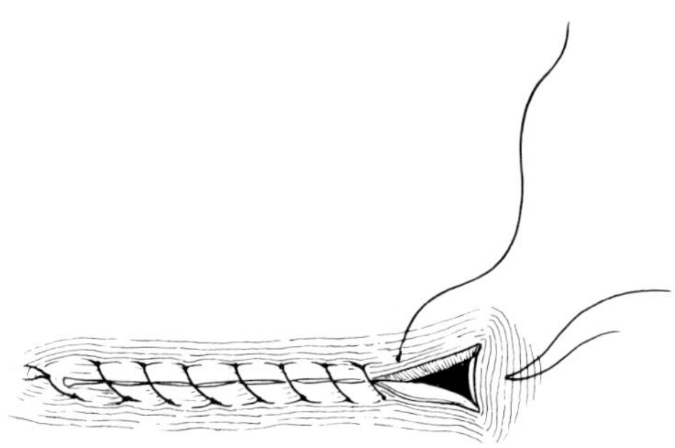

7-11e

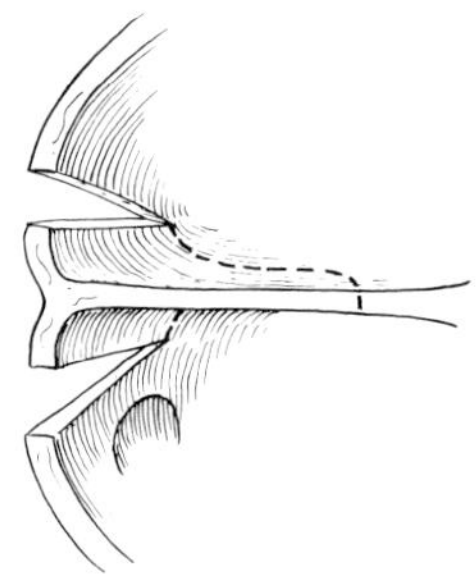

7-11f

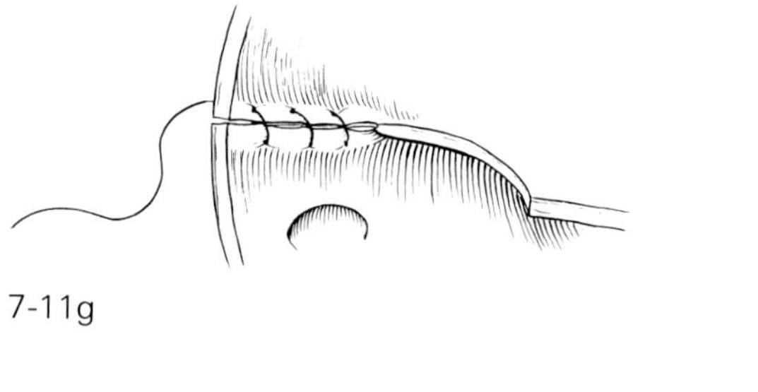

7-11g

Once the endothelium is *clearly* seen, the exposed edge of the atrial septum is grasped with another straight hemostat (Figure 7-11c). Initial incisions are made at each end of the septum. Then the clamp is loosened, allowing additional septum to be withdrawn and excised (Figure 7-11d). Care must be taken not to withdraw so much septum that the left atrial wall is imbricated and perforated.

Finally, the incision is rapidly closed with sutures preplaced at either end of the incision (Figure 7-11e). The clamp and the occlusive ligatures are removed. Now blood is able to pass freely between right and left atria (Figure 7-11f, g).

A chest tube is inserted, and the wound is closed in layers.

Speed is of the essence in this procedure. These babies are often extremely unstable and often do not tolerate clamping for more than five minutes. Before starting, the surgeon is wise to rehearse every move with his nurse and assistant to eliminate delays.

Postoperative Care Following Atrial Septectomy

The postoperative problems encountered following atrial septectomy usually are related to the patient's preoperative condition. Vigorous babies, operated upon electively, usually require little special care. Those who are profoundly acidotic and moribund preoperatively, however, should be ventilated initially, have arterial pressures and blood gases monitored, and be closely observed for hypoglycemia and for hypocalcemia. Some require catecholamine support for a few days. Of the 48 infants who have had atrial septectomy at the University of Michigan, 19 have required postoperative ventilatory support, 17 have had major postoperative complications, and 3 have required catecholamine infusions.

Results

Most patients have improved dramatically following septectomy for transposition. They show an increase in atrial Po_2 from preoperative levels averaging from 25 mm Hg to postoperative levels averaging 37 mm Hg, with substantial improvement of cardiac output, and with relief of left atrial hypertension. This improvement has been well maintained until the time of total correction, and there have been few late deaths or complications.

The mortality from this operation remains high—21 percent in our hands—mainly because of the poor preoperative condition of the patients. As mentioned above, some cardiologists prefer to perform atrial septostomy by rupturing the septum with a balloon-tipped catheter at the time of catheterization (Rashkind procedure). This procedure has had about the same immediate mortality rate as surgical septectomy in most hands in the past, but the long-term results may be less reliable, with an appreciably high incidence of late deaths, strokes, and inadequate oxygenation.

We prefer to carry out definitive repair of transposition at about one year of age following initial palliation. If a balloon atrial septostomy has been performed and palliation is inadequate, it may be necessary to carry out total repair earlier. We and others have carried out total correction primarily in a few neonates, and we have been discouraged by the excessive incidence of complications, such as obstruction of the superior vena cava and leaks about the patch.

We have performed very few atrial septectomies for tricuspid atresia. Most infants with this anomaly have required only a shunting procedure and have survived for many years. Total repair of tricuspid atresia is now possible in some cases by the Fontan procedure, which has been carried out in later childhood but has not been attempted in infants.

The mortality for operative procedures in pulmonary atresia with intact ventricular septum has been very high. Because of the great anatomic variability in these infants, it is hard to determine an overall prognosis. In general, when the right ventricle and tricuspid valve are fairly normal, some patients may survive ultimate total correction. Only short-term follow-up is available in infants who have had the staged approach outlined above, but there is evidence that the right ventricle can develop with time—thus raising the hope that ultimately total correction may be possible.

Pulmonary Artery Banding

In a patient with a large intraventricular defect (VSD), blood shunts from the left ventricle into the right ventricle and pulmonary circulation because the systemic resistance exceeds the pulmonary resistance. When the VSD is large, as it usually is in symptomatic infants, the pulmonary blood flow is huge, and the pressures are equal in the right ventricle, left ventricle, aorta, and pulmonary artery.

In 1952 Muller and Damman [4] showed that pulmonary artery pressure and blood flow in patients with intraventricular left-to-right shunts could be reduced by constricting the pulmonary artery. By means of serial lung biopsies, they demonstrated also that the histologic damage associated with pulmonary hypertension may regress.

Banding the pulmonary artery adds an additional resistance to the pulmonary resistance, so that, ideally, these two together equal the systemic resistance, and there is no net left-to-right shunt. The ventricular pressures remain equal as the band is tightened while the pulmonary artery pressure beyond the band falls toward normal levels.

The wall of the pulmonary artery beneath the band is compressed by the band and becomes fibrotic, so that usually the pulmonary artery must be reconstructed at the time of total correction. Some band materials excite more inflammatory reaction than others and cause even greater scarring. Because the band obstructs right ventricular emptying, right ventricular and infundibular hypertrophy progresses following banding, which may further complicate the subsequent total repair.

Indications

This operation has proved valuable in relieving congestive heart failure in infants with uncomplicated VSD or with VSD and associated endocardial cushion defect, transposition of the great vessels, double-outlet right ventricle, or other conditions in which pulmonary blood flow is excessive. In general, these infants have dyspnea, respiratory infections, and poor feeding because of their overwhelming pulmonary blood flow. When the congestive failure cannot be managed with drugs and salt restriction, operation is indicated.

Diagnosis

The intracardiac anatomy must be delineated by cardiac catheterization and angiography, at which time the pulmonary artery pressure and pulmonary blood flow are measured. It is most important to determine if a patent ductus arteriosus is also present because, if so, this further increases pulmonary blood flow. The ductus arteriosus must be closed at the time of pulmonary banding.

Preparation for Operation

Blood loss from this procedure should be minimal; so only one unit need be crossmatched. A secure intravenous cannula must be inserted. A recording system is prepared to allow intraoperative pressure measurements to be made of pulmonary artery and ventricular pressures during the banding.

Operative Technique

The patient is positioned for a left thoracotomy, and the fourth intercostal space is entered (see Chapter 6). The ductus arteriosus is identified and ligated or divided if it is patent or suspected of being patent (Figure 7-12a). Then the pericardium is opened longitudinally anterior to the phrenic nerve.

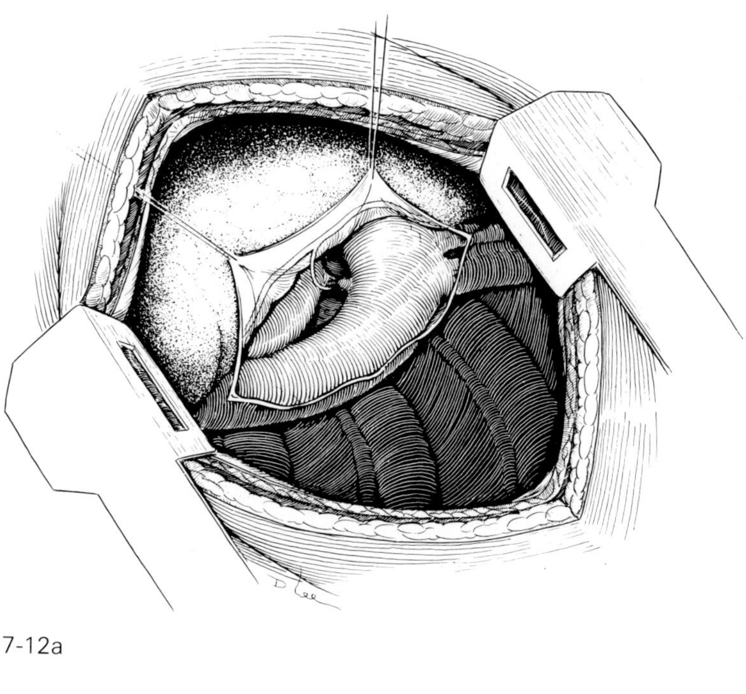

7-12a

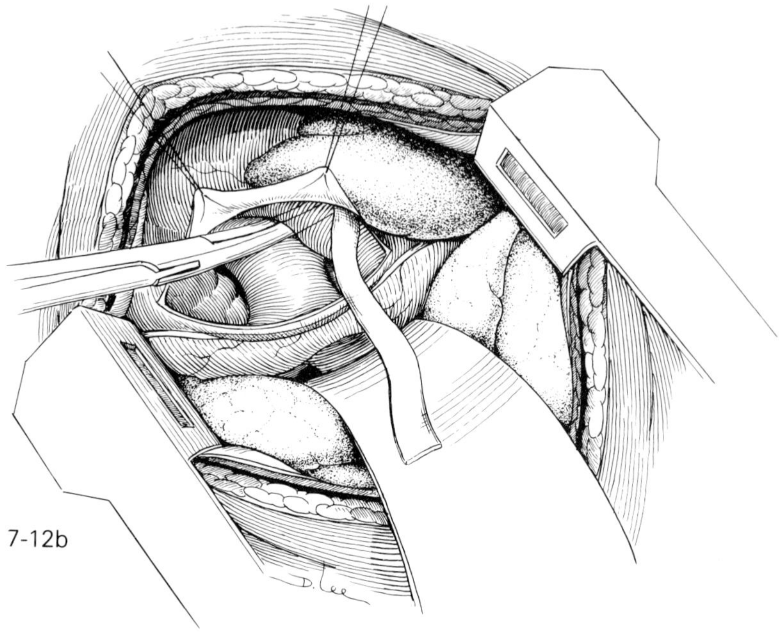

7-12b

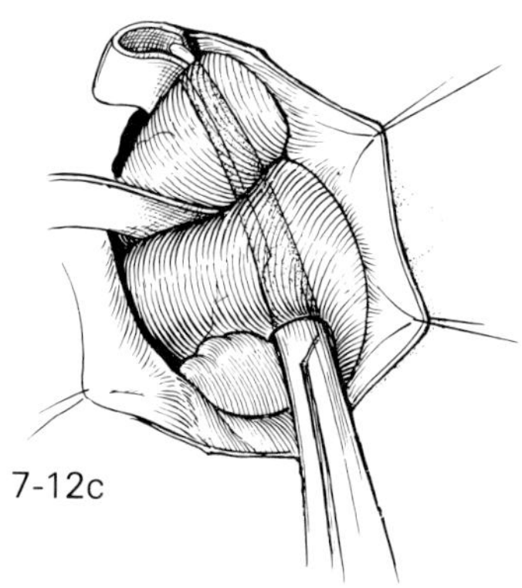

7-12c

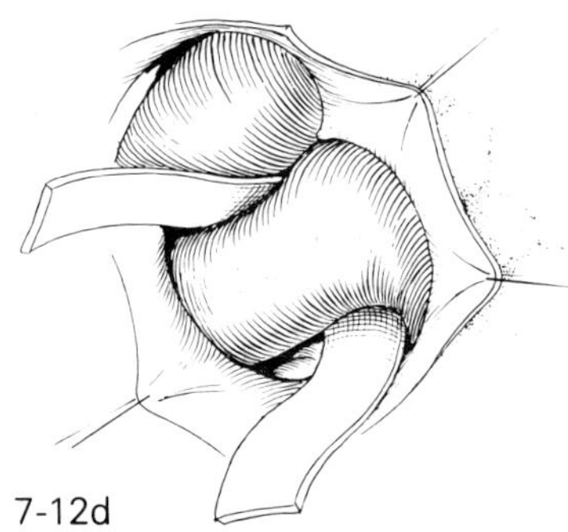

7-12d

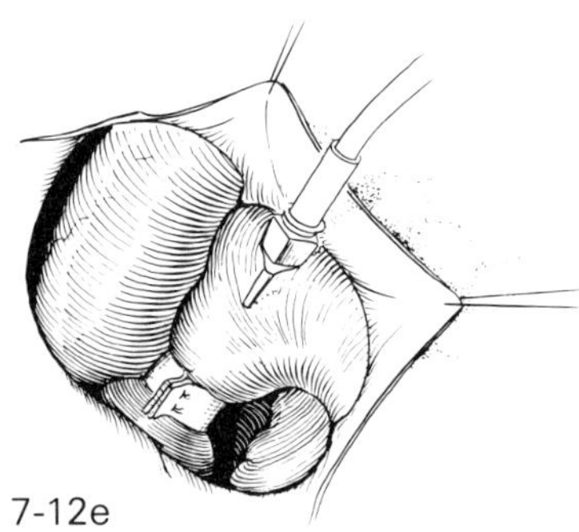

7-12e

The pulmonary artery is separated from the aorta and circumscribed with a band. Sometimes it is difficult to draw the band directly around the pulmonary artery; it may be easier to draw it first around the aorta (Figure 7-12b) and then around the entire root of the heart through the transverse pericardial space (Figure 7-12c) to "subtract the aorta," leaving just the main pulmonary artery circumscribed (Figure 7-12d).

The choice of band material is a matter of debate. In emergency situations we have used a heavy silk ligature (number 5 plaited silk) because this can be applied rapidly with a minimum of adjustment. In more elective situations we prefer a tightly woven Teflon tape, which is sutured to itself after tightening (Figure 7-12e). This is easier to remove at the time of eventual reconstruction.

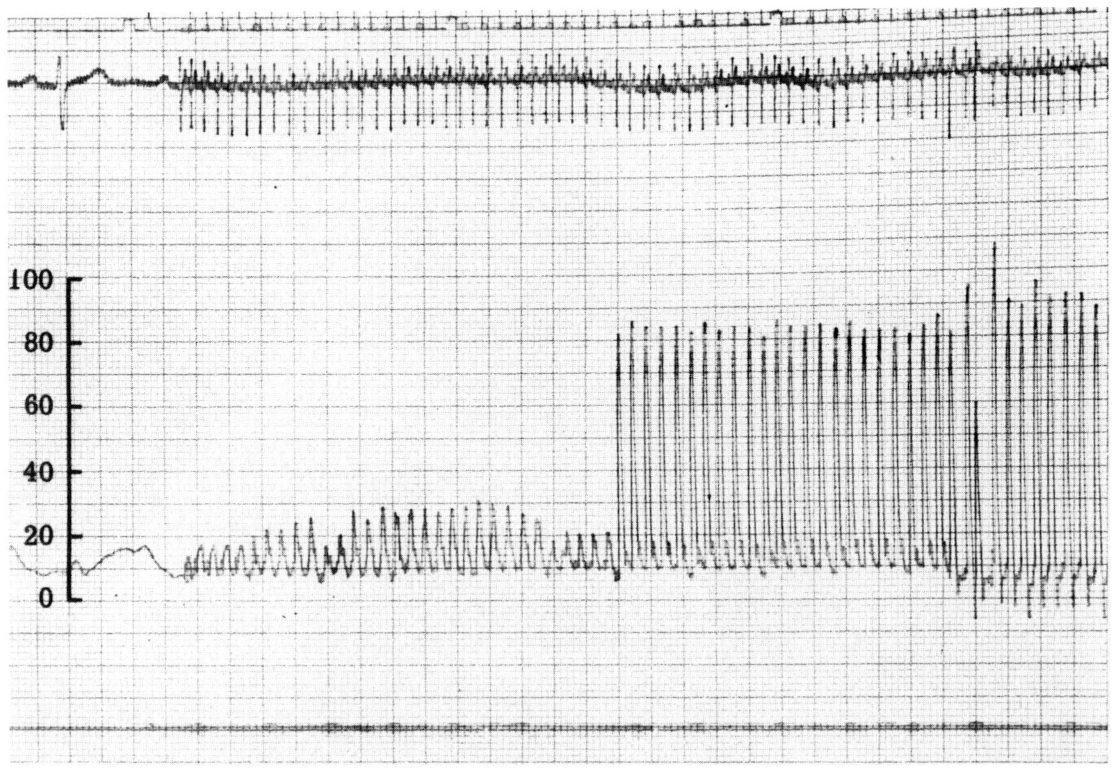

7-13. Pressure withdrawal tracing from patient with pulmonary artery band. The pressure distal to the band is normal, while proximal to the band it is elevated to systemic levels.

The band is progressively tightened until the distal pulmonary artery pressure falls to normal levels, if this pressure can be tolerated (Figure 7-13). Dilatation or slowing of the heart indicates that less constriction must be accepted. As the band is tightened, the interventricular and systemic arterial pressures generally increase.

When banding is carried out in transposition with ventricular septal defect, an additional problem arises. The patient's systemic arterial oxygen saturation depends in part upon the ratio of pulmonary to systemic blood flow. As the pulmonary blood flow is reduced during banding, the patient becomes more cyanotic. Thus, to determine how tightly a band can be applied, arterial oxygen saturations must be determined as well as pulmonary artery pressures.

Postoperative Care Following Banding

These patients usually require no more than the usual care afforded sick patients who undergo operation. Some have such severe pulmonary edema that positive-pressure ventilation and diuresis will be required postoperatively until the edema is resolved.

Results

The mortality from pulmonary artery banding in infants with uncomplicated ventricular septal defect has been low—below 10 percent—compared with approximately 50 percent in patients with more complex lesions. How severely the ultimate total correction is complicated by the debanding depends on many factors, such as the type of material used, the location of the band, and the length of time it has been in place. In general, we have found that the additional problems created at the time of total correction are sufficiently troublesome so that we do not recommend pulmonary artery banding if primary total correction is feasible. Thus at our institution primary total repair has been preferred for uncomplicated VSD; we reserve banding for more complex anomalies.

Selected References

1. Blalock, A., and Hanlon, D. R. The surgical treatment of complete transposition of the aorta and the pulmonary artery. *Surg. Gynecol. Obstet.* 90:1, 1950.
2. Daicoff, G. R., Aslami, A., Victorica, B. E., and Schiebler, G. L. Ascending aorta-to-pulmonary artery anastomosis for cyanotic congenital heart disease. *Ann. Thorac. Surg.* 18:260, 1974.
3. Laks, H., and Castaneda, A. R. Subclavian arterioplasty for the ipsilateral Blalock-Taussig shunt. *Ann. Thorac. Surg.* 19:319, 1974.
4. Muller, W. H., Jr., and Damman, J. F., Jr. The treatment of certain congenital malformations of the heart by the creation of pulmonic stenosis to reduce pulmonary hypertension and excessive pulmonary blood flow. *Surg. Gynecol. Obstet.* 95:213, 1952.
5. Rashkind, W. J., and Miller, W. W. Transposition of the great arteries. Results of palliation by balloon atrioseptostomy in thirty-one infants. *Circulation* 38:453, 1968.
6. Waterston, D. J., Stark, J., and Ashcraft, K. W. Ascending aorta-to-right pulmonary artery shunts: Experience with 100 patients. *Surgery* 72:897, 1972.

8

Patent Ductus Arteriosus and Aortic Arch Anomalies

Patent Ductus Arteriosus

Most infants born with patent ductus arteriosus remain asymptomatic. Their anomalies are discovered in later childhood at physical examination. For them, surgery can be carried out electively to prevent occurrence of later complications. Another group show symptoms early in infancy, with severe congestive heart failure, so that surgery becomes a lifesaving maneuver. Most infants with patent ductus arteriosus also have a coarctation of the aorta, an intracardiac defect—such as ventricular septal defect, atrial septal defect, aortic or mitral valve anomaly, or hypoplastic left heart syndrome—or a combination of these conditions. It is the high incidence of associated defects that sets this group apart from the group who remain asymptomatic, and it is the associated defects that are responsible for the very high mortality attending operation.

Premature infants have persistent patent ductus arteriosus in from 7 percent to 38 percent of cases. At least 60 percent of these patients also have respiratory distress syndrome (RDS). The causative relationship between patent ductus and RDS is not clear, but it is certain that infants with a large left-to-right shunt may have their respiratory problems worsened, and operation in such patients may be beneficial if the ductus does not close spontaneously. The problem is to separate patients with congestive heart failure caused by large left-to-right shunts from those patients with predominant bronchopulmonary dysplasia, who are unlikely to benefit from operation. Some infants clearly have large left-to-right shunts with cardiomegaly and pulmonary plethora on chest film (Figure 8-1). Others have a radiographic pattern more typical of the respiratory distress syndrome with a normal heart size (Figure 8-2). Unfortunately, in many cases the radiographic pattern falls between these extremes.

Diagnosis

The diagnosis of patent ductus arteriosus is suspected in the neonate who has a systolic murmur, a wide arterial pulse pressure, and increased pulmonary vascularity on chest film. The characteristic continuous murmur may not be present in neonates because their elevated pulmonary vascular resistance inhibits diastolic flow.

Because of the high incidence of associated anomalies, complete cardiac catheterization should be carried out in full-term infants. This will reveal the characteristic oxygen step-up in the pulmonary artery. Angiography will show dye escaping from the aorta into the pulmonary artery (Figure 8-3). In premature infants cardiac catheterization is technically difficult; the patient's physiologic state may vary rapidly, limiting the usefulness of this diagnostic procedure. Other techniques such as aortography, dilution curves from ear oximetry, echocardiography, and radionuclide scanning have

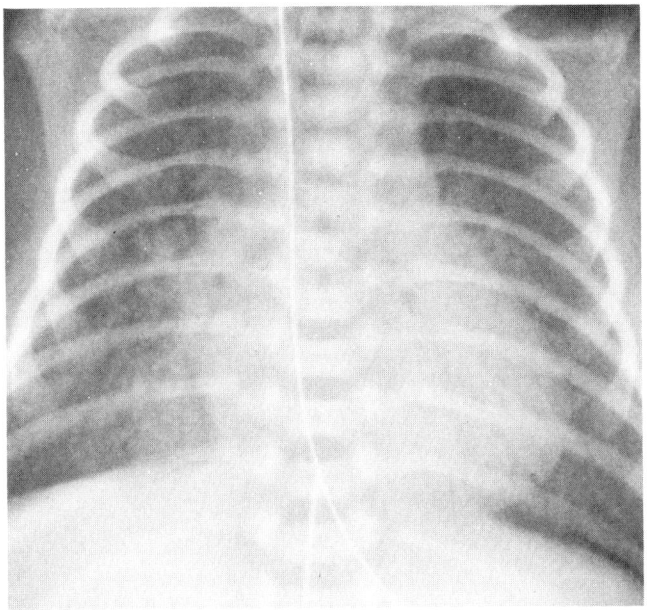

8-1. Chest roentgenogram of premature infant with patent ductus and pulmonary plethora.

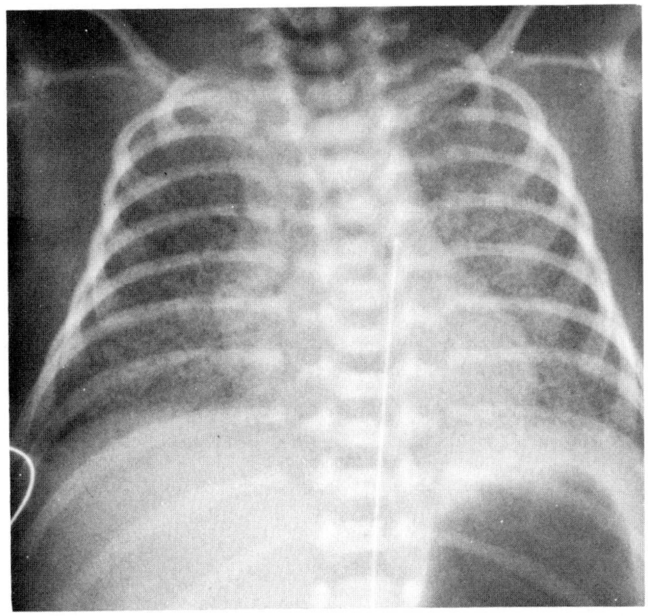

8-2. Chest roentgenogram of premature infant with predominant respiratory distress syndrome and small left-to-right shunt.

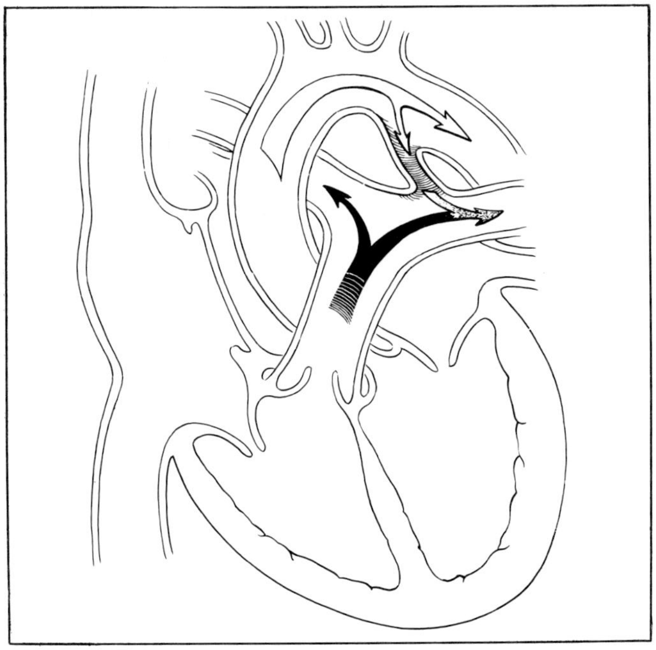

A

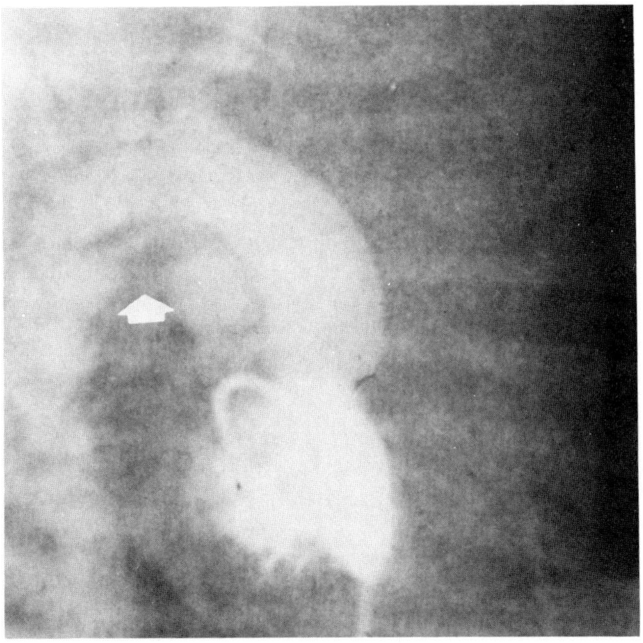

B

8-3. (A) Diagram of anatomy in persistent patent ductus arteriosus. (B) Angiogram revealing (arrow) escape of contrast from aorta into pulmonary artery through patent ductus.

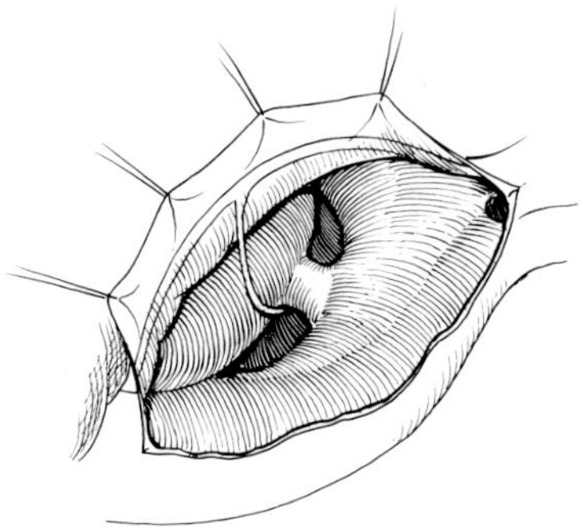

8-4a

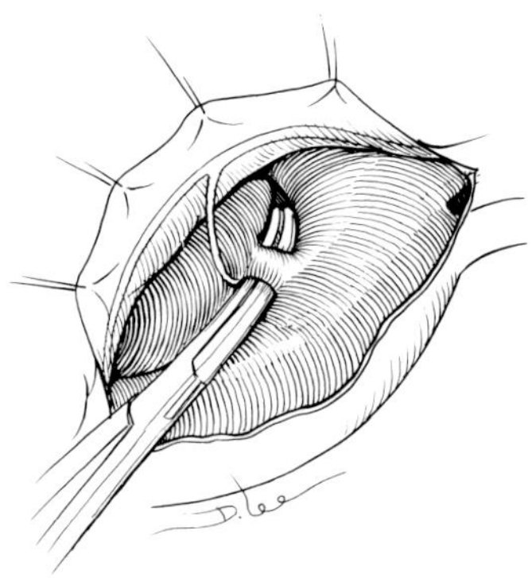

8-4b

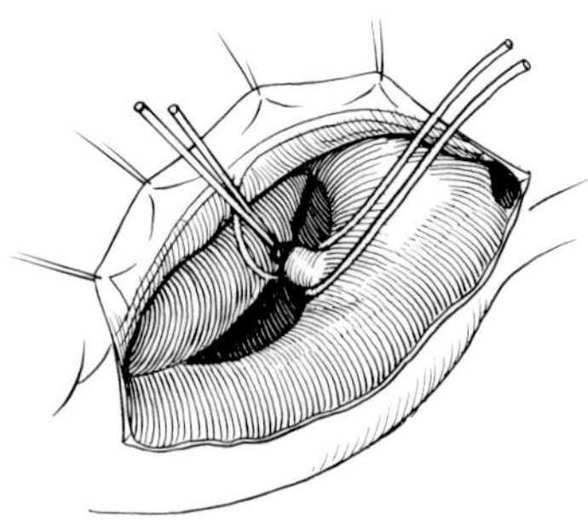

8-4c

been used to estimate the shunt size and to help exclude associated abnormalities. Recently we have come to rely on the echocardiogram in quantitating the amount of left-to-right shunting. The ratio between left atrial diameter and aortic diameter is determined. If this exceeds 1.15, the patent ductus probably is important. Contrast enhancement may further improve the precision of echocardiography and make this an even more valuable screening tool.

Preparation for Operation

Major blood loss should rarely occur during operation, but a unit of blood should be crossmatched. A reliable intravenous cannula must be inserted. It is not necessary to use an arterial line unless correction of associated intracardiac defects is contemplated.

Preparation for temperature control and humidification of inspired gases should be made, especially for premature infants (see Chapter 2).

Operative Technique

The patent ductus can be either divided or ligated with excellent results, but in these sick neonates we prefer ligation because it is simpler and quicker.

A left thoracotomy is performed (see Chapter 6). An incision in either the third or fourth interspace provides adequate exposure. In premature infants we sometimes use an extrapleural approach because of the slight protection it may afford the lung, and because we prefer not leave in a chest tube postoperatively.

The mediastinal pleura is incised over the aorta. It is most important to carry this incision right down to the adventitia of the aorta. Then the mediastinal soft tissues and recurrent laryngeal nerve will be readily retracted medially by traction sutures while the ductus is sharply and bluntly cleared of areolar tissue (Figure 8-4a).

The ductus must not be lifted or handled roughly while it is circumscribed with an angled clamp (Figure 8-4b). The ductus is especially vulnerable to being torn on its undersurface, which is the surest way to turn a small operation into a big one!

Two heavy (number 4 silk) ligatures are gently drawn under the ductus, with care taken not to saw the back of it. It is wise at this point to occlude the ductus temporarily to be sure that closure is tolerated, especially when no cardiac catheterization has been done and unrecognized cardiac anomalies may be present.

As the ligatures are tied down, care is again taken *not* to lift the ductus and *not* to allow the ligatures to overlap each other (Figure 8-4c). A 4- to 5-mm segment of ductus must be compressed within the ligatures to assure that recanalization cannot occur. The mediastinal pleura is reapproximated, a chest tube is inserted if the pleural space has been entered, and then the wound is closed in layers.

Results

Although closure of a patent ductus in an older infant or child carries little risk, mortality is high in neonates because of the associated anomalies. For example, in the past three years at our institution these associated defects have included:

Transposition	3	Coarctation	4
Aortic stenosis	1	Ventricular septal defect	5
Atrial septal defect	3	Double-outlet right ventricle	1
Respiratory distress syndrome	19	Tetralogy of Fallot	2
Truncus type 1	1		

Of these patients, nine had total correction of the associated intracardiac anomalies, with two survivors. Four had also pulmonary artery banding or a Blalock-Hanlon procedure, and three of these survived. Of the 19 patients with RDS, 11 survived and were discharged home.

Coarctation of the Aorta

Many infants born with uncomplicated coarctation of the aorta remain asymptomatic until their upper-extremity hypertension or diminished femoral pulses are discovered in later childhood. A substantial number, perhaps half of the total, however, develop heart failure in infancy. This group is distinguished by the high incidence of associated anomalies (89 percent in one series), usually a patent ductus arteriosus but also sometimes a ventricular septal defect or aortic or mitral valve anomaly.

Coarctations may be classified according to their relationship to the patent ductus (or ligamentum arteriosum). In the uncomplicated postductal (postligamental) variety, the only physiologic abnormality is increased afterload to left ventricular ejection (Figure 8-5).

Conversely, the physiologic relationships of the preductal form are much more complex because the descending aorta is perfused by the right ventricle through the ductus. It is this form that occurs most commonly in neonates and that is usually complicated by other anomalies (Figure 8-6).

When congestive heart failure does not promptly respond to vigorous medical therapy, operation should be undertaken.

Diagnosis

The classic diagnostic signs of coarctation are weak, delayed femoral pulses and upper-extremity hypertension. In the preductal form, however, the femoral pulses may be present, obscuring the diagnosis. An important diagnostic clue is that femoral pulses may vary in strength as the pulmonary artery pressure varies, appearing when the baby cries and disappearing when he relaxes. Another clue is that arterial blood from the lower half of the body is more desaturated than that in the upper half.

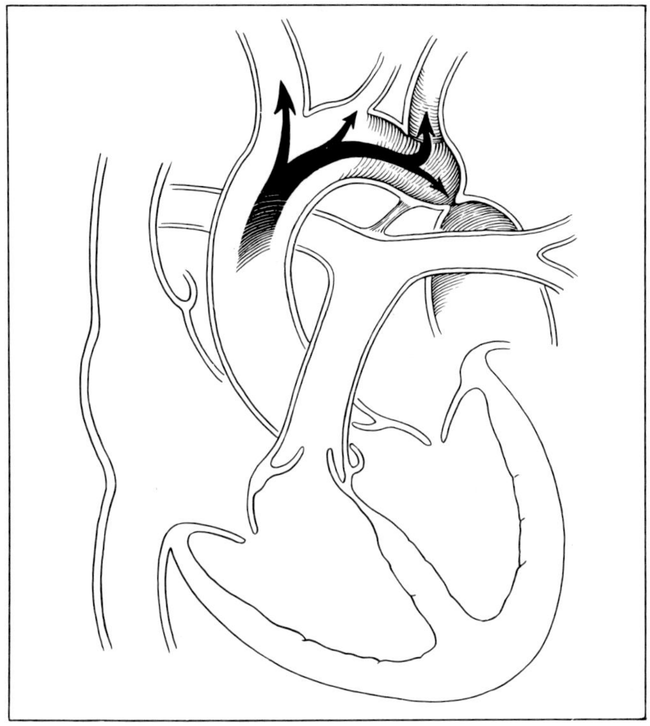

A

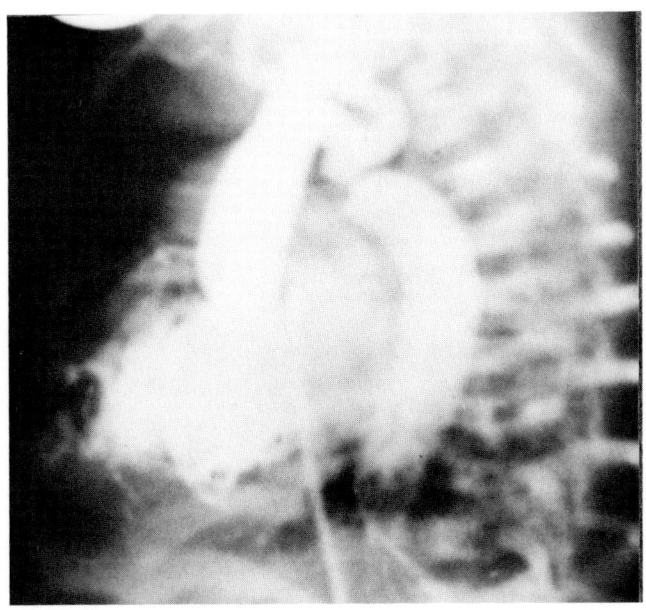

B

8-5. (A) Diagram of anatomy in postligamental coarctation. (B) Typical angiogram.

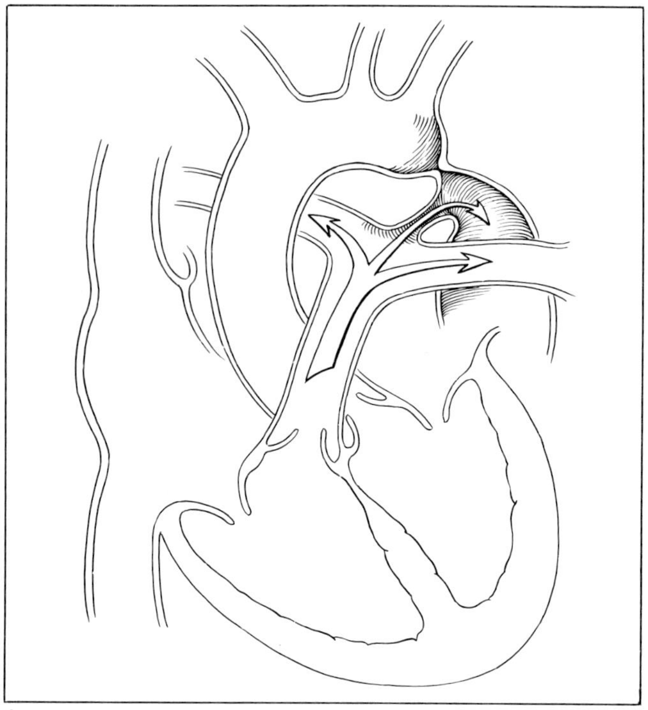

A

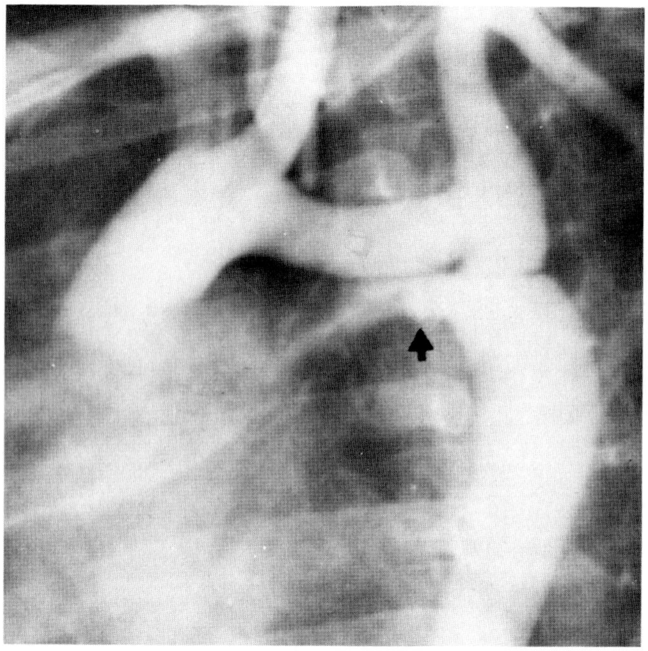

B

8-6. (A) Diagram of anatomy in preductal coarctation. (B) Typical angiogram. Arrow indicates patent ductus.

Because the diagnosis of coarctation can sometimes be made with certainty on clinical grounds and because the most commonly associated anomaly (patent ductus) can be diagnosed and corrected by the same operative approach, we occasionally perform operations without catheterization. In neonates, however, it is certainly preferable to have an accurate preoperative assessment of the anatomy and of associated anomalies. The anatomy of the coarctation itself and its relationship to the ductus arteriosus are defined by an aortogram as part of this study.

The importance of a complete study in neonates who have coarctation is exemplified by the combination of coarctation, patent ductus arteriosus, and ventricular septal defect that is frequently encountered in this group. When the ventricular septal defect is large, we believe that a primary total correction of all three defects, using hypothermic arrest, is most likely to be successful.

Preparation for Operation

The infant should be digitalized and the electrolyte and acid-base status normalized if possible. Unless repair of an associated intracardiac defect is planned, only one unit of whole blood need be crossmatched.

A central venous line is inserted through which blood, bicarbonate, and cardiotonic drugs can be reliably administered if necessary. An arterial line should be inserted in the right arm. (An infant who is not sick enough to require close monitoring probably should not be undergoing operation as a neonate!)

Operative Technique

Either of two techniques of repair may be chosen. In the past we performed the more conventional resection and end-to-end anastomosis. Recently we have preferred the subclavian patch angioplasty first described by Waldhausen and Nahrwold [9].

A left-lateral thoracotomy is performed entering the pleural space through the third interspace (see Chapter 6). The mediastinal pleura is incised and reflected medially, with traction sutures used to expose the aortic arch, subclavian artery, and ductus arteriosus (Figure 8-7a). Particularly in infants for whom the data may be incomplete, it is essential to visualize clearly the anatomy of the arch.

In performing resection and anastomosis the surgeon must mobilize enough aorta proximally and distally to allow primary anastomosis. Synthetic grafts are not used in neonatal coarctation. Often one or two pairs of intercostal arteries must be divided. Aneurysms of these collateral vessels may be encountered, even in neonates. These aneurysms are likely to rupture if not handled with extreme care. Often the aorta between the origin of the left subclavian artery and the ductus (the so-called isthmus of the aorta) is hypoplastic even if uninvolved in the actual coarctation. If this

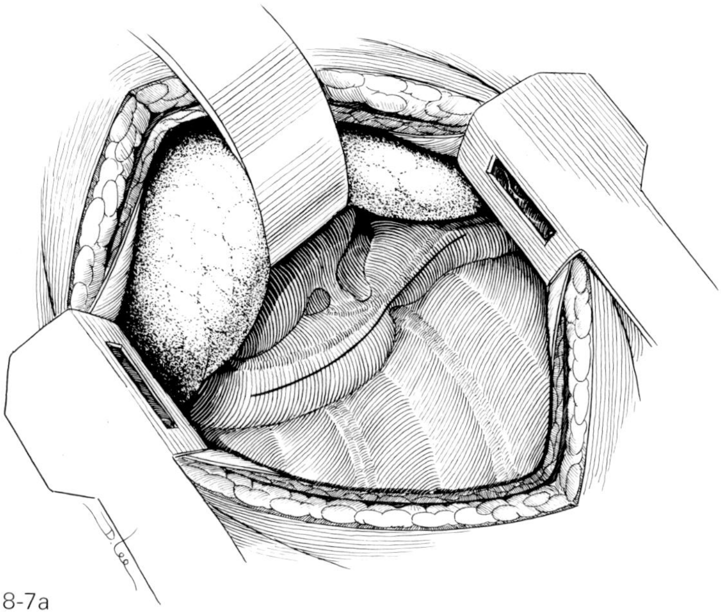

8-7a

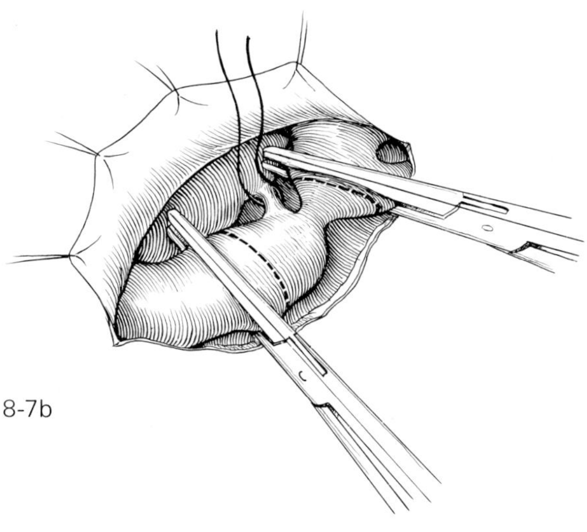

8-7b

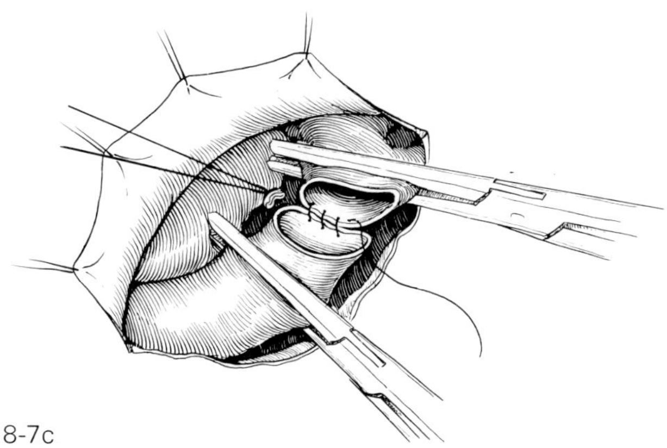

8-7c

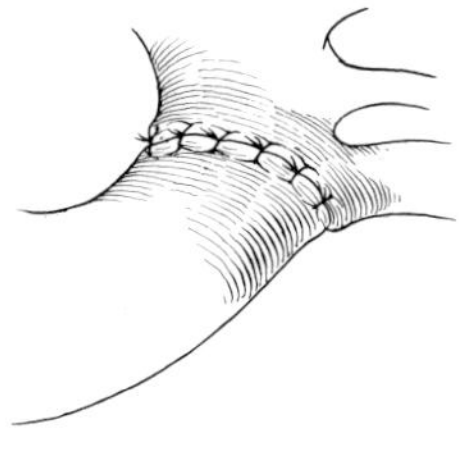

8-7d

is the case, it should be excised and the poststenotic segment should be brought up to the base of the subclavian artery.

Parallel straight vascular clamps are placed above and below the coarctation. Often the proximal clamp must be placed across the origin of the subclavian artery to provide an adequate proximal cuff (Figure 8-7b). The ductus is ligated, and a segment of aortic wall is left attached to it and oversewn after the specimen has been excised. The anastomosis is begun on the back row with a simple running 5-0 suture (Figure 8-7c). The suture line on the anterior surface is interrupted two or three times to allow growth later (Figure 8-7d).

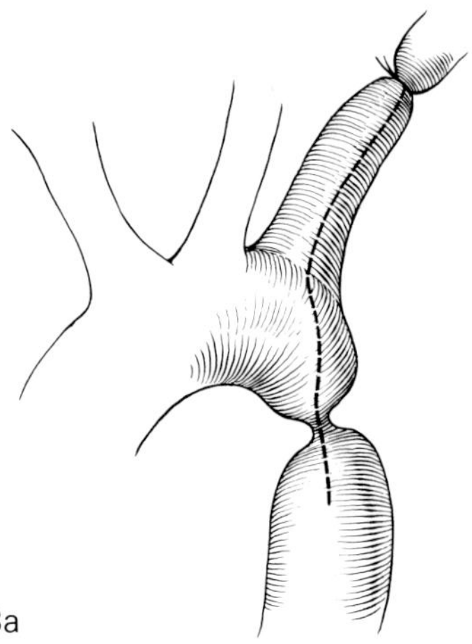

8-8a

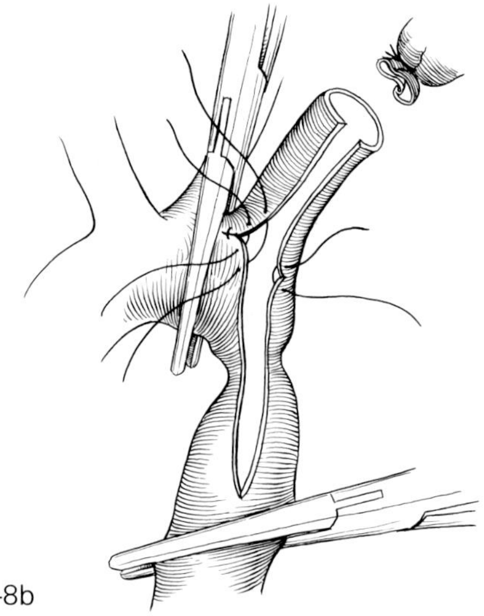

8-8b

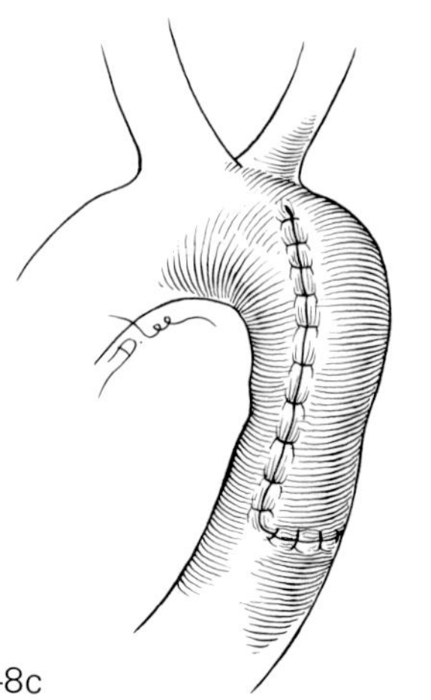

8-8c

Any bleeding that occurs following clamp removal can usually be controlled with local pressure until clotting seals the needle holes.

Sometimes it is difficult to achieve an adequate reconstruction after coarctation resection in small babies. The technique of subclavian patch angioplasty obviates many of the technical problems of resection and anastomosis in neonates. The patent ductus is first ligated in situ. The aorta is clamped. Then the subclavian artery is divided at the apex of the chest following ligation of its branches, just as in a Blalock-Taussig shunt (Figure 8-8a). Then the subclavian artery is split longitudinally, and this incision is carried down the aorta itself, well into the area of poststenotic dilatation (Figure 8-8b). If there is a diaphragm of the coarctation, it is excised. Finally, the subclavian flap is folded down and sutured in place with a 6-0 continuous suture (Figure 8-8c).

Sick small babies tend to show sudden deterioration, especially within a few minutes after clamp removal. The anesthetist must be particularly alert, ready to give blood or cardiotonics as appropriate.

Results

A high operative mortality (50 percent to 70 percent) has followed repair of coarctation by resection and anastomosis in neonates. Almost all these deaths occur in patients with associated anomalies, but a few are related to the technical difficulty of achieving a good anastomosis. Our experience confirms these observations. Associated defects in our group have included patent ductus (most often), ventricular septal defect, transposition, and atresia of the aortic valve. In this group with refractory failure, however, persistent medical therapy alone rarely succeeds; so operation should be attempted in spite of the risk.

Recurrence of coarctation is likely in a number of these patients—as many as 34 percent in one series. In a sense, this is a sign of success, as suggested by Tawes and associates [7], because one must have a live patient to have a recoarctation; but recurrence is one good reason to undertake coarctation repair in infants only when it is essential.

Because of these poor results, we have recently employed the subclavian patch angioplasty in all neonates. Certainly the procedure itself is easier than resection and anastomosis. Whether the long-term results will be improved remains to be determined. During the period of aortic crossclamping one generally relies upon the collateral vessels around the coarctation to prevent ischemic damage to the spinal cord. Although neonates usually have poorly developed collaterals, paraplegia has been reported only once. Another complication of coarctation repair—paradoxical hypertension with mesenteric vasculitis—is rarely seen in neonates.

Aortic Arch Interruption

Fortunately rare, complete interruption of the aortic arch is a rapidly lethal congenital abnormality. Of affected children, 80 percent die within the first month of life. In 43 percent of cases the interruption occurs just distal to the left subclavian artery—Type A; in 53 percent of cases, between the left carotid and left subclavian arteries—Type B; or, in 4 percent of cases, between the innominate and left carotid arteries—Type C (Figure 8-9). Virtually all these patients have also a ventricular septal defect and a patent ductus arteriosus, providing blood flow from the right ventricle to the aortic segment distal to the interruption. This anomaly may be part of the so-called hypoplastic left heart complex, which includes aortic and mitral valve hypoplasia, underdevelopment of the left ventricle, and endocardial fibroelastosis. In this instance, no therapy is likely to succeed.

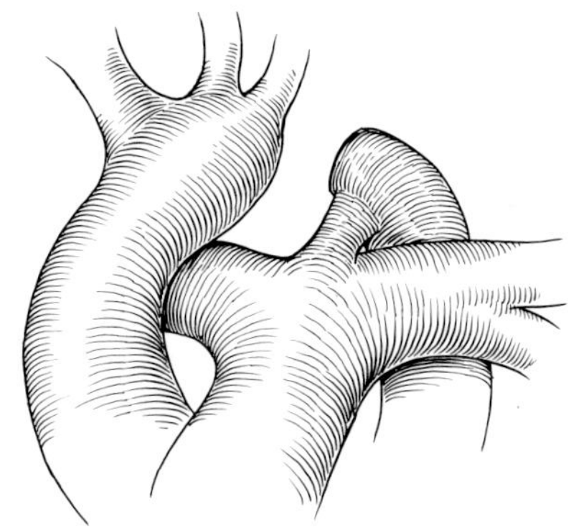

8-9a

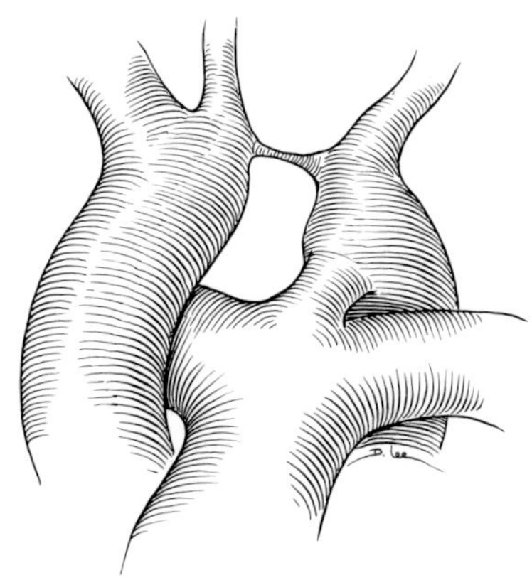

8-9b

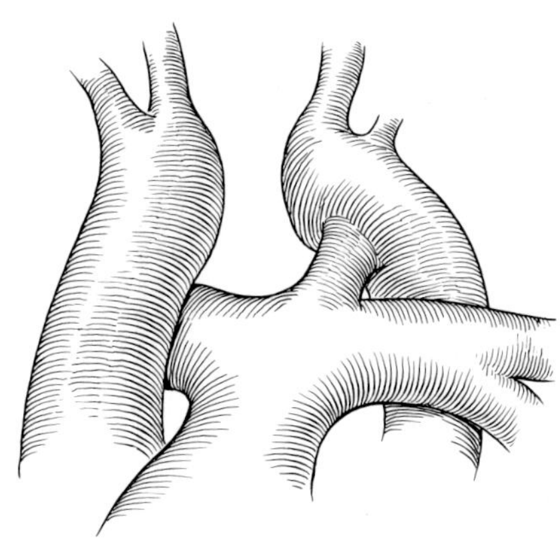

8-9c

Choice of Operation

Because of the anatomic variability of this rare anomaly, it is difficult to recommend any one operation. Lesions of type A are best treated as one would treat a preductal coarctation, as discussed previously in this chapter. Some surgeons have used the subclavian artery plus or minus the left carotid artery to restore aortic continuity. One of our patients survived a total repair under hypothermic arrest, which included repair of the aortic interruption and division of the ductus through a left thoracotomy followed by closure of the VSD and atrial septal defect (ASD) through a sternotomy. An alternative approach would be to repair the aorta, divide the ductus, and band the pulmonary artery. A very high mortality must be expected.

One approach for lesions of types B and C makes use of the fact that adequate blood flow through the distal aortic segment depends upon wide patency of the ductus arteriosus as well as a high pulmonary vascular resistance. This operation involves creating an artificial ductus by placing a ¼-inch to ⅜-inch Dacron graft between the pulmonary artery and the descending aorta and then banding the main pulmonary artery distally. This ensures continued good blood flow to the distal aortic segment even if the natural ductus arteriosus closes or the pulmonary vascular resistance falls. Two of four infants treated in this manner at Boston Children's Hospital [3] survived operation and have remained relatively well for several years; all other approaches have failed in neonates. Definitive repair has not yet been undertaken in these two patients.

Recently the successful primary definitive repair of a defect of type B with associated VSD was reported by Murphy [4] and Trusler [10] and their associates.

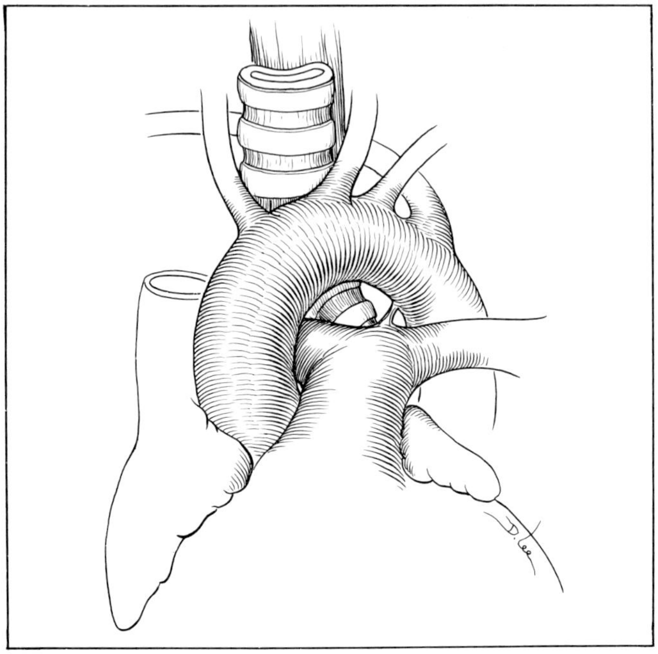

A

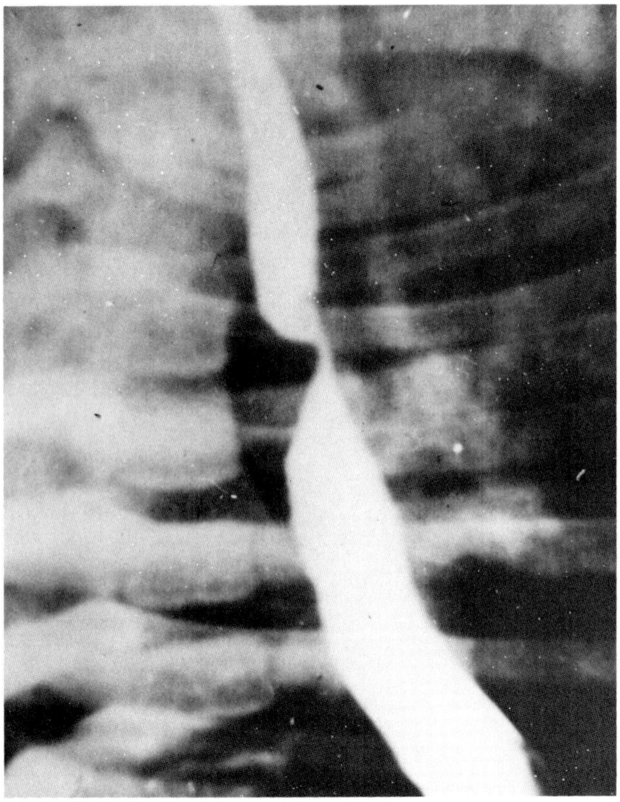

B

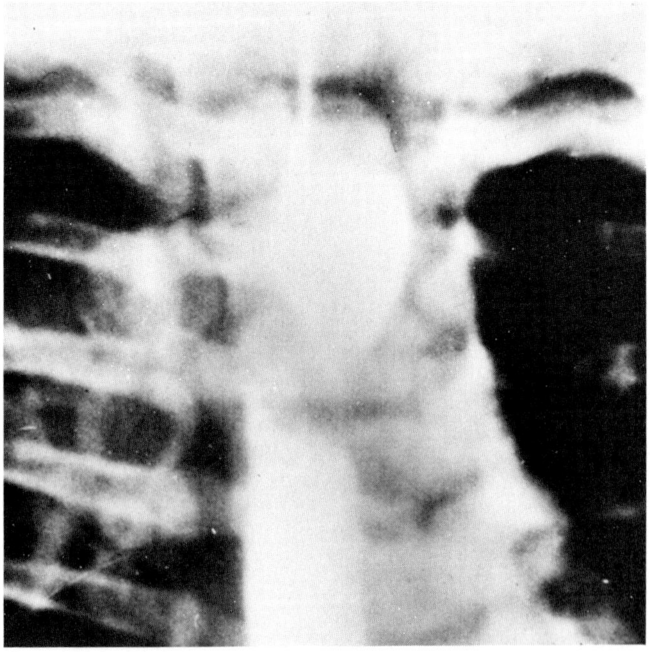

C

8-10. (A) Typical anatomy in aberrant right subclavian artery. (B) Barium swallow showing posterior indentation of esophagus by aberrant subclavian artery. (C) In frontal view, the aberrant vessel causes an oblique filling defect in the esophagogram.

Vascular Ring

Anomalies of the aortic arch and its major branches can result in the formation of vascular rings about the esophagus and trachea, causing stridor and dysphagia [11]. Most common is the aberrant right subclavian artery from a left descending aorta, but this rarely causes serious symptoms in infancy (Figure 8-10). Double aortic arch is the most important of these anomalies, often causing serious respiratory distress in young infants (Figure 8-11).

Diagnosis

The diagnosis of vascular ring is suspected when feeding difficulty, coughing during feeding, or stridor is present. The infant tends to hold his neck extended to relieve the compression. Plain chest roentgenograms are rarely helpful, but a barium swallow will reveal the characteristic filling defect. Cardiac catheterization and angiography may be done, primarily to establish the presence of associated abnormalities, but rarely do these procedures provide any additional useful information about the vascular ring itself.

Operation

No matter what the anatomy of the ring may be, it is best approached through a left thoracotomy. The entire aortic arch and its branches must first be dissected free so that the anatomy of the ring can be clearly understood. In the usual case of double arch, the right arch is posterior to, and higher and larger than, the left arch, which forms the anterior portion of the ring. The smaller of the two arches is generally divided to interrupt the constricting ring. It is wise to occlude the vessel temporarily at the site of intended division, to be sure flow to the carotids and descending aorta is not compromised by an inapparent stricture in the other arch. In addition, it is essential to divide the ligamentum arteriosum or patent ductus and to dissect the esophagus and trachea free to the apex of the chest, dividing any constricting bands.

When the posterior arch is divided, further decompression of the trachea can sometimes be achieved by anchoring with sutures the major anterior arch to the back of the sternum.

Aberrant subclavian arteries may be simply divided and other forms of rings may be treated by interruption of the ring at an appropriate site, in all cases with care taken to free the trachea and esophagus completely.

Results

In many cases stridor will not be immediately relieved because there may be tracheomalacia at the site of compression. In some instances, in fact, prolonged tracheostomy may be required until tracheomalacia resolves itself with growth of the child. In all cases, careful attention should be given to full humidification of the inspired gases, frequent suctioning, and chest physiotherapy.

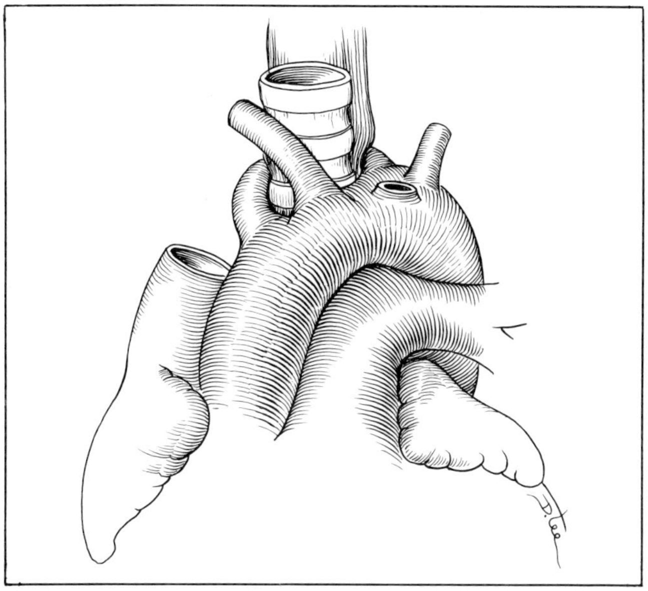

A

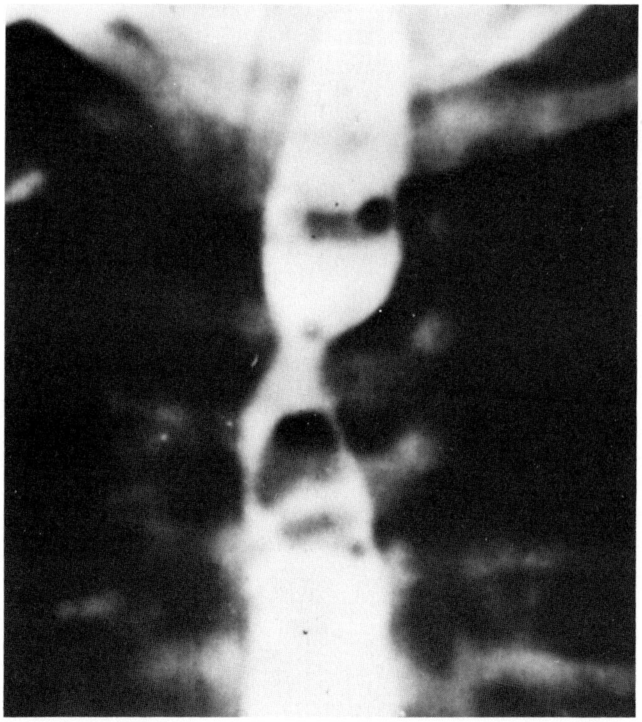

B

8-11. (A) Typical anatomy in double aortic arch. Here the anterior arch is larger, but in some instances the posterior is more important. (B) Barium esophagogram reveals typical lateral indentations.

Selected References

1. Coran, A. G., Cabal, L., Siassi, B., and Rosenkrantz, J. G. Surgical closure of patent ductus arteriosus in the premature infant with respiratory distress. *J. Pediatr. Surg.* 10:399, 1975.
2. Lincoln, J. C. R., Deverall, P. B., Stark, J., et al. Vascular anomalies compressing the oesophagus and trachea. *Thorax* 24:295, 1969.
3. Litwin, S. B., Van Praagh, R., and Bernard, W. F. A palliative operation for certain infants with aortic arch interruption. *Ann. Thorac. Surg.* 14:369, 1972.
4. Murphy, D. A., Lemire, G. G., Tessler, I., and Dunn, G. L. Correction of type B aortic arch interruption with ventricular and atrial septal defects in a three-day-old infant. *J. Thorac. Cardiovasc. Surg.* 65:882, 1973.
5. Panagopoulos, PH. G., Tatooles, C. J., Aberdeen, E., et al. Patent ductus arteriosus in infants and children. A review of 936 operations (1946–69). *Thorax* 26:137, 1971.
6. Shuford, W. H., and Sybers, R. G. *The Aortic Arch and Its Malformations.* Springfield, Ill.: Charles C Thomas, 1974.
7. Tawes, R. L., Jr., Aberdeen, E., Waterston, D. J., and Bonham-Carter, R. E. Coarctation of the aorta in infants and children. A review of 333 operative cases, including 179 infants. *Circulation* 39(suppl. I): 1–173, 1969.
8. Tyson, K. R. T., Harris, L. C., and Nghiem, Q. X. Repair of aortic arch interruption in the neonate. *Surgery* 67:1006, 1970.
9. Waldhausen, J. A., and Nahrwold, D. L. Repair of coarctation of the aorta with a subclavian flap. *J. Thorac. Cardiovasc. Surg.* 51:532, 1966.
10. Trusler, G. A., and Izukawa, T. Interrupted aortic arch and ventricular septal defect. *J. Thorac. Cardiovasc. Surg.* 69:126, 1975.
11. Gross, R. E. The Surgery of Infancy and Childhood. Chapter 65 in *Vascular Anomalies in the Thorax Producing Compression of the Trachea or Esophagus.* Philadelphia: W. B. Saunders Co., 1953.

9

Open-Heart Procedures

In general, open-heart procedures in neonates have been reserved for those conditions allowing no palliative operation, such as total anomalous pulmonary venous drainage, critical aortic valve stenosis, and critical pulmonary valve stenosis with intact ventricular septum. Management of each of these conditions is discussed in this chapter. As technical expertise has improved, it has become possible to perform total correction of many other cardiac anomalies primarily in the neonate, avoiding the added risk of palliative operations. The psychological, sociological, and economic advantages offer compelling arguments in favor of primary early total correction even if the immediate mortality is somewhat greater than it might be with the staged approach. It is not yet proved, however, that this will yield better long-term results than the traditional staged approach. Furthermore, it is probably wise to restrict these innovations to a few highly specialized centers where a substantial volume of neonatal open-heart surgery is done, at least until the short-term and long-term problems have been worked out.

Preparation for Operation

Six units of blood are crossmatched. Citrate-phosphate-dextrose-preserved blood may be used in neonates for five days after donation. Two fresh platelet packs are ordered as well.

Serum electrolyte, blood urea nitrogen (BUN), and hematocrit levels are measured. Blood coagulation is not assessed in small babies until after perfusion, because preoperative values are rendered meaningless by the exchange transfusion provided by the pump prime.

Conduct of the Operation

The patient is anesthetized and arterial and venous cannulations are performed (see Chapter 2). Most open-heart operations in neonates are performed through a median sternotomy, which allows the greatest flexibility in dealing with all possible eventualities.

Because thorough cardiac catheterization in these babies is technically difficult, the surgeon must remain alert to the possibility of unrecognized defects. Upon opening the pericardium he should inspect the external cardiac anatomy, measure the pressures and oxygen saturations within all cardiac chambers and great vessels, note the location of any systolic or diastolic thrills, and determine how the location of the coronary arteries might affect placement of incisions in the heart.

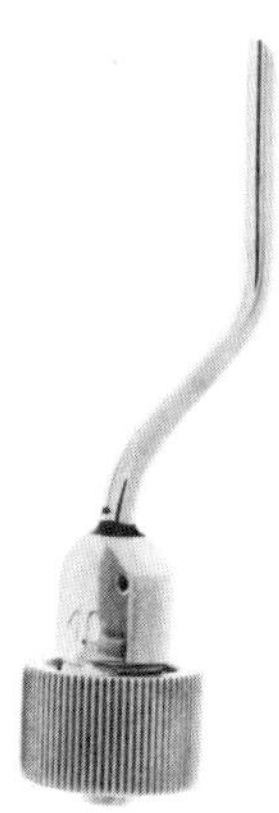

9-1. Femoral artery perfusion cannula available in sizes from 2.0 to 6.5 mm from Sarns, Inc. (6200 Jackson Road, Ann Arbor, Michigan 48103).

Cannulations

The ascending aorta is usually cannulated for arterial input from the pump. It is perfectly possible, however, to perfuse a neonate through the femoral artery with a small metal cannula when this will facilitate the cardiac repair (Figure 9-1). A

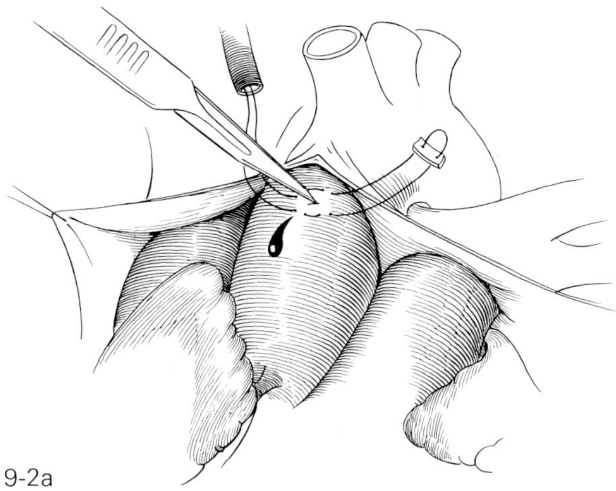

9-2a

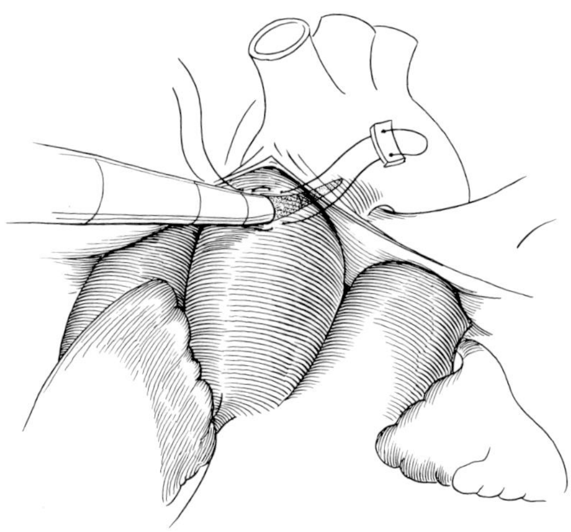

9-2b

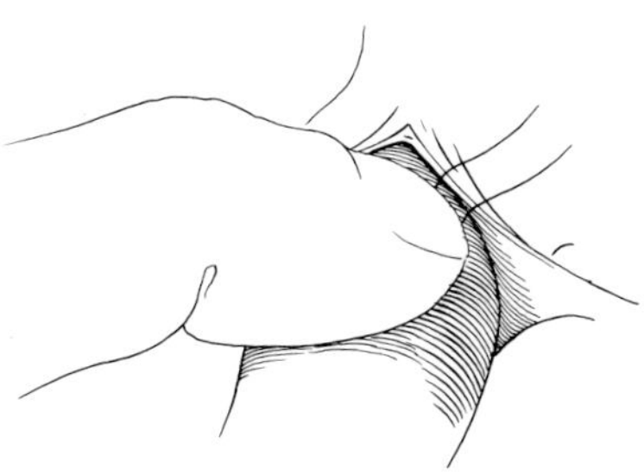

9-2c

pursestring suture is placed on the ascending aorta as high as is convenient and passed through a tourniquet. The adventitia is excised, and a 2-mm stab wound is made (Figure 9-2a). This is dilated enough to accept the aortic cannula (Figure 9-2b) yet left small enough to seal by elasticity around the cannula. During these steps, bleeding is controlled by light digital pressure (Figure 9-2c). Then the cannula is slipped into the aorta and secured to the tourniquet (Figure 9-2d).

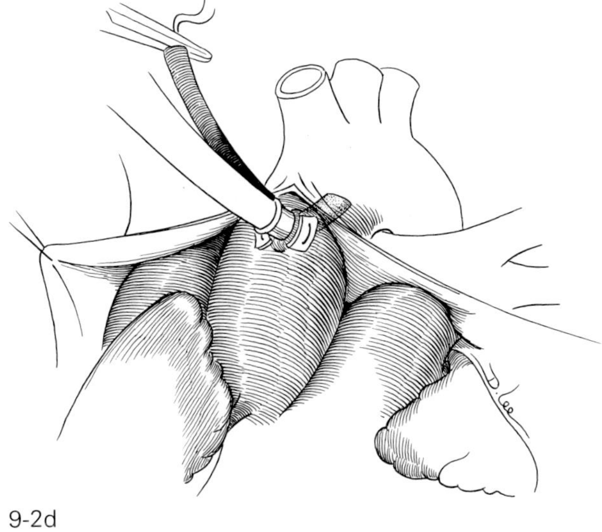

9-2d

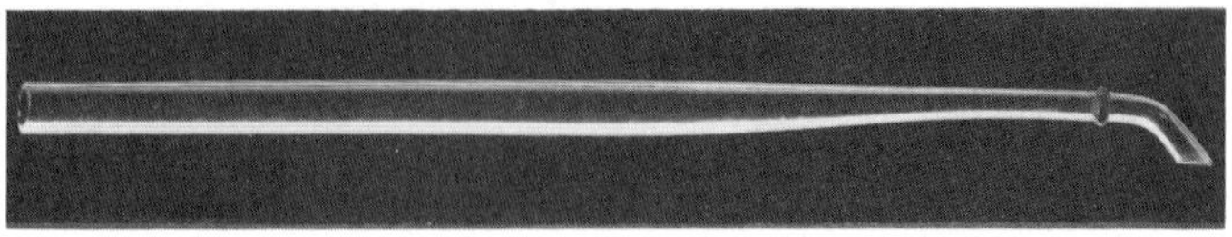

9-3. Flexible plastic aortic arch cannula (manufactured by Sherwood Medical, 11802 West Line Industrial Drive, St. Louis, Missouri).

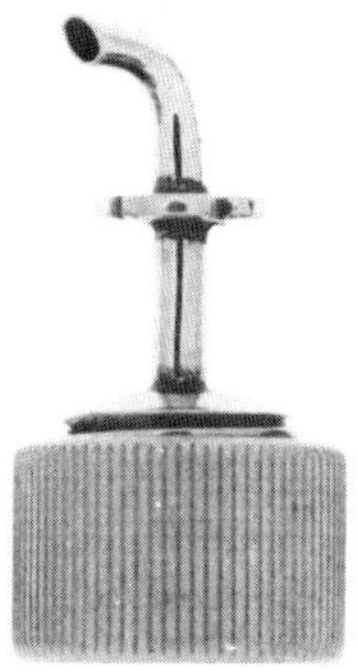

9-4. Aortic perfusion cannula available in sizes from 2.0 to 6.5 mm from Sarns, Inc.

The disposable THI aortic perfusion cannula is satisfactory for infants who weigh over 3 kg (Figure 9-3), but a smaller right-angled metal cannula is preferable for smaller infants (Figure 9-4). The tip of the cannula is palpated to ascertain that it is in the aortic lumen and not directed up the innominate artery.

The vena cavae are cannulated with right-angled plastic cannulas through pursestring sutures on the right atrium, positioned with a view toward the exposure required for the repair (Figure 9-5). Considerable care should be exercised in avoiding damage to the sinoatrial node at the junction of the superior vena cava and right atrium. The tourniquet on the superior vena cava, particularly, must be placed high enough to avoid crushing the sinus node, but not above the azygous vein.

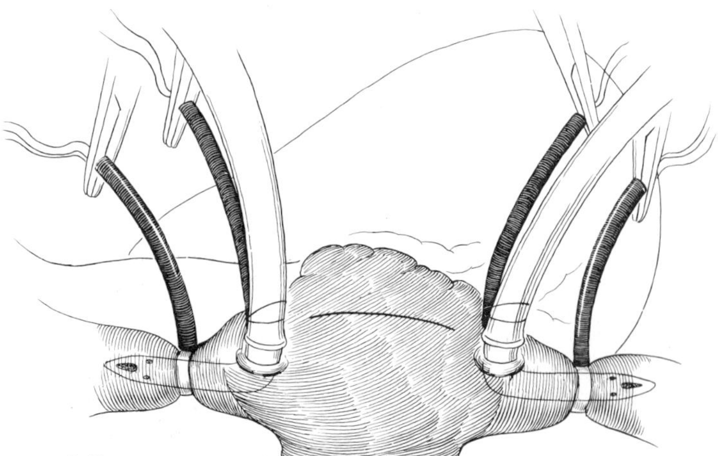

9-5

Perfusion Technique

Open-heart surgery can be performed safely in neonates with standard extracorporeal circulation techniques and miniaturized equipment. In spite of theoretical advantages, more complex systems such as membrane oxygenators have not proved to be superior. We utilize a standard Sarns roller pump and heat exchanger with a Bentley* infant oxygenator, a bubble trap, and arterial and pericardial suction filters. This system requires 1300 ml of priming volume.

It has been our experience that extreme hemodilution is tolerated poorly by neonates during conventional bypass operations of usual duration. Ascites develops rapidly, and all tissues, including the heart, promptly become edematous, especially if the venous return is impeded in any way. Therefore our prime consists of:

1000 ml	whole fresh citrate-phosphate-dextrose (CPD) blood reconstructed with 3000 units of heparin
1 g	dextrose
1 g	calcium chloride
134 mg	potassium chloride
200 ml	Ringer's lactate
	sodium bicarbonate to correct base deficit measured after recirculating prime through pump

Perfusion is initiated at a rate of 150 ml per kg of body weight and then is adjusted as the operation proceeds to maintain a mean arterial pressure of between 60 and 100 mm Hg. Superior vena cava pressure, or, sometimes, the inferior vena cava pressure, or both, must be monitored continuously to verify adequate venous drainage.

Because the pump volume is large relative to the infant's blood volume, it is easy to overfill or underfill the circulation drastically with very little change in the oxygenator level. Thus perfusion is instituted and discontinued gradually as the surgeon communicates to the perfusionist the degree of distention of the heart.

When the left side of the heart is open or when the ventricles are fibrillating, a vent should be placed in the left ventricle to remove blood from the operative field and to prevent left ventricular distention and ejection of air into the aorta. We insert the vent through the left ventricular apex, right upper pulmonary vein, or foramen ovale (when the right atrium is open).

Before the heart is allowed to eject blood into the aorta, care must be taken to evacuate *all* residual air from the left-sided chambers. The left ventricular vent will evacuate most of the air (Figure 9-6). A few other maneuvers are useful:

1. The aortic valve can be rendered incompetent with a clamp before completing a ventricular septal defect (VSD)

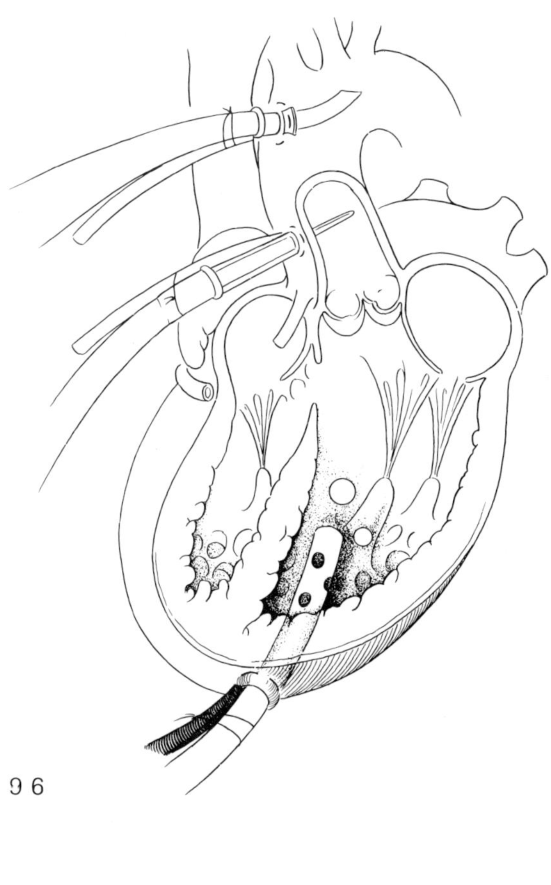

9 6

* Bentley Laboratories, Inc., 17502 Armstrong Avenue, Irvine, California 92705.

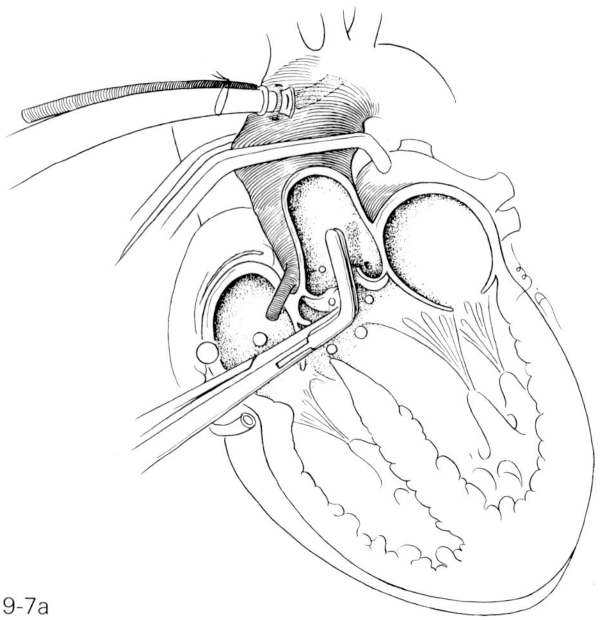

9-7a

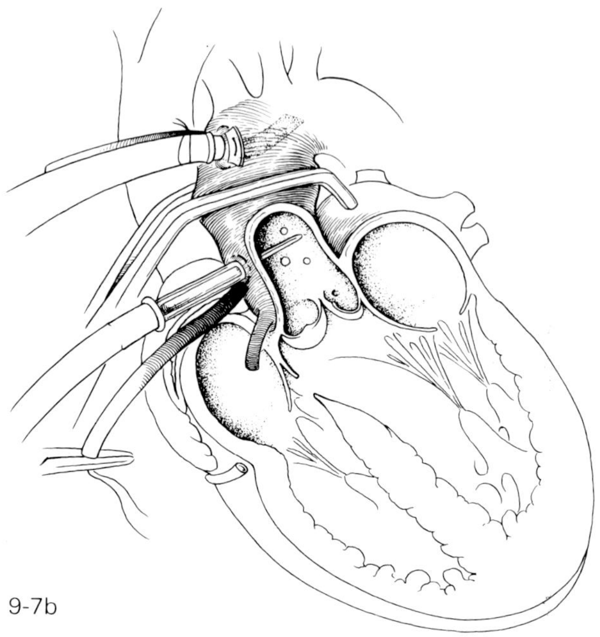

9-7b

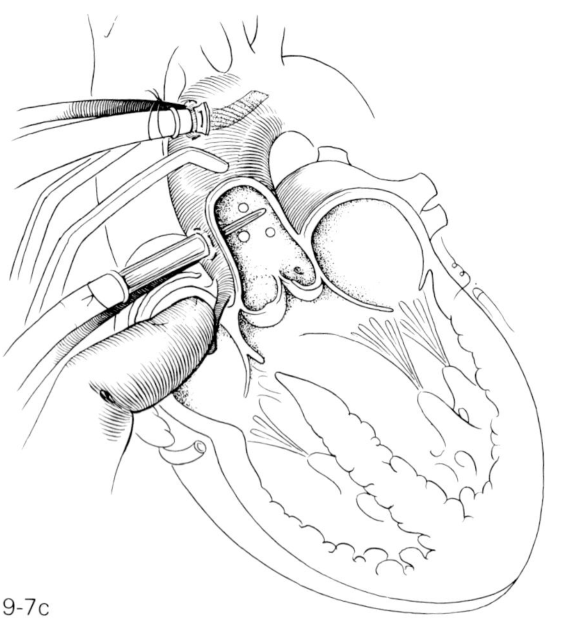

9-7c

patch, to allow air in the aortic root to flush back into the heart, where it can be removed (Figure 9-7a).

2. A slotted needle can be placed in the aortic root and connected to gentle suction to remove trapped air (Figure 9-7b).
3. The right coronary artery can be compressed while the aortic crossclamp is removed, so that air cannot be forced down it (Figure 9-7c).

The temperature at which perfusion is carried out is dictated by the technical demands of the operation being performed. It is often desirable to clamp the aorta to relax the heart so that exposure within the heart can be optimized without damage by retraction. The myocardium must be protected during this period of ischemic arrest. Reducing the body temperature to 28 C (82.4 F) and further cooling the heart by irrigation with ice-cold Ringer's lactate has provided satisfactory myocardial protection for periods of up to two hours of continuous aortic crossclamping. Recently, we and others have found that administration of cold cardioplegic solution into the coronary arteries provides even better myocardial protection. This has become our standard technique. There are instances where these methods do not provide sufficient exposure, such as when there is copious venous return from bronchial collaterals or during the repair of total anomalous pulmonary venous return—in which situations the patient may be further cooled to 20 C (68 F), so that the perfusion rate may be reduced to 25 ml per kg of body weight or even suspended completely for periods of up to an hour.

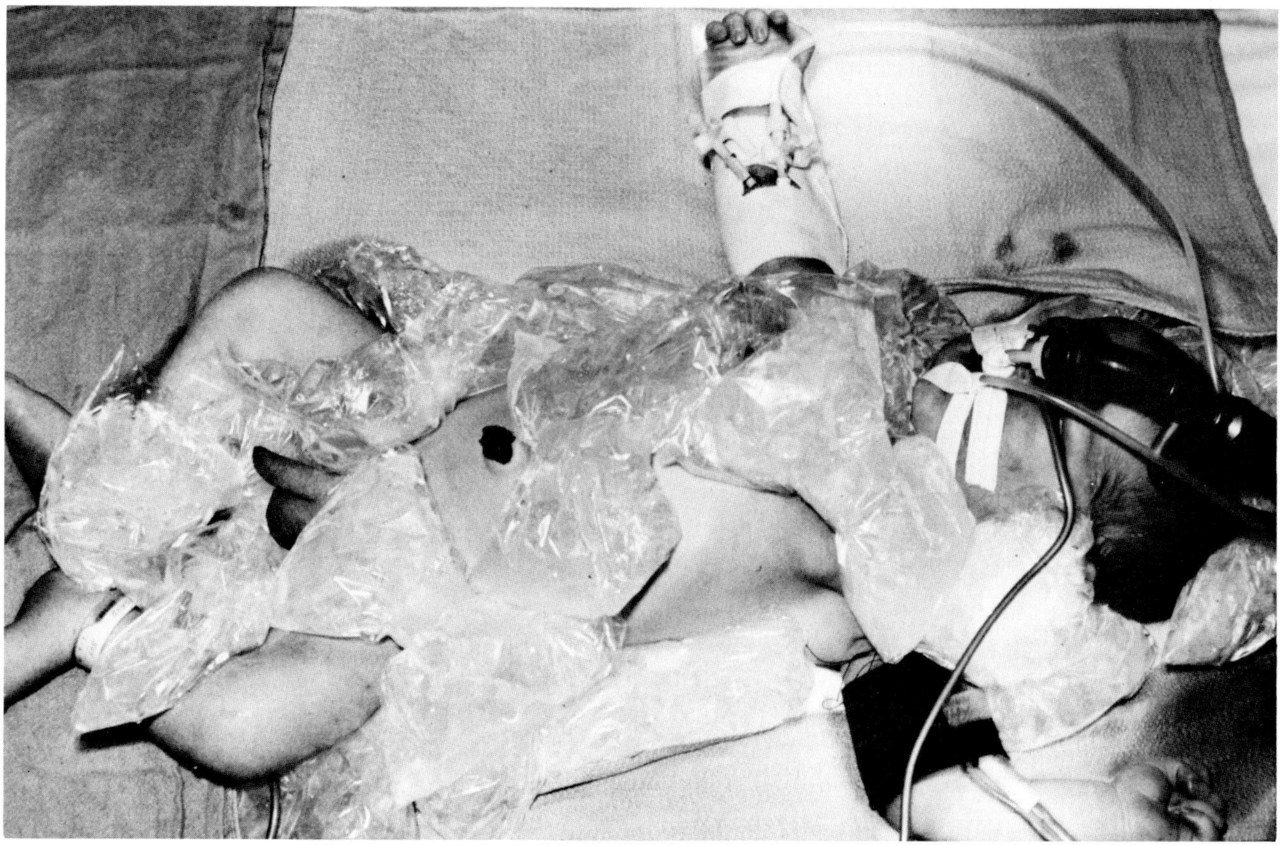

9-8. Infant undergoing surface cooling.

Deep Hypothermia with Total Circulatory Arrest

Deep hypothermia with total circulatory arrest, which has been used since the inception of open-heart surgery, has recently been popularized for intracardiac repairs in infants. Ideal operating conditions are provided. If the patient sustains a cardiac arrest while the chest is being opened, the hypothermia allows an extra margin of time to make the cannulations and initiate perfusion. The cannulations are simple—a major advantage in small neonates.

Initial surface cooling is carried out for about one hour (Figure 9-8) to reduce the esophageal temperature to 28 C (82.4 F). During this time the venous and arterial cutdowns are performed. The rate of ventilation is gradually reduced, and 5% carbon dioxide is added to the inspired gases to prevent respiratory alkalosis. A near-normal P_{CO_2} should be maintained because this is a main determinant of cerebral blood flow.

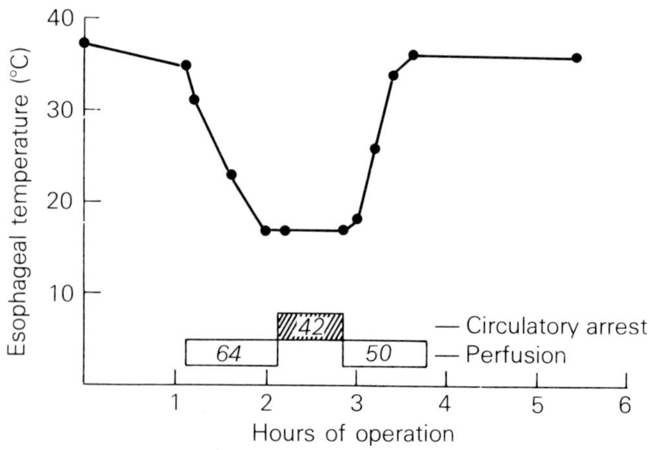

9-9. Course of operation for total correction of transposition with hypothermic circulatory arrest.

At 28 C (82.4 F) the patient is prepared and draped, and a sternotomy is performed. The aorta and right atrium are cannulated. Then perfusion is begun at 100 ml per kg of body weight, and the patient is rapidly cooled to 20 C (68 F) by keeping the blood temperature 7 C (12.6 F) less than the esophageal temperature (Figure 9-9). Circulation is then suspended; the blood is allowed to drain from the venous line into the pump; the cavae, aorta, and perfusion lines are clamped and the intracardiac repair is undertaken. Following repair, perfusion is resumed at 100 ml per kg of body weight, and the patient is rapidly rewarmed, with the blood temperature kept 7 C (12.6 F) above the esophageal temperature. Spontaneous cardiac action usually resumes promptly, and defibrillation is rarely necessary. When the heart resumes vigorous contraction, the venous pressure is increased to 10 mm Hg by partly occluding the venous drainage. This allows the heart to fill and add its pulsatile output to the pump flow. The lungs are gently ventilated. Finally, perfusion is discontinued in the usual manner at an esophageal temperature of 35 C (95 F).

Bicarbonate should be administered sparingly during rewarming to correct any major metabolic acidosis that may have been incurred during the arrest.

A number of physiologic changes occur during cooling. The pulse rate gradually slows, cardiac output falls, and peripheral vascular resistance rises. Left ventricular dp/dt falls, coincident with the fall in heart rate and cardiac output. All patients become hyperglycemic. Although this condition corrects itself spontaneously in the 12 hours or so after rewarming, it presents a hazard of brain damage caused by the attendant hyperosmolarity. The rise in blood glucose can be limited by avoiding glucose-containing intravenous solutions. Concerns remain about the possibility of long-term brain damage, as evidenced by the relatively high incidence of postoperative seizures in many series. It is not known whether these imply long-term damage.

Acute renal failure has occurred, and some of our patients have had transient increases in blood urea nitrogen and creatinine. Believing that this might be the result of the increased viscosity and sludging of blood that accompany cooling, we now use hemodilution. A diuresis is initiated during the surface-cooling phase by administering a water load and Lasix (1 mg per kg). The pump is initially primed with 400 ml plasma, 400 ml Ringer's lactate, and 12.5 g mannitol, which reduce the patient's hematocrit value to 10 percent to 15 percent during cooling. During the period of circulatory arrest the oxygenator is drained and reprimed with whole blood, which restores the hematocrit reading to 30 percent to 35 percent for rewarming. With these precautions, our results have been much improved.

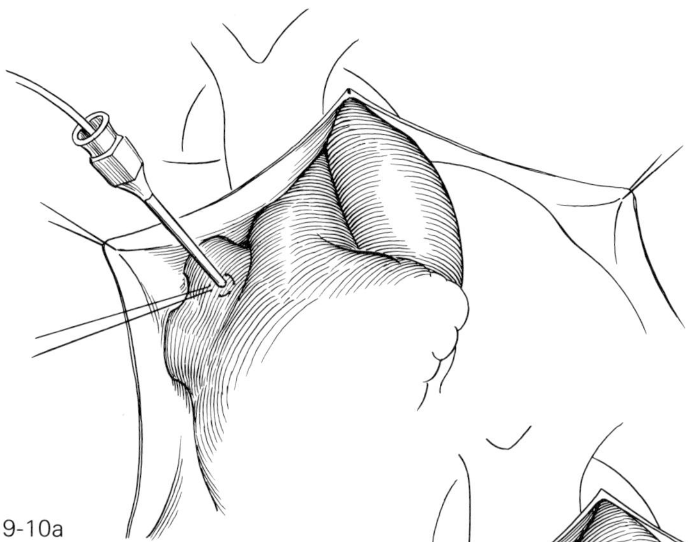

9-10a

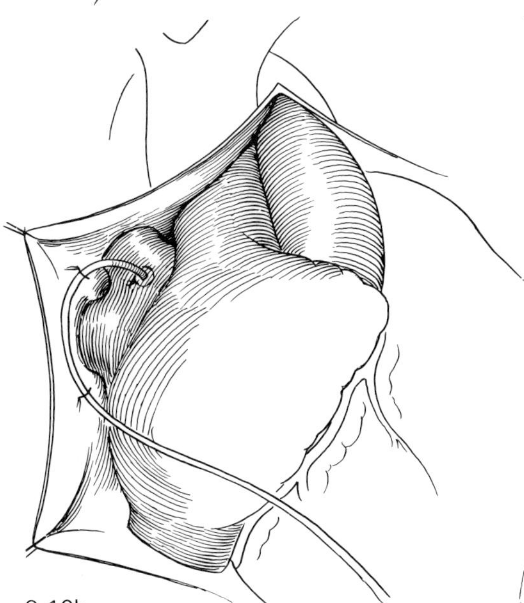

9-10b

Preparation for Postoperative Care

At the completion of every open-heart procedure in sick infants a left atrial pressure monitor is inserted. We use a Deseret Intracath* inserted through the left upper pulmonary vein (Figure 9-10a). The tubing is secured to the pericardium with 4-0 catgut (Figure 9-10b) and is passed through the chest wall (Figure 9-10c). The hub is cut off, the needle is removed, and a blunt needle is used to make connection to the transducer line (Figure 9-10d). Extreme care must be taken not to allow air bubbles or clots to be flushed into the left atrium. The line is kept open with a continuous slow infusion of heparinized saline solution when pressure recordings are not being taken (Figure 9-11).

* Manufactured by Deseret Pharmaceutical Company, Sandy, Utah 84070.

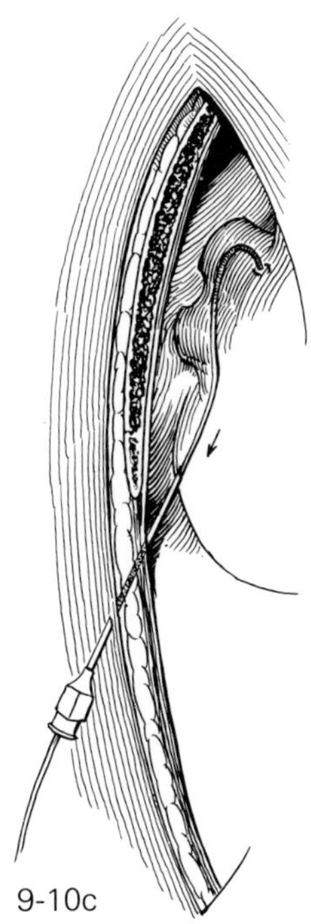

9-10c

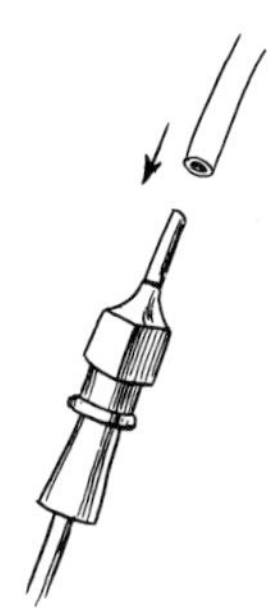

9-10d

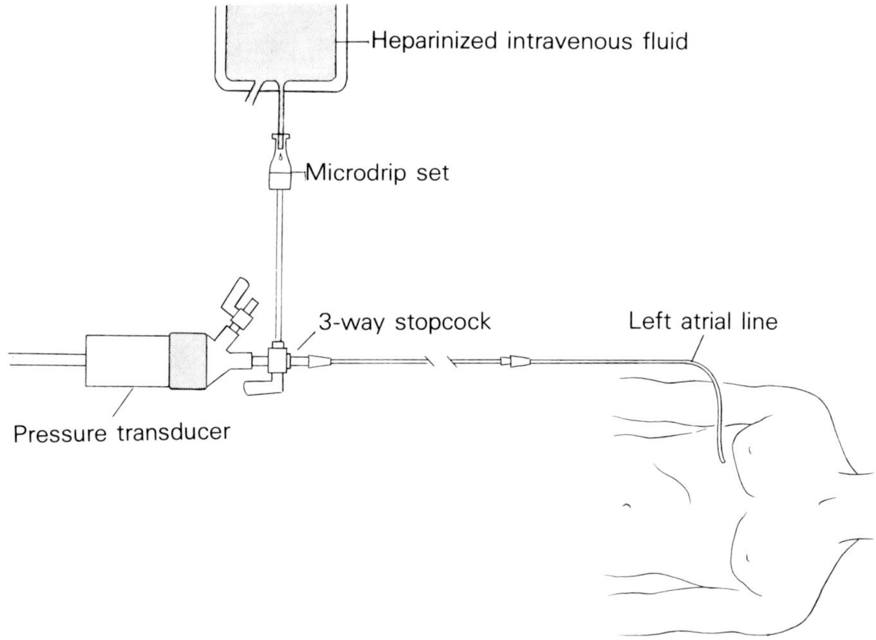

9-11. Airtight system for maintaining left atrial line patency. Fluid infusion (2 ml per hour) is briefly interrupted to record pressure by turning stopcock.

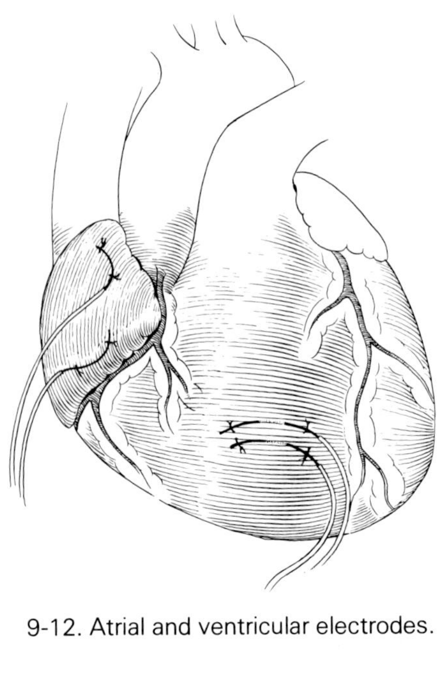

9-12. Atrial and ventricular electrodes.

Atrial and ventricular pacing wires are sutured to the myocardium (Figure 9-12), the former for recording atrial activity to diagnose postoperative arrhythmias and the latter for pacing if heart block occurs.

Total Anomalous Pulmonary Venous Drainage

Total anomalous pulmonary venous drainage (TAPVD) is a rare condition among the general population, but it is encountered several times a year in hospitals that care for many infants with heart disease. In this anomaly all four pulmonary veins fail to connect with the left atrium and drain into the right atrium, either

1. by means of a persistent left anterior cardinal vein to the innominate vein (Figure 9-13)—*supracardiac type*—55 percent of our cases;
2. directly into the right atrium or into the coronary sinus (Figure 9-14)—*cardiac type*—21 percent of our cases;
3. by means of a descending vertical vein that connects with the portal system or inferior vena cava (Figure 9-15)—*infracardiac type*—16 percent of our cases;
4. by a combination of the above—*mixed type*—8 percent of our cases.

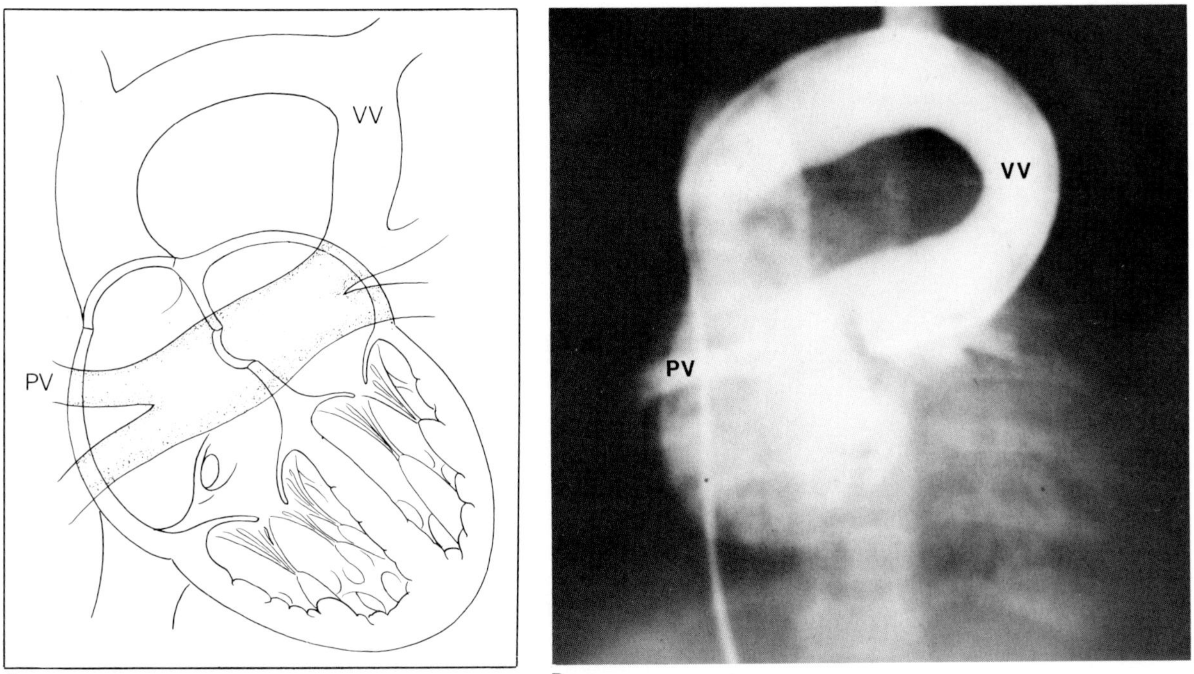

A B

9-13. In the supracardiac type of total anomalous pulmonary venous drainage the pulmonary veins (PV) drain into the innominate vein through a vertical vein (VV)—a persistent left anterior cardinal vein, sometimes called a left vena cava.

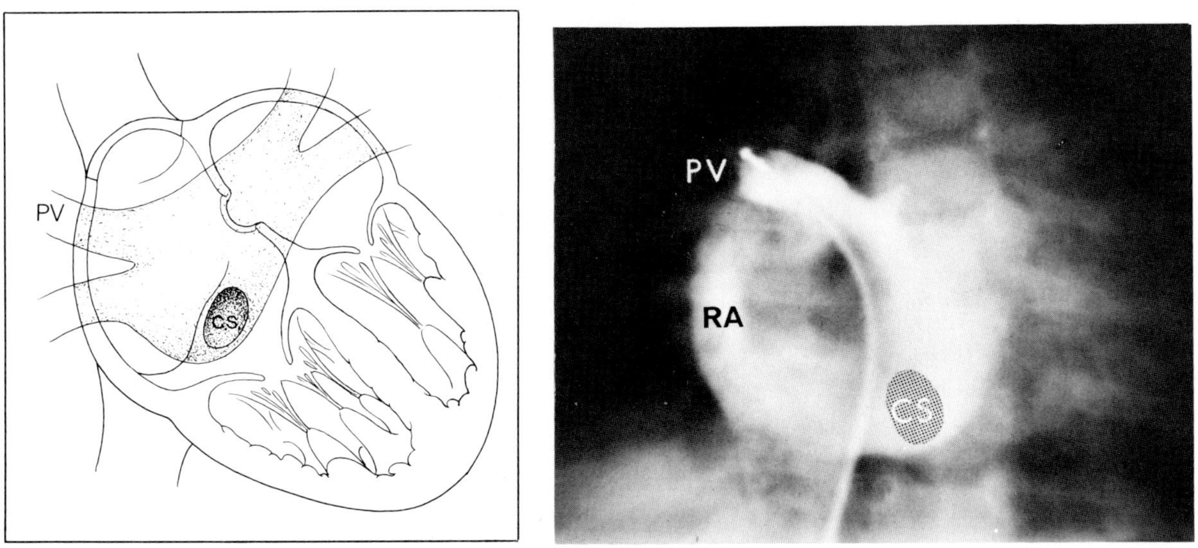

9-14. In the cardiac type of total anomalous pulmonary venous drainage the pulmonary veins (PV) drain into the right atrium (RA) through the coronary sinus (CS).

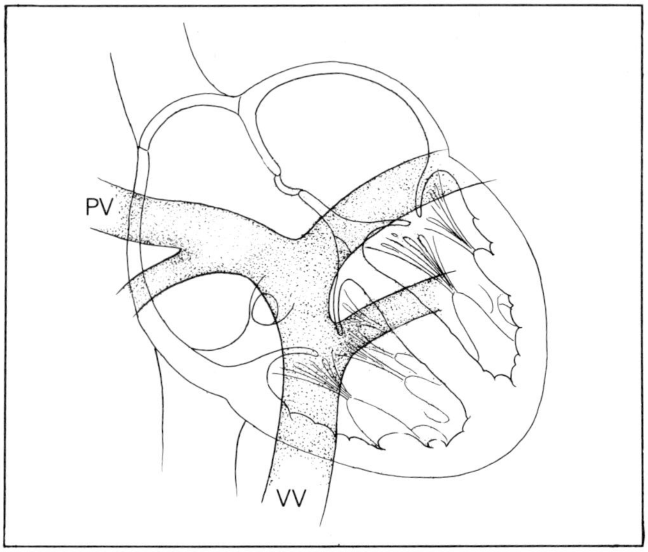

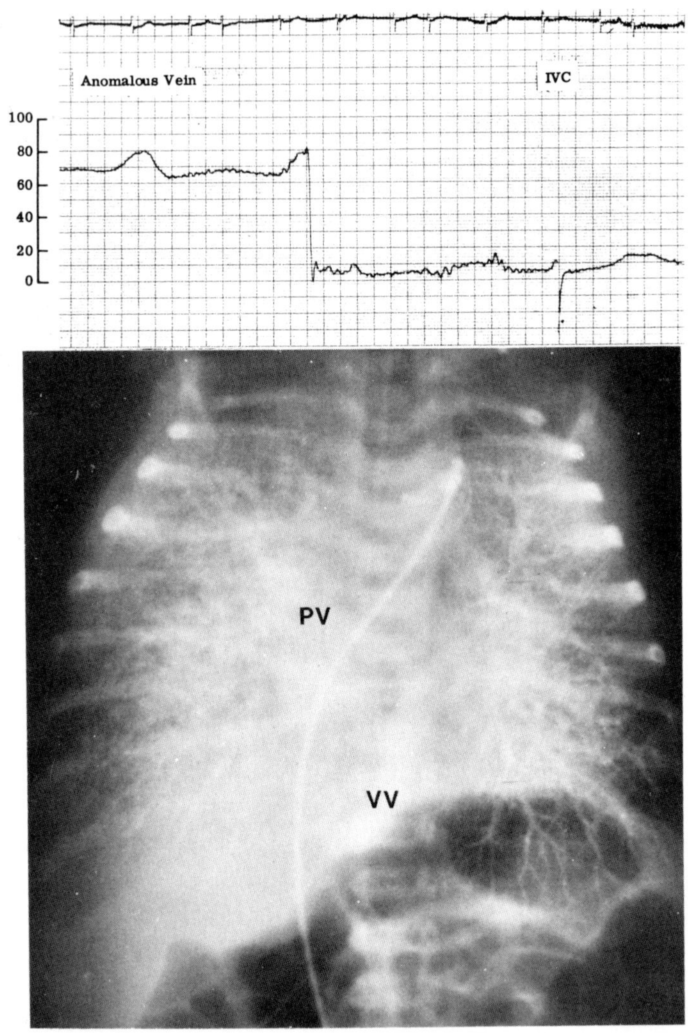

9-15. In the infracardiac type of total anomalous pulmonary venous drainage the pulmonary veins (PV) drain into the inferior vena cava through a vertical vein (VV), which usually connects with the portal vein. There is invariably severe hypertension in the anomalous veins, as the pressure recording shows, because of the resistance to flow created by the capillary bed of the liver.

All types share the same physiologic abnormalities. (1) There is a volume overload of the right ventricle and pulmonary circulation, resulting in congestive cardiac failure and right ventricular hypertrophy. (2) There is complete mixing of systemic and pulmonary blood within the right atrium, resulting in systemic arterial desaturation. (3) The entire systemic blood flow must traverse an atrial septal patency and its adequacy depends on the size of that patency (usually a foramen ovale). (4) In addition, there is sometimes obstruction to pulmonary venous flow, which further increases the burden on the right ventricle and restricts cardiac output. This obstruction is most often caused by compression of the vertical vein between the left bronchus and the pulmonary artery (Figure 9-16).

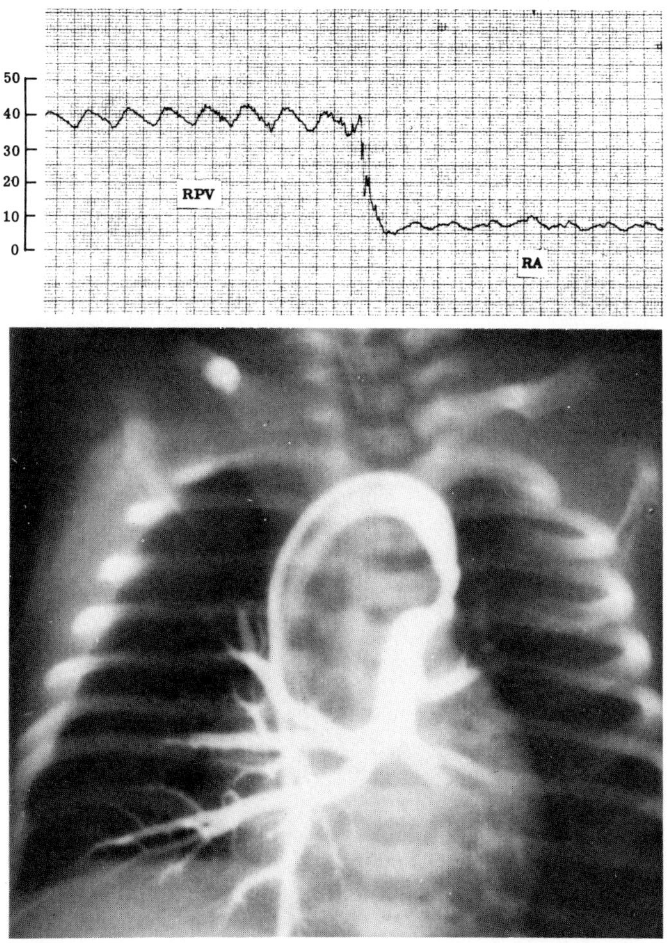

9-16. Angiogram and pressure recordings in supracardiac TAPVD with obstruction of vertical vein as it passes between pulmonary artery and bronchus.

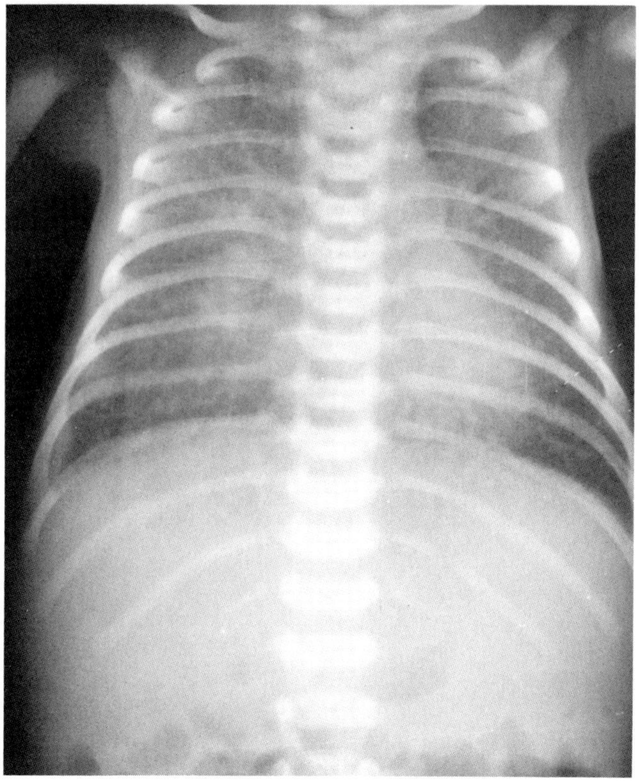

9-17. Chest roentgenogram of infant with total anomalous pulmonary venous drainage and obstructed pulmonary venous flow.

More than 75 percent of patients with TAPVD die during infancy, often following sudden deterioration during the neonatal period. To achieve an appreciable salvage, therefore, diagnosis and operation must often be undertaken urgently. Since no palliative procedure is possible, this means that a total repair must be carried out.

Diagnosis

The diagnosis of TAPVD must be considered in any cyanotic infant with plethoric lung fields on chest x-ray and right ventricular hypertrophy. When pulmonary venous flow is obstructed, the heart may be small, and the lungs may have a ground-glass appearance radiographically (Figure 9-17). The diagnosis is proved and the anatomy is delineated by means of cardiac catheterization and angiography. At catheterization the foramen ovale is sometimes found to be small, preventing free flow of blood into the left atrium. In this situation a Rashkind balloon atrial septostomy may be of benefit; this will allow more blood to enter the left heart and permit operation to be temporarily deferred. We prefer to operate immediately.

Operative Technique, Supracardiac and Infracardiac Types

Following surface cooling a median sternotomy is performed. Perfusion is instituted, the patient is cooled, and the circulation is arrested (see pages 107–108). The advantage of circulatory arrest in this operation is that it allows a precise, open anastomosis to be made without backbleeding from the pulmonary veins.

In all cases the four pulmonary veins form a retropericardial confluence, which can be dissected with the heart elevated cranially (Figure 9-18a).

A transverse incision is made in the confluence of the veins, followed by a parallel incision across the full width of the adjacent left atrium extending into the base of the appendage. An anastomosis is then made with a simple one-layer suture line (Figure 9-18b).

The ascending or descending trunk is ligated (Figure 9-18c). The atrial septal defect is closed. Usually this is a foramen ovale that can be sutured directly through a right atriotomy (Figure 9-18d). When the left atrium appears small, it may be preferable to enlarge it by excising the residual atrial septum and placing an interatrial patch to the right of its usual position.

Perfusion is resumed, the patient is rewarmed, and the operation is completed as described above.

Operative Technique, Cardiac Type

After preliminary surface cooling, perfusion is instituted, cooling is completed, and the circulation is arrested. We use a median sternotomy incision.

The right atrium is opened wide, and the sites of entrance of each of the four pulmonary veins are identified. Usually

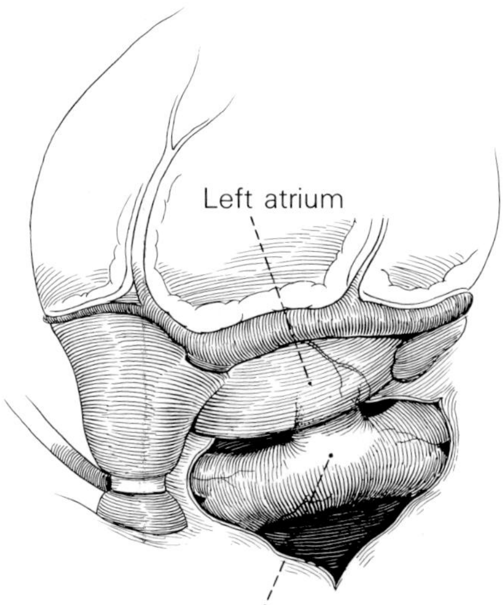

9-18a

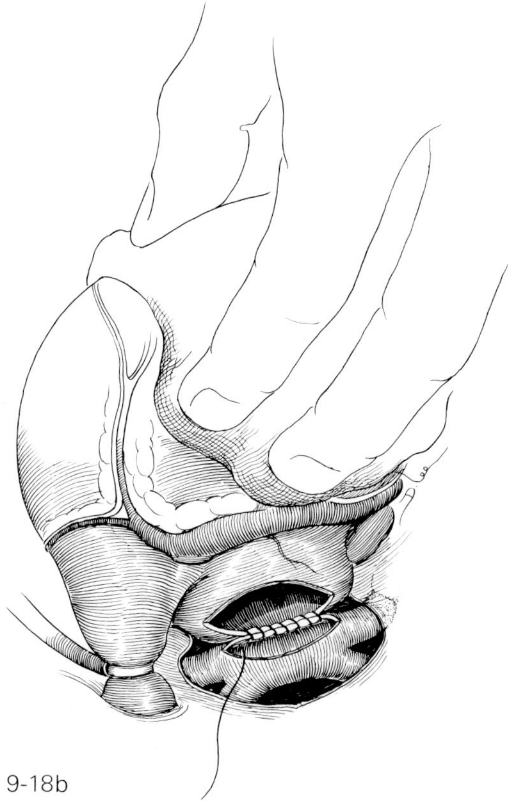

9-18b

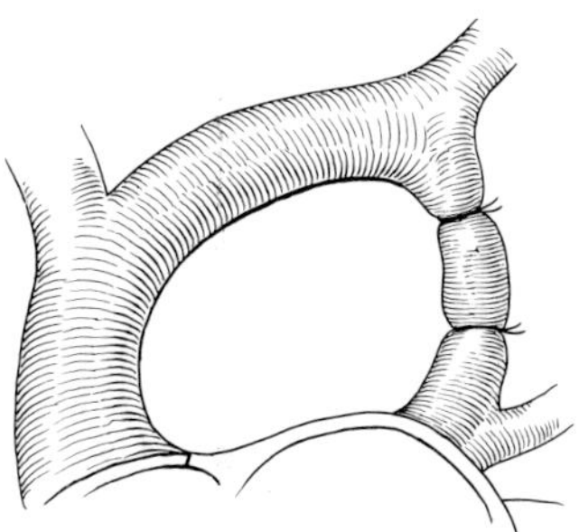

9-18c

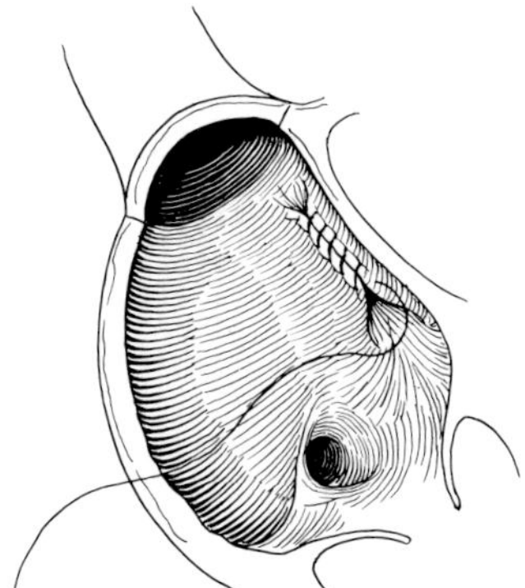

9-18d

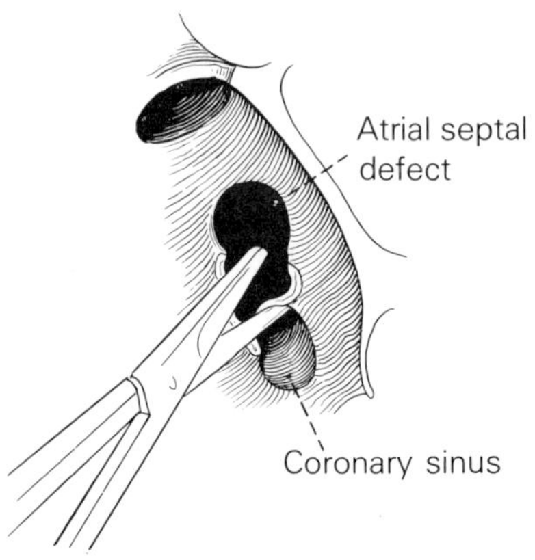

9-19a

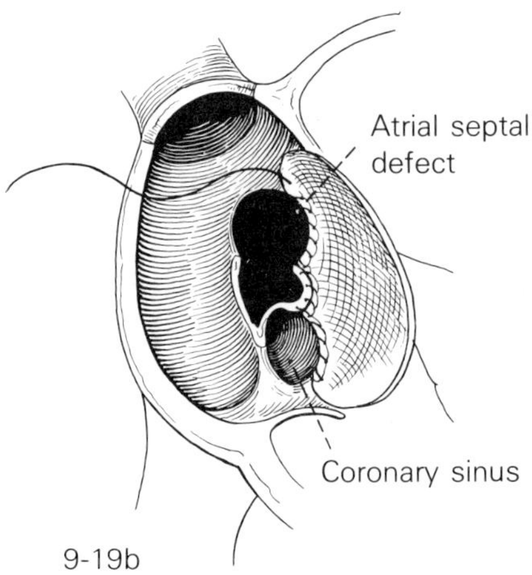

9-19b

the entrances are into a huge coronary sinus, but each may drain directly into the right atrium. The atrial septal defect is enlarged toward the pulmonary vein orifices by cutting away the intervening atrial septum (Figure 9-19a).

Finally, a large Dacron patch is inserted, to divert the pulmonary venous blood into the left atrium (Figure 9-19b).

The atrium is closed, the patient is rewarmed, and the operation is completed.

Comments

The results of TAPVD repair in neonates have been poor, usually because of the poor preoperative condition of the patients. Infants with the most abnormal physiology are brought to the hospital earliest in life in the most severe distress. As might be expected, the mortality has been highest in this group (Figure 9-20).

Recently, earlier referral and the use of deep hypothermia have improved the outlook considerably.

Some surgeons prefer to stage the operation for the supracardiac and infracardiac types in the sickest patients. The anastomosis is created, but the atrial septal defect is left open and the vertical vein is left unligated for subsequent operation at an older age. Often the atrial defect closes spontaneously when this is done.

Long-term follow-up reveals that, in general, patients develop normally following repair of TAPVD, and that the repair withstands the test of time and growth.

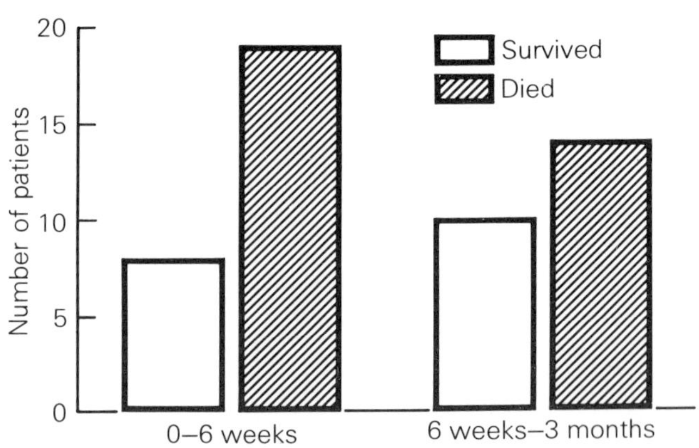

9-20. Results of TAPVD repair in neonates, 1963–1975. Data pooled from available large series from University of Michigan, Columbia-Presbyterian Medical Center, and the Hospital for Sick Children, London.

Aortic Valve Stenosis

Critical aortic stenosis or even aortic valvular atresia, although rare, produces acute left ventricular failure and a high mortality among affected infants. Unfortunately, aortic valve stenosis or aortic valvular atresia is often part of the so-called hypoplastic left-heart syndrome, which may include, in varying degrees, (1) hypoplasia of the left atrium, ventricle, or aorta; (2) hypoplasia of the mitral valve; (3) right-to-left shunting through a patent ductus; and (4) endocardial fibroelastosis.

In its severe form, this syndrome is at present untreatable. Even when only the aortic valve is involved, surgical therapy is often of limited value because the valve annulus is hypoplastic or the leaflets are severely malformed (Figure 9-21).

Diagnosis

Aortic valve stenosis is suspected in a neonate who has uniformly diminished peripheral pulses in addition to left ventricular hypertrophy as shown by electrocardiography. The characteristic aortic ejection murmur may be difficult to appreciate, especially when the cardiac output is diminished. The chest film may show evidence of pulmonary venous hypertension.

A definitive diagnosis of aortic stenosis is made, and associated lesions are delineated by cardiac catheterization and angiography. The sine qua non is the demonstration of a pressure gradient between the left ventricle and the aorta. In sick small babies it can be difficult and hazardous to manipulate a catheter across the aortic valve to obtain these data. Thus the diagnosis often rests on the angiographic appearance of the valve.

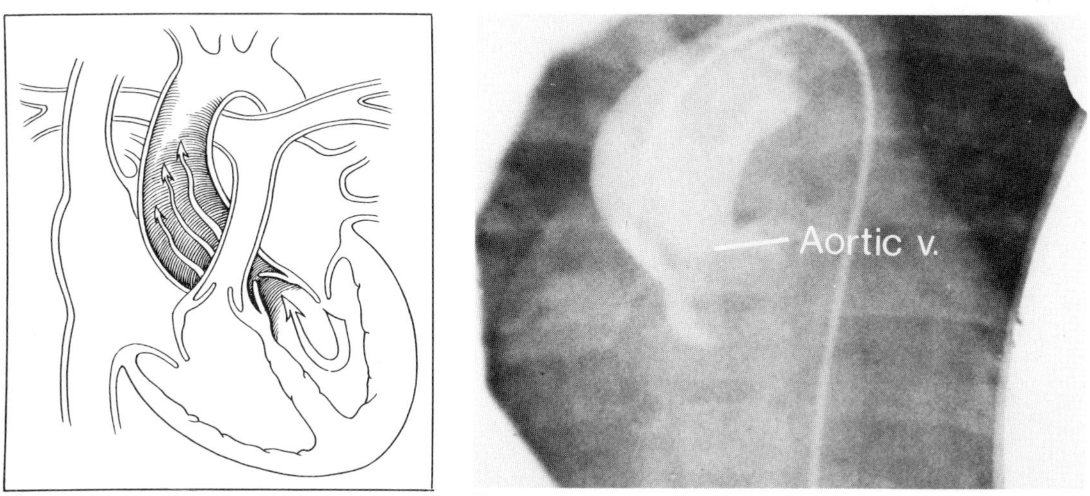

A B

9-21. (A) Diagram of anatomy in congenital aortic stenosis. (B) Typical angiogram showing domed aortic valve.

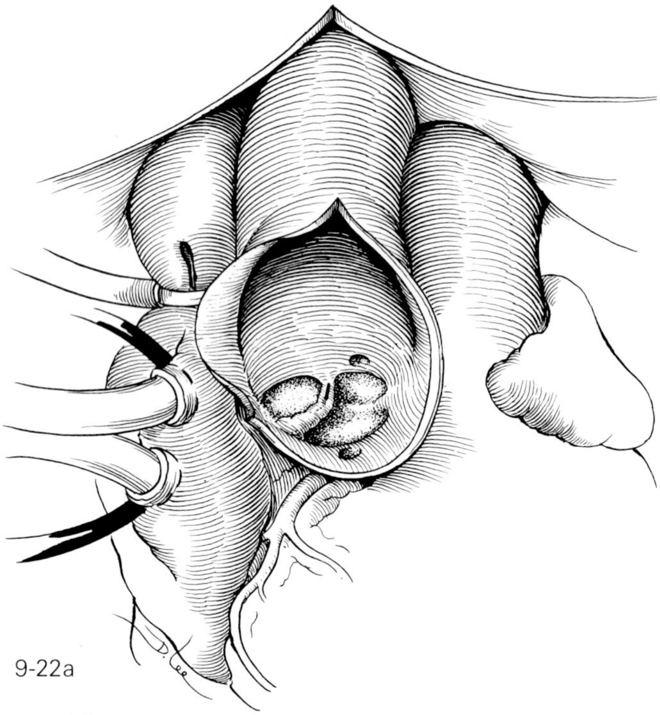

9-22a

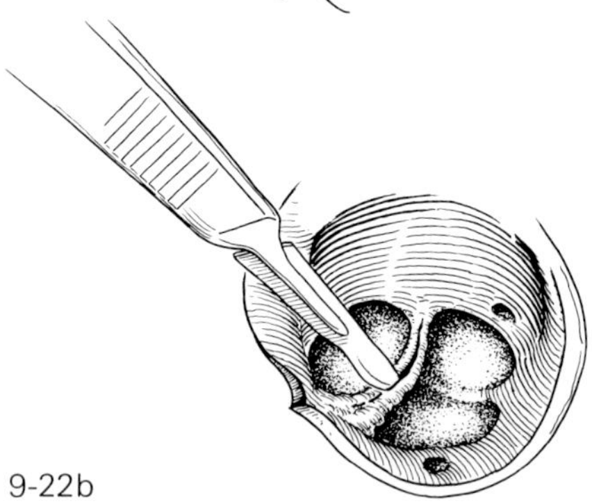

9-22b

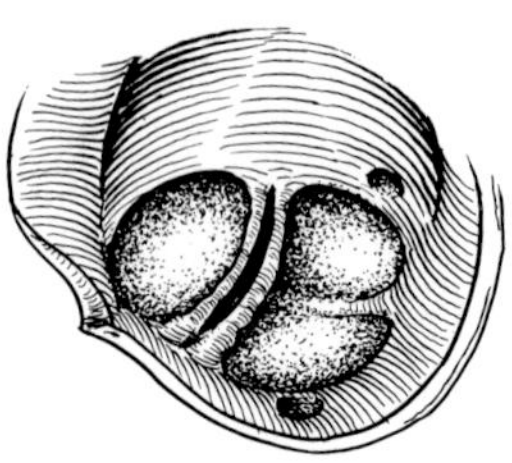

9-22c

Operative Technique

Operation is performed through a median sternotomy. The aorta is opened obliquely, and the aortic valve is inspected. The true commissures (if there are any) must be differentiated from false commissures. A true commissure extends all the way to the edges of the leaflets and sweeps up onto the wall of the aorta above the valve plane (Figure 9-22a). In general, the true commissures are located anteriorly and posteriorly, resulting in a bicuspid valve with right and left leaflets. Occasionally the commissures of a bicuspid valve may be oriented toward the right and left. A tricuspid valve may be found with normally oriented, fused commissures. Rarely, the valve may be unicuspid.

The fused commissures are opened to 1 mm from the annulus (Figure 9-22b). Overcorrection or incision of a false commissure will result in severe valvular regurgitation. A small incision will result in a large increase in valve orifice area (Figure 9-22c). There may be a significant residual pressure gradient, but the improvement may be enough to allow survival of the patient.

Rarely, commissures cannot be identified in very dysplastic valves. In this situation incisions are made 180 degrees apart through the valve tissue, with little hope for success.

The aortotomy is closed with a continuous suture, and air is evacuated from the aortic root and left ventricle. During the period of aortic crossclamping, the myocardium is protected by systemic and local hypothermia. After the patient has been rewarmed, bypass is discontinued and the incisions are closed.

Comments

Because operation for aortic stenosis is undertaken infrequently in neonates, it is difficult to generalize about the results. From 1959 to 1974 at Boston Children's Hospital, 28 infants less than six months of age were operated on for critical aortic stenosis (many with hyperbaric inflow occlusion), with eight deaths [9]. In the past five years we have operated on two neonates with this condition, and they both survived.

Because of poor results with open valvuloplasty, some surgeons have carried out closed dilatations of the valve, with success. We have no experience with this approach.

Pulmonary Valve Stenosis or Atresia

Stenosis of the pulmonary valve occurs in all degrees of severity, from a mild form, in which a gradient of 40 to 60 mm Hg or less is produced (which is well tolerated into adult life), to complete obstruction, which produces a surgical emergency in the neonate.

When critical pulmonary valve stenosis or actual valve atresia occurs in the neonate who does not have a ventricular

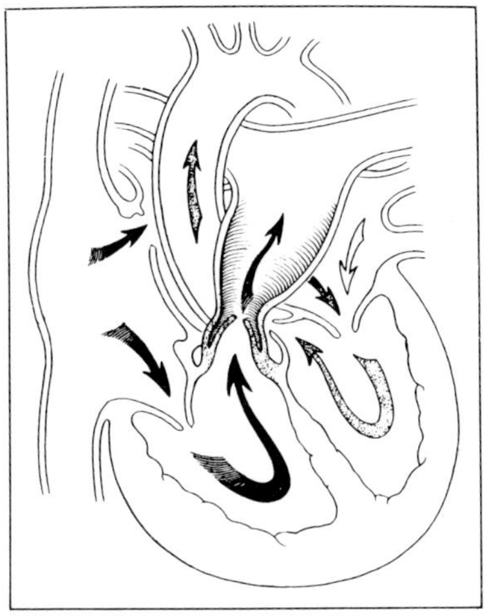

A

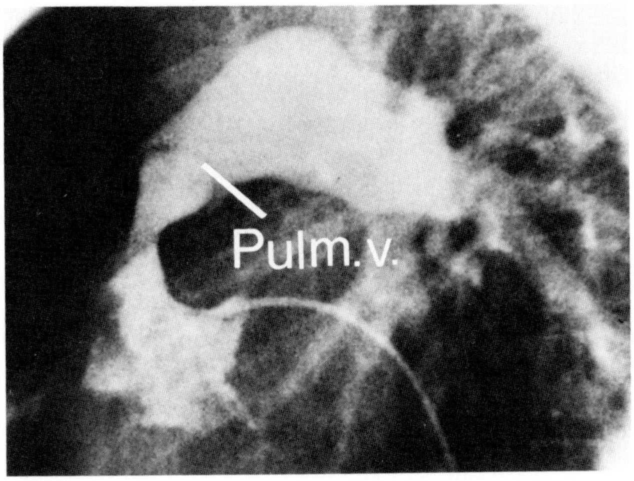

B

9-23. (A) Diagram of anatomy in pulmonary valve stenosis. (B) Angiogram reveals thickened, domed pulmonary valve.

septal defect, acute right ventricular failure occurs, with obligatory right-to-left shunting of blood across the foramen ovale.

In pulmonary stenosis the valve appears to be a dome with a small apical opening (Figure 9-23a, b). There may be two or three commissures, often poorly formed in the neonate. The leaflets themselves are usually formed of markedly thickened, immobile, and dysplastic tissue. The annulus itself may be small.

In pulmonary valvular atresia there is usually only a fibrous membrane separating the right ventricular infundibulum from the main pulmonary artery. The pulmonary blood flow depends on a patent ductus arteriosus or bronchial collateral circulation (Figure 9-24a, b).

Pulmonary atresia can be further subdivided into two types, on the basis of right ventricular size:

I. The right ventricle has severe wall hypertrophy, a small chamber size, and prominent intramyocardial sinusoids.
II. The right ventricular chamber is normal or dilated in size. Often there is massive tricuspid valve insufficiency and the right ventricular wall may be thinned out.

Diagnosis

Stenosis of the pulmonary valve is suspected clinically in a cyanotic infant with right ventricular hypertrophy and decreased pulmonary vascularity on chest film (Figure 9-25).

Cardiac catheterization reveals elevated right atrial pressures and right-to-left atrial shunting. The right ventricular

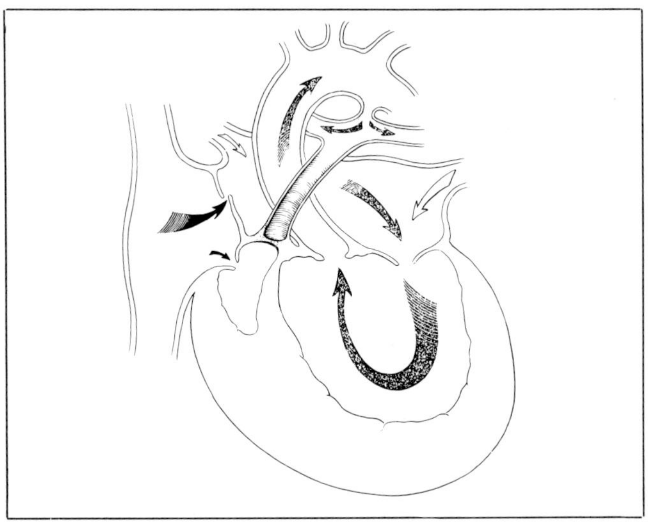

A

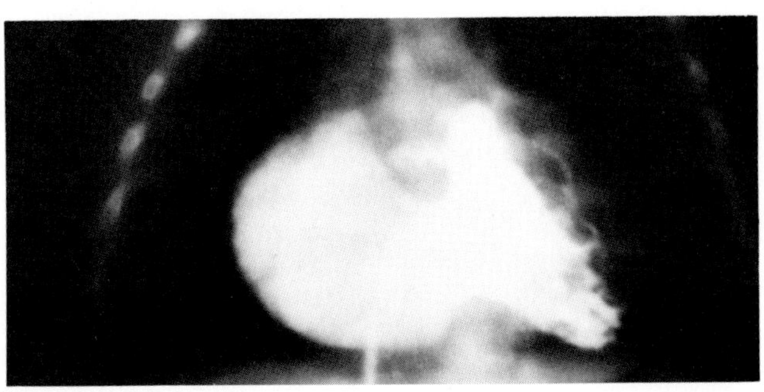

B

9-24. (A) Diagram of typical anatomy in pulmonary valve atresia with intact ventricular septum. (B) Angiogram reveals blind right ventricular outflow tract.

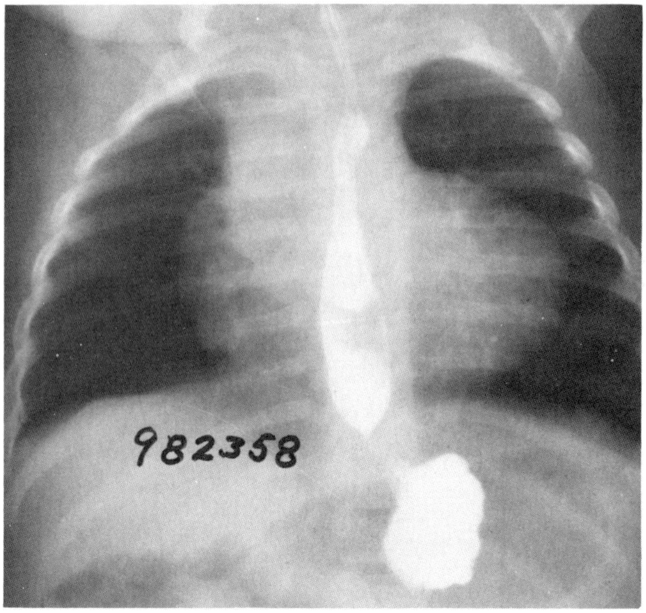

9-25. Chest roentgenogram of infant with pulmonary atresia and intact ventricular septum.

pressure is elevated, often to levels above systemic when it has not decompensated. A right ventricular angiogram is the definitive diagnostic study.

Choice of Operation

There is no question that pulmonary valvulotomy is the procedure of choice in treating severe pulmonary stenosis when the right ventricle and tricuspid valve are basically normal. We prefer to do this by an open technique with circulatory arrest.

The proper surgical therapy for pulmonary atresia, however, is not established. In atresia of type I, the right ventricle usually cannot eject a normal stroke volume, especially into a pulmonary vascular bed with high resistance (which neonates have); therefore the mortality in valvulotomy alone has been very high. Better results have been obtained with a systemic-to-pulmonary shunt coupled with an atrial septectomy or septostomy (see Chapter 8). This effectively bypasses the right ventricle and assures an adequate pulmonary blood flow. Then, to allow for development of the right ventricle and pulmonary valve, an open or closed valvotomy is performed at the same operation or as a second stage.

Patients with atresia of type II may be treated with primary pulmonary valvotomy when the right ventricle is of normal size and appears to contract well and when the tricuspid valve functions well. Otherwise these defects are probably best treated the same way as defects of type I.

Technique of Pulmonary Valvuloplasty

A variety of techniques have been advocated for pulmonary valvuloplasty. We prefer to perform an open valvuloplasty with perfusion and circulatory arrest because:

1. The preliminary surface cooling affords a measure of protection in event of cardiac arrest while the pericardium is being opened, a frequent occurrence with this anomaly.
2. A period of good tissue oxygenation is provided during the perfusion.
3. An unhurried, careful valvuloplasty can be performed, and outflow patching or infundibular resection can be performed if necessary.
4. The foramen ovale can be closed, to prevent postoperative right-to-left shunting.

Surface cooling, a median sternotomy, and perfusion are carried out, and the circulation is arrested as described previously.

The main pulmonary artery is brought into view by caudal retraction on the right ventricle (Figure 9-26a).

A longitudinal arteriotomy is made and the edges are held apart with stay sutures (Figure 9-26b).

The valve commissures are usually found plastered up onto the pulmonary artery wall. They are sharply freed to

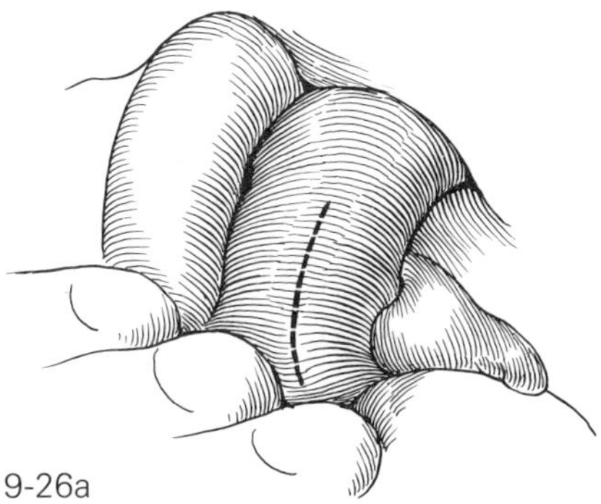

9-26a

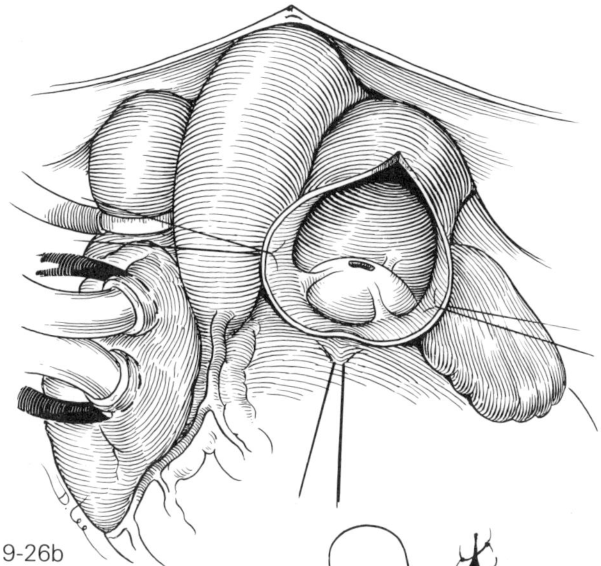

9-26b

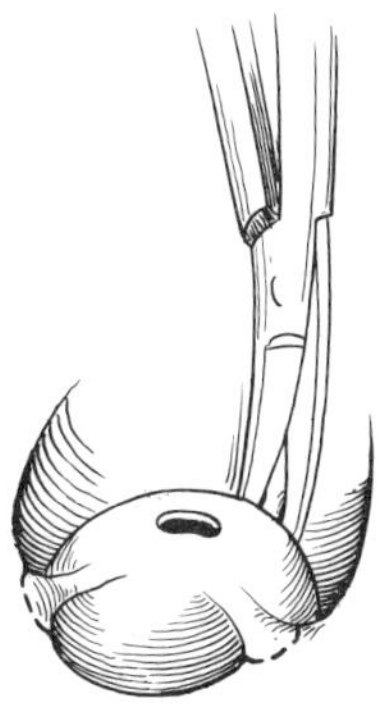

9-26c

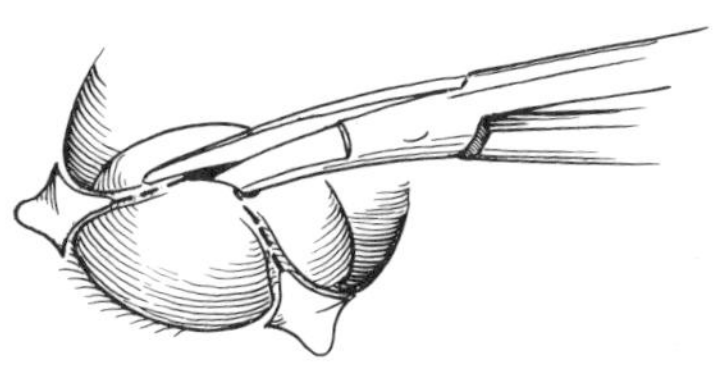

9-26d

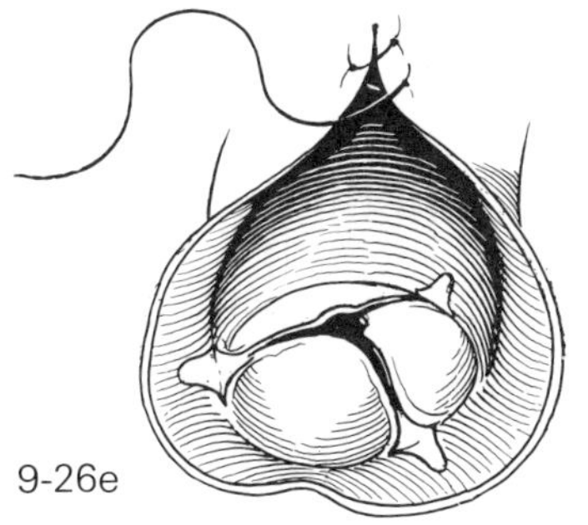

9-26e

elongate the edges of the cusps (Figure 9-26c). Then the commissures are themselves incised to the annulus (Figure 9-26d). If the annulus is narrow, cuts are made into it and it is forcibly dilated (Figure 9-26e). Pacifico and associates [12] have provided guidelines as to what orifice size is acceptable following valvuloplasty. Based on these data our aim would be to achieve an orifice diameter of 5 to 6 mm in neonates. If the right ventricular pressure is 60 percent or less of left ventricular pressure at the completion of the repair and if the right ventricle appears to be contracting well and is not dilated, we would be satisfied. Otherwise, perfusion would be resumed, and a large oval patch would be placed across the valve ring and across any areas of stenosis in the pulmonary artery (Figure 9-27). One must remember that stenosis in the right or left pulmonary artery is commonly associated with valve stenosis, and this condition must be searched for also and corrected if it is severe.

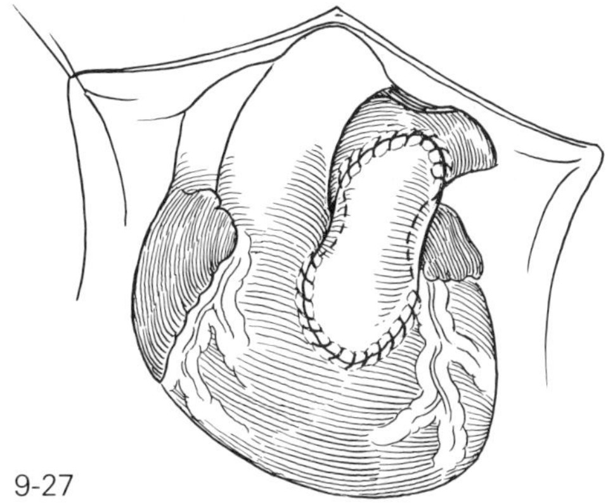

9-27

Comments

Because of the rarity of critical stenosis of the pulmonary valve in neonates and the variability of the anatomy of these lesions, only small series of patients have been reported, and comparisons are hard to make. In general, the approach of an initial systemic-to-pulmonary shunt with or without an atrial septectomy followed by a pulmonary valvotomy has met with most success in treating patients with pulmonary valve atresia with severely hypoplastic right ventricles. Growth of the diminutive right ventricle has been demonstrated in some survivors. Direct pulmonary valvuloplasty has been successful in some patients, particularly infants with good-sized right ventricles and normal tricuspid valves.

The long-term results of these operations are unknown. One would expect many of the survivors to have sufficiently severe residual obstruction so that reoperation would be necessary.

Other Anomalies of the Heart Amenable to Total Repair

Virtually all congenital cardiac anomalies potentially are totally correctable in neonates. Until more experience has been gained, however, most surgeons will prefer to carry out preliminary palliative procedures when these can be expected to yield reasonable results in neonates.

In some complex situations we have found palliative procedures to be generally unsatisfactory, and we believe an attempt at primary total correction should be made. Such conditions include:

1. the combination of large ventricular septal defect, patent ductus, and coarctation or arch atresia;
2. complete endocardial cushion defect with refractory congestive heart failure:
3. truncus arteriosus type I, II, or III with excessive pulmonary blood flow, and refractory congestive heart failure;
4. transposition with large ventricular septal defect.

Descriptions of these total repairs are not included in this book because they will be performed rarely in neonates, even in centers performing a large volume of heart surgery for congenital conditions.

Selected References

1. Barratt-Boyse, B. G., Simpson, M., and Neutze, J. M. Intracardiac surgery in neonates and infants using deep hypothermia with surface cooling and limited cardiopulmonary bypass. *Circulation* 43, 44(suppl. I):1–25, 1971.
2. Breckenridge, I. M., deLeval, M., Stark, J., and Waterston, D. J. Correction of total anomalous pulmonary venous drainage in infancy. *J. Thorac. Cardiovasc. Surg.* 66:447, 1973.

3. Burroughs, J. T., and Edwards, J. E. Total anomalous pulmonary venous connection. *Am. Heart J.* 59:913, 1960.
4. Castaneda, A. R., Lamberti, J., Sade, R. M., et al. Open-heart surgery during the first three months of life. *J. Thorac. Cardiovasc. Surg.* 68:719, 1974.
5. Fisher, R. D., Mason, D. T., and Morrow, A. G. Results of operative treatment in congenital aortic stenosis. *J. Thorac. Cardiovasc. Surg.* 59:218, 1970.
6. Freed, M. D., Rosenthal, A., Bernhard, W. F., et al. Critical pulmonary stenosis with a diminutive right ventricle in neonates. *Circulation* 48:875, 1973.
7. Graham, T. P., Jr., Bender, H. W., Atwood, G. F., et al. Increase in right ventricular volume following valvulotomy for pulmonary atresia or stenosis with intact ventricular septum. *Circulation* 49, 50 (suppl. II):11–69, 1974.
8. Hikasa, Y., Shirotarii, H., Satomura, K., et al. Open heart surgery in infants with an aid of hypothermic anesthesia. *Arch. Jpn. Chir.* 36:495, 1967.
9. Keane, J. F., Bernhard, W. F., and Nadas, A. S. Aortic stenosis surgery in infancy. *Circulation* 52:1138, 1975.
10. Krous, H. F., Tenckhoff, L., Gould, N. S., and Stamm, S. J. Subdural hematoma following open-heart operations. *Ann. Thorac. Surg.* 19:269, 1975.
11. Oberman, H. A. Transfusion of the neonatal patient. Special report by The Committee on Standards of the American Association of Blood Banks. *Transfusion* 14:183, 1974.
12. Pacifico, A. D., Kirklin, J. W., and Blackstone, E. A. Surgical management of pulmonary stenosis in tetralogy of Fallot. *J. Thorac. Cardiovasc. Surg.* 74:382, 1977.
13. Rittenhouse, E. A., Mohri, H., Dellard, D. H., and Merinding, K. A. Deep hypothermia in cardiovascular surgery. *Ann. Thorac. Surg.* 17:63, 1974.
14. Silove, E. D., Behrendt, D. M., Aberdeen, E., and Bonham-Carter, R. E. Total anomalous pulmonary venous drainage. II. Spontaneous functional closure of interatrial communication after surgical correction in infancy. *Circulation* 46:357, 1972.
15. Sinha, S. N., Rusnak, S. L., Sommers, H. M., et al. Hypoplastic left ventricle syndrome. Analysis of thirty autopsy cases in infants with surgical considerations. *Am. J. Cardiol.* 21:166, 1968.
16. Trinkle, J. K., Norton, J. B., Richardson, J. D., et al. Closed aortic valvotomy and simultaneous correction of associated anomalies in infants. *J. Thorac. Cardiovasc. Surg.* 69:758, 1975.
17. Venugupal, P., Olszowka, J., Wagner, H., et al. Early correction of congenital heart disease with surface-induced deep hypothermia and circulatory arrest. *J. Thorac. Cardiovasc. Surg.* 66:375, 1973.

10

Diaphragmatic Hernia

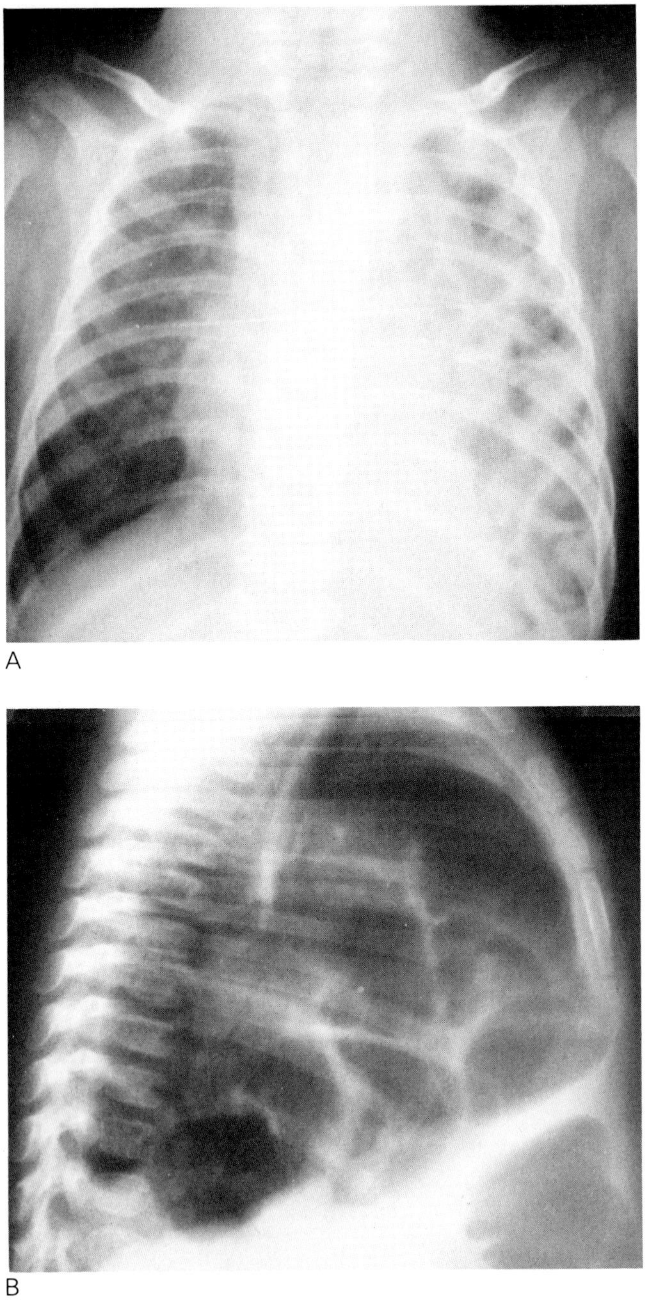

A

B

10-1. (A) Posteroanterior and (B) lateral roentgenograms of infant with left diaphragmatic hernia through the foramen of Bochdalek.

Congenital diaphragmatic hernia through the posterolateral portion of the diaphragm (foramen of Bochdalek) is one of the acute emergencies in pediatric surgery. Children born with this abnormality almost always have severe respiratory distress, either at birth or shortly thereafter. The clinical findings can be diagnostic, and both the pediatrician and the surgeon should be familiar with the steps necessary to make the diagnosis. The newborn with a diaphragmatic hernia has dyspnea, tachypnea, bowel sounds audible over the chest, and a scaphoid abdomen. The severe respiratory embarrassment results in a respiratory acidosis (increased Pco_2) as well as a metabolic acidosis (decreased tissue oxygenation). A chest x-ray should be taken at once to confirm the diagnosis of diaphragmatic hernia (Figure 10-1).

As soon as the diagnosis is suspected, a 12 French nasogastric tube should be placed into the stomach and kept on suction to reduce the amount of air getting into the intestines. This air dilates the loops of bowel that are in the chest, causing, in turn, a shift of the mediastinum to the other side, which results in obstruction of the vena cava as well as compression of the contralateral lung. Respiratory assistance may be necessary for these infants, and it must be given with a minimal amount of inspiratory pressure, by means of a mask or an endotracheal tube, because higher pressure can rupture the opposite lung, resulting in a pneumothorax of the only functioning lung.

Of hernias of the foramen of Bochdalek, 85 percent occur on the left side (perhaps because the liver protects the right diaphragm). Most of the abdominal contents are found in the left chest, whereas right-sided hernias often contain only liver. Thus more severe clinical symptoms occur with left-sided defects. However, the treatment of diaphragmatic hernia on either side is essentially the same. In general, infants with smaller hernias have fewer symptoms, develop symptoms later, and have a better prognosis.

Differential Diagnosis

The presence of bowel sounds in the chest, a scaphoid abdomen, and a typical x-ray film are indications for surgery. Occasionally, the x-ray picture must be differentiated from cystic adenomatoid malformation of the lung (Figure 10-2). Roentgenograms of the chest in cystic adenomatoid malformation can look similar to those in diaphragmatic hernia, but a scaphoid abdomen is not present, and one usually sees a stomach bubble below the diaphragm on the x-ray. Preoperatively, severe eventration of the diaphragm is essentially impossible to differentiate from diaphragmatic hernia (Figure 10-3). However, the treatment of a symptomatic eventration in the newborn is identical to that of a diaphragmatic hernia with a sac. Therefore the differentiation preoperatively is not essential.

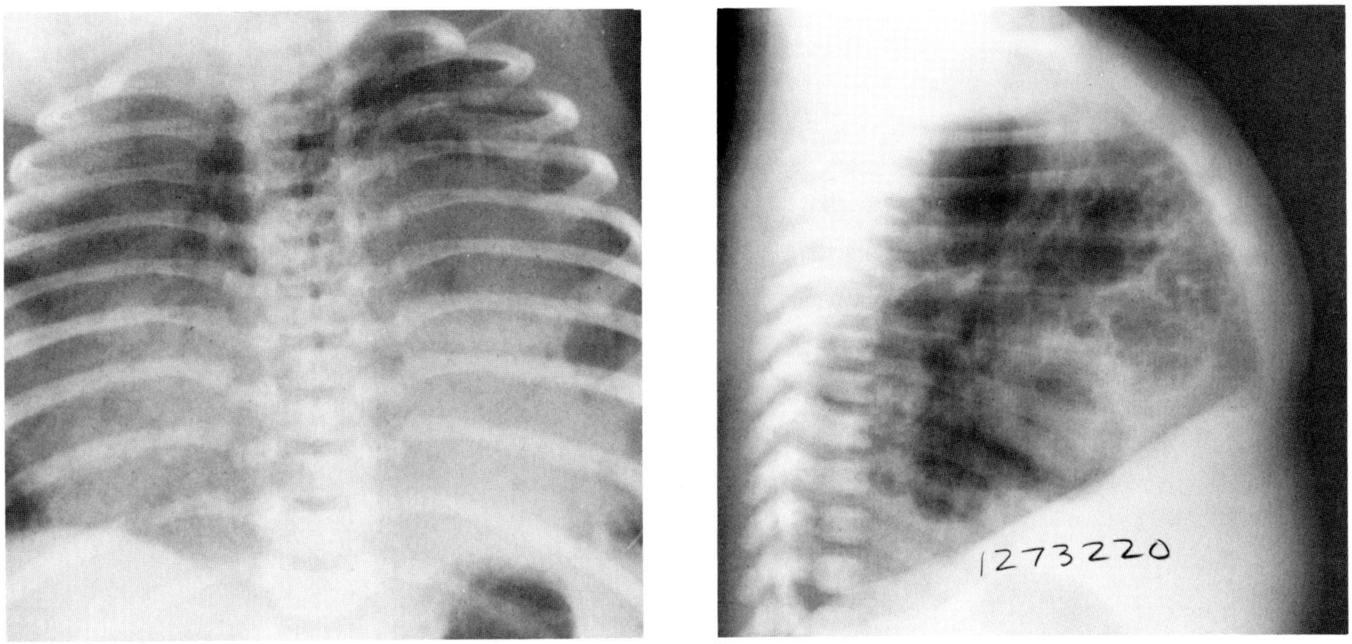

A

B

10-2. (A) Posteroanterior and (B) lateral roentgenograms of child with cystic denomatoid malformation of the right lung. Note the normal stomach bubble.

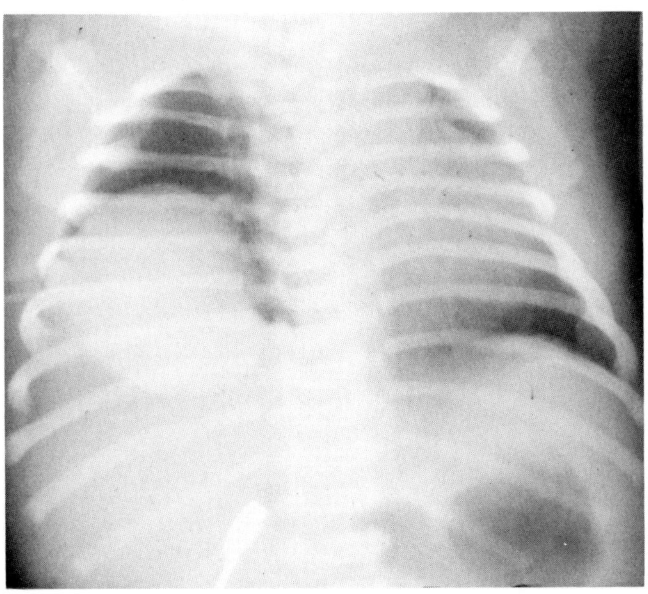

10-3. Eventration of right diaphragm. A small right-sided diaphragmatic hernia might look identical on x-ray.

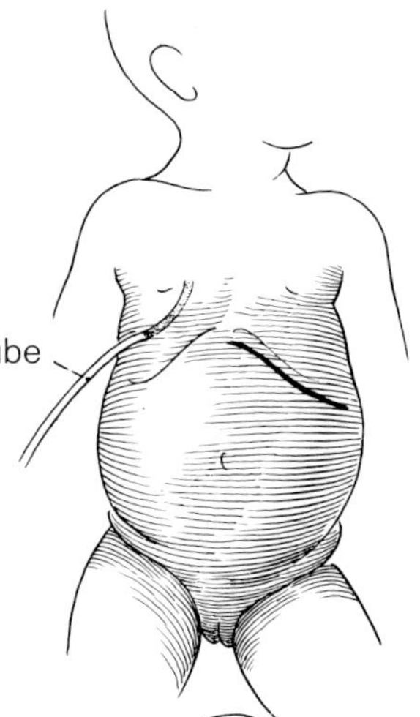

10-4a

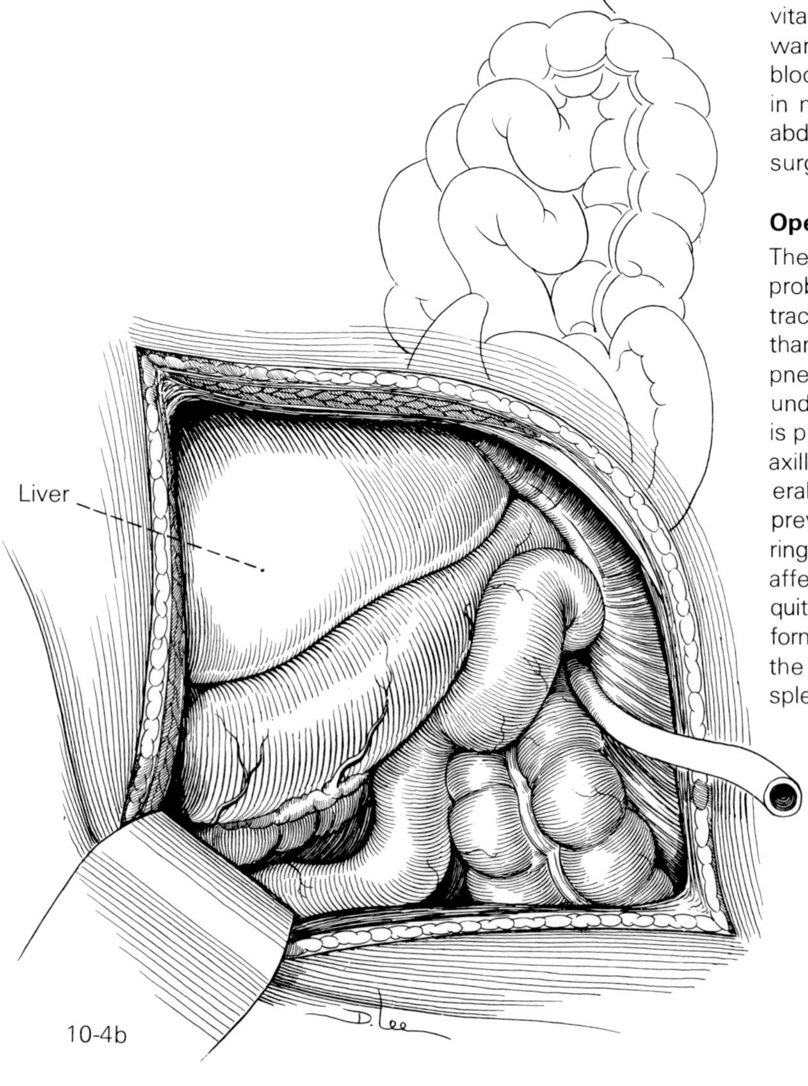

10-4b

Preoperative Preparation

An infant with a diaphragmatic hernia must be taken to the operating room quickly, because the exchange of gases may not improve until the bowel is reduced from the chest. The severe metabolic derangements, however, markedly increase the risk of anesthesia. One hour of preoperative preparation may therefore improve the clinical status considerably. As soon as the condition is suspected, a nasogastric tube should be passed, a large-bore catheter should be placed into a vein, and the acidosis should be corrected, starting with an initial dose of three milliequivalents per kilogram of body weight of sodium bicarbonate. Blood gases should be obtained immediately and followed closely. Gentle mechanical ventilation with oxygen may be required. The patient should be started on broad-spectrum antibiotics, have a blood type and crossmatch sent, be given 1 mg of vitamin K intramuscularly, and be placed in an open infant warmer. If the previously described measures correct the blood gases to normal, the prognosis is good. Unfortunately, in most babies the acidosis will not be corrected until the abdominal viscera are reduced from the thoracic cavity at surgery. Excessive delay should therefore be avoided.

Operative Technique

The patient is placed supine on an infant warmer with a rectal probe and electrocardiographic leads in place. Careful endotracheal anesthesia with inspiratory pressures no higher than 20 cm of water is instituted. Because a contralateral pneumothorax can occur during positive-pressure ventilation under anesthesia and it can be fatal, shortly after the patient is prepped a 14 French chest tube is placed into the anterior axillary line of the second intercostal space on the contralateral side (Figure 10-4a). This is done under direct vision to prevent an unsuspected tension pneumothorax from occurring during surgery. A subcostal incision is then made on the affected side, going through all muscle layers with cautery quite expeditiously. Meticulous hemostasis should not be performed at this time. The bowel should be rapidly removed from the thoracic cavity, with care taken to avoid injury to the spleen. A 14 French rubber catheter placed into the chest

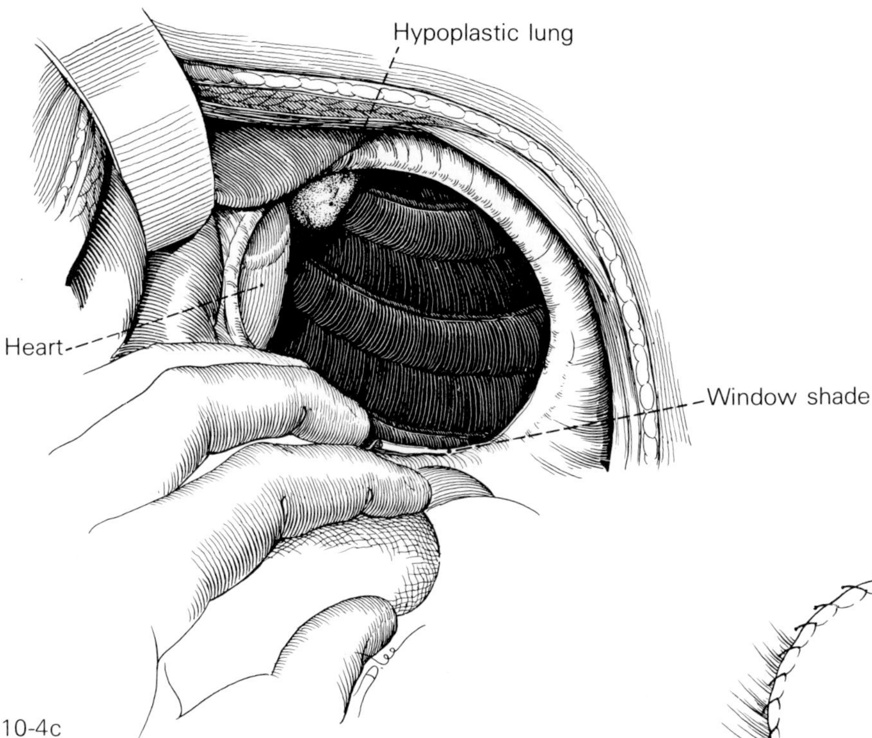

10-4c

through the abdominal incision will release the suction and facilitate removal of the intestinal contents from the chest (Figure 10-4b). The organs are then placed on a moist warm laparotomy pad while the defect in the diaphragm is evaluated. Care must be taken to search for a hernia sac. A sac is present in fewer than 5 percent of the cases, but if it is missed before the diaphragm is closed, the lung may not be able to expand postoperatively. If a sac or severe eventration is found, it is usually excised. Before excision, however, the surgeon should be certain that he does not need a rim of this tissue for his repair.

Before the defect is closed, the surgeon should inspect the lung on the ipsilateral side. Usually the lung is small and hypoplastic. If it is not, the prognosis is better. Under no circumstances should the anesthesiologist attempt to expand the lung forcibly. Expansion may result in rupture of the opposite lung, which can be fatal. It may be days or even weeks before the lung fully expands. An intercostal chest tube is placed in the ipsilateral pleural cavity before the diaphragm is closed.

In patients without a sac, a search of the posterior thoracic wall will usually reveal a rim of diaphragm that is rolled up like a window shade (Figure 10-4c). It is thin and not very muscular but will usually hold sutures. Most often there is a good rim of tissue anteriorly (Figure 10-4d). The diaphragm is closed with horizontal mattress sutures of 2-0 or 3-0 silk.

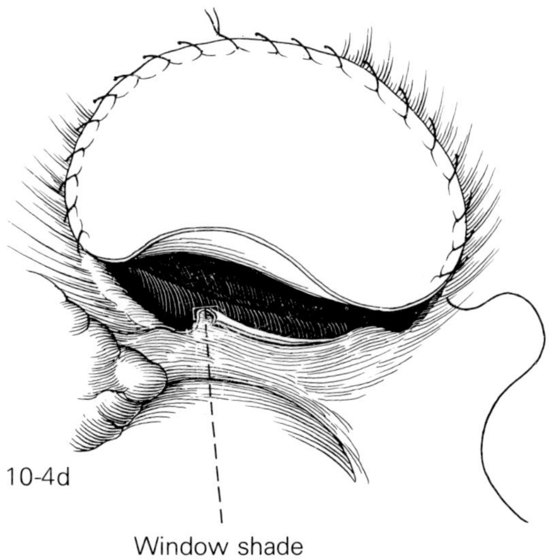

10-4d

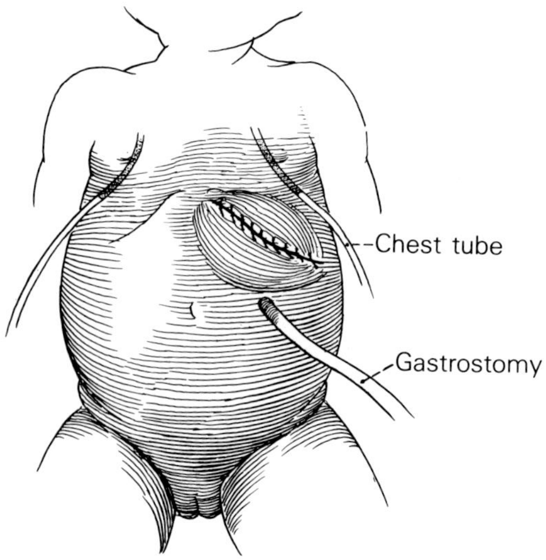

10-5. Postoperatively the child has bilateral chest tubes connected to underwater seal, a gastrostomy, and perhaps a ventral hernia.

Frequently simple sutures of 2-0 or 3-0 silk are necessary because the rim of tissue is too small for mattress sutures. Occasionally there is not sufficient anterior or posterior diaphragm to perform a primary closure, and a patch of appropriate size must be fashioned out of Dacron-reinforced Silastic sheeting (Dow-Corning number 501-3). (Figure 10-4d). Flaps of abdominal musculature can also be rotated to replace the diaphragm if necessary. Posteriorly it may be necessary to place the stitches through a rib in order to provide a firm holding point for the mesh or diaphragm.

Attention is then directed to the bowel. Most infants with diaphragmatic hernia have an associated malrotation of the intestine. A search for this entity must be made and the defect must be corrected (see Chapter 12). A Stamm gastrostomy with a number 12 or 14 Malecot catheter is performed and is brought out through a separate stab wound below the skin incision.

Because the intestinal contents have not been in the abdomen during intrauterine life, the size of the peritoneal cavity is small, making it difficult to close the abdominal incision once the intestines have been placed back in the peritoneal cavity. Stretching the abdomen by placing one's fingers inside the lateral aspects of the abdominal cavity and forcibly stretching the abdominal wall may help. If the abdomen can be closed without tension it is done with interrupted 2-0 or 3-0 silk in layers. If it is obvious that primary closure would create undue tension, the fascia can be left open and just the skin closed with a running 2-0 nylon, creating a ventral hernia (Figure 10-5). If the clinical course has been good, a patient with a ventral hernia is returned to the operating room five to seven days later, at which time the fascia is closed with interrupted 3-0 silk. After ten days the ventral hernia repair becomes more difficult because of denser adhesions between the undersurface of the skin and the intestines.

Right-sided diaphragmatic hernias are often clinically less significant (Figure 10-6a). The contents are more easily reduced (Figure 10-6b) and the defect can often be closed primarily (Figure 10-6c, d), because there is usually a good rim of tissue posteriorly. A contralateral chest tube and gastrostomy may not be needed.

Postoperative Care

The baby is best cared for on an open warmer in the neonatal intensive care unit. The infant can remain intubated at the discretion of the anesthesiologist and surgeon; mechanical ventilation is frequently required. Once again, in order to prevent a pneumothorax in the contralateral chest, the inspiratory pressure should not be greater than 20 cm of water. The gastrostomy is placed on gravity drainage, and intravenous fluids and antibiotics are continued. Blood gas determinations are performed at frequent intervals. The chest tubes are placed to underwater seal only. Occasionally

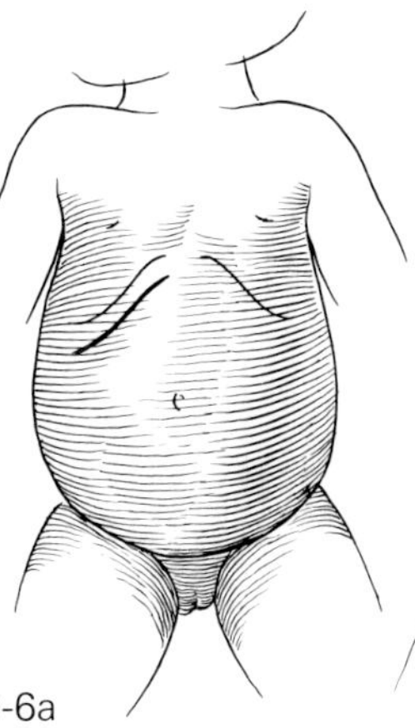

10-6a

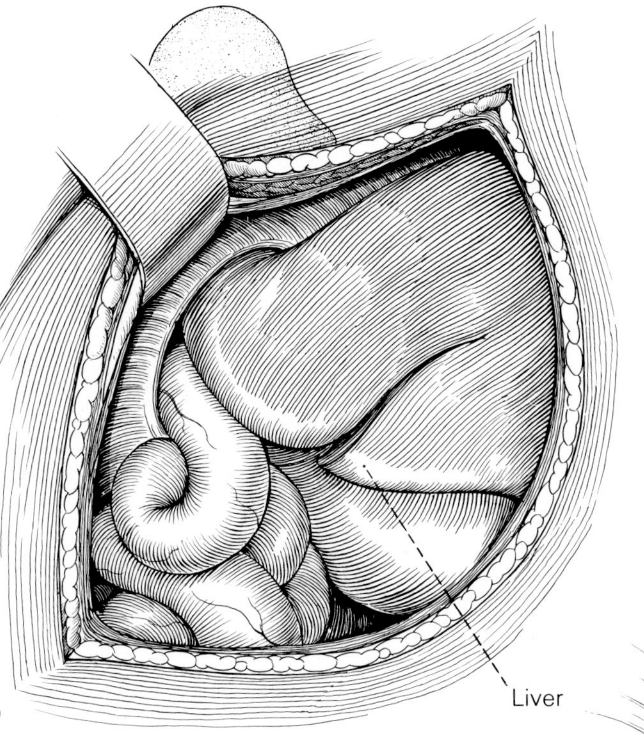

10-6b

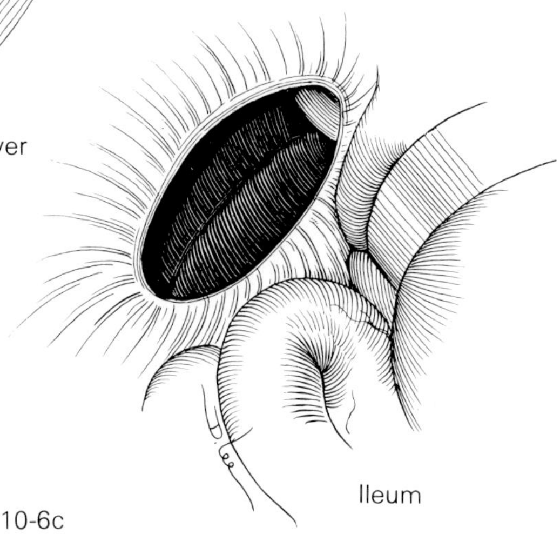

10-6c

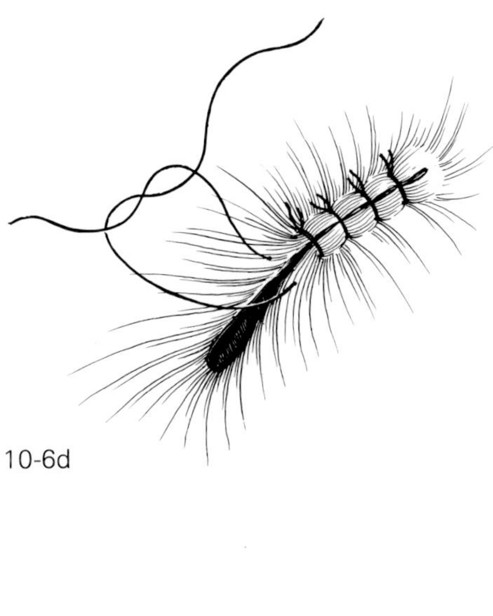

10-6d

negative pressure of one to three centimeters of water may be used. Suction of higher pressure can result in shifting of the newborn's mediastinum, which is not fixed, resulting in acute emphysema of the contralateral lung, with a resultant pneumothorax and possible obstruction of the vena cava. Frequent chest films are needed to be certain that the mediastinum has not shifted significantly. Adding and subtracting small amounts of negative pressure to either tube will allow the surgeon to keep the mediastinum near the midline.

Despite careful attention to details, about half of these patients do not survive. The final determinant of success is the total amount of functioning lung tissue available for gas exchange. Until such time as extracorporeal oxygenation becomes available for neonates, a significant percentage of these infants will not survive.

Complications

Poor lung function is responsible for both the respiratory acidosis (from CO_2 retention) and metabolic acidosis (from tissue anoxia) that recur postoperatively. Constant observation is necessary to provide these babies with the best chance of survival. Dehiscence of the single-layer skin closure has been reported. Careful observation of the skin closure and emergency repair if dehiscence occurs will eliminate deaths from this problem. A Silastic silo as is used in repair of omphaloceles may be needed to close a dehiscence (see Chapter 17). Antibiotics should be continued for at least ten days. Contralateral tension pneumothorax is common. This can best be prevented by the prophylactic insertion of a contralateral chest tube, as described earlier. If such a chest tube is not used, any sudden worsening of the infant's clinical course should make the surgeon suspicious of pneumothorax. The possibility of obstruction from incompletely lysed Ladd's bands or from a postoperative volvulus (because of malrotation) must always be considered. A recurrent diaphragmatic hernia is rare but possible; if found, it must be repaired.

Hernias of the Foramen of Morgagni

Medial hernias through the anterior aspect of either diaphragm near the sternocostal junction are not common. They are rarely if ever discovered during the first month of life because the hernia is usually small and asymptomatic. These hernias, which have true membranous sacs and do not cause pulmonary compression, most commonly contain a lobe of the liver or part of the transverse colon (Figure 10-7a). The

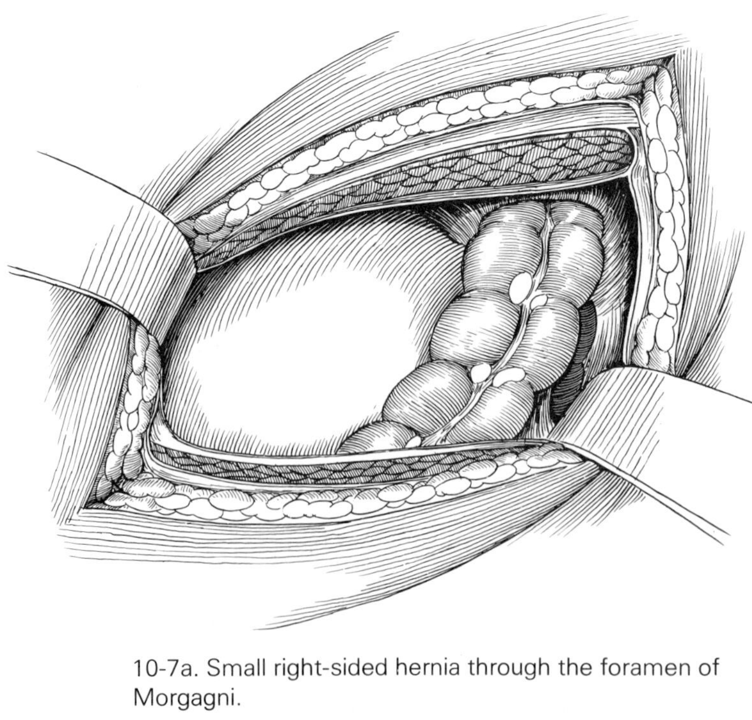

10-7a. Small right-sided hernia through the foramen of Morgagni.

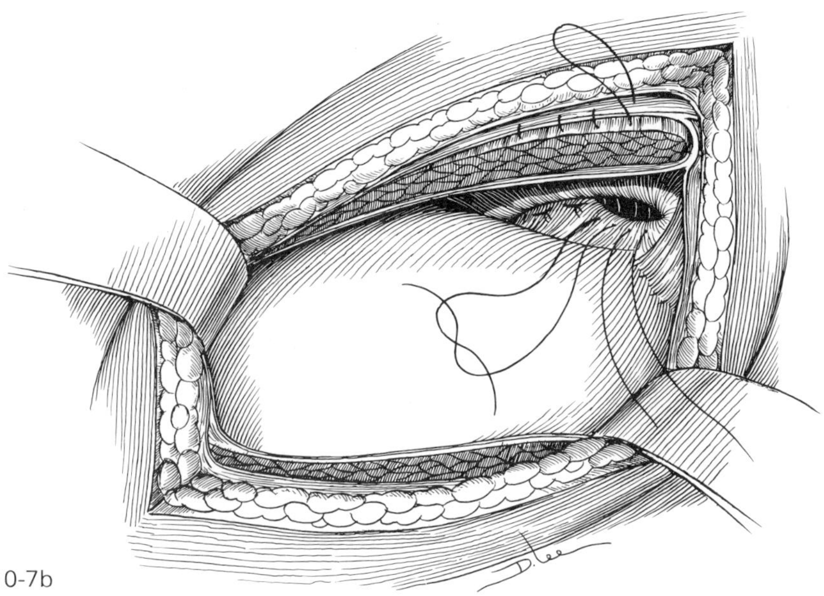

10-7b

diagnosis is usually made by an x-ray film of the chest. Instillation of radiopaque dye into the intestinal tract may help to confirm the diagnosis. The surgical treatment is similar to that described for the more common Bochdalek hernias except that the sac must be excised before the defect is closed (Figure 10-7b). Because the hernia is small, abdominal-wall closure is rarely a problem.

Esophageal Hiatus Hernia and Chalasia

Hiatus hernias are rare in the newborn, but they become more common after the first month of life. One must differentiate hiatus hernia from chalasia. This can be done easily with a barium swallow (see Chapter 11, on pyloric stenosis). Treatment of either consists of feeding the baby in the erect position and maintaining the infant in that position for one to two hours after each feeding. It also helps to thicken the child's formula with cereal. Surgery is rarely necessary for chalasia and, in fact, is not usually necessary for hiatus hernia. On some occasions, however, the symptoms of hiatus hernia are so severe that failure to thrive results, in which case a Nissen fundoplication is required at a few months of age.

Selected References

1. Baffes, T. G. Diaphragmatic Hernia. In W. T. Mustard, M. M. Ravitch, W. H. Snyder, Jr., et al. (eds.). *Pediatric Surgery*. Chicago. Year Book Medical Publishers, 1969, pp. 342–56.
2. Dibbins, A. W., and Wiener, E. S. Mortality from neonatal diaphragmatic hernia. *J. Pediatr. Surg.* 9:653–62, 1974.
3. Orringer, M. B., Kirsh, M. M., and Sloan, H. Congenital and traumatic diaphragmatic hernias exclusive of the hiatus. *Curr. Probl. Surg.* March 1975.
4. Prinsen, J. E. Hiatus hernia in infants and children: A long-term follow-up of medical therapy. *J. Pediatr. Surg.* 10:97–103, 1975.
5. Wayne, E. R., Campbell, J. B., Burrington, J. D., and Davis, W. S. Eventration of the diaphragm. *J. Pediatr. Surg.* 9:643–52, 1974.

11

Pyloric Stenosis and Spontaneous Gastric Perforation

Hypertrophic pyloric stenosis is a benign overgrowth of the pyloric musculature of unknown cause. The typical patient develops symptoms at three weeks of age with a history of progressively more frequent, nonbilious, projectile vomiting. In an occasional patient there will be a delay in presentation and significant dehydration and weight loss may result. Hypochloremic, hypokalemic alkalosis and shock may be seen in advanced stages, and occasionally blood may be present in the vomitus secondary to reactive gastritis.

Preoperative Evaluation

Fortunately, in most cases the history is typical and the patient is referred to the surgeon early in the course of the disease. The surgeon should make a careful effort to feel the olive-shaped tumor. This is possible in more than 90 percent of cases. To find the so-called olive, the right-handed surgeon should be on the baby's left side. First he should observe the abdomen to see if peristaltic waves can be seen going across the abdomen from left to right. Then the stomach should be decompressed with a nasogastric tube. (Frequently, three to four ounces of undigested formula will be found in the stomach despite the fact that the child may not have been fed for four hours.) The surgeon then places his left hand under the child's buttocks and flexes the abdomen. With a nipple in the baby's mouth to quiet him, the right hand of the surgeon is gently placed near the umbilicus and rocked cephalad and caudad with increasing pressure until the mass is felt squirting under the surgeon's fingertip. It is important that the surgeon be sitting or in a comfortable position because, even with experience, it may be several minutes before the olive can be palpated. There are no other structures in the abdomen that feel like a wet olive squirting under the surgeon's fingers. If the history is suggestive but a careful examination does not reveal a palpable mass, then a small amount of barium can be placed into the stomach under fluoroscopic control, and the classic string-shaped defect of the pyloric lesion can be seen (Figure 11-1). The fluoroscopist should be alerted to check for the presence of chalasia (free esophageal reflux) because this is another common cause of vomiting in infants in the first month of life; thickened feedings and propping up in an infant seat will cure this problem without surgery (Figure 11-2).

An occasional patient with pyloric stenosis will have jaundice. Recent studies have shown that this may be related to a decrease in hepatic glucuronyl transferase. The jaundice disappears following surgical correction of the pyloric stenosis.

The treatment of pyloric stenosis is surgical. The surgeon is cautioned to wait, however, until any metabolic alkalosis has been corrected before undertaking operation. There is no harm in delaying the operation, and the infant faces an obvi-

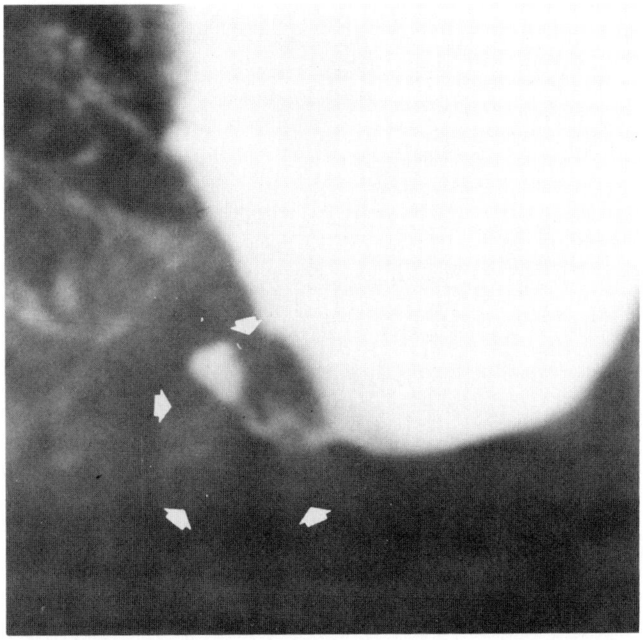

11-1. Classic x-ray sign of pyloric stenosis. Arrows outline the pyloric olive, through which the narrowed pyloric lumen is visualized.

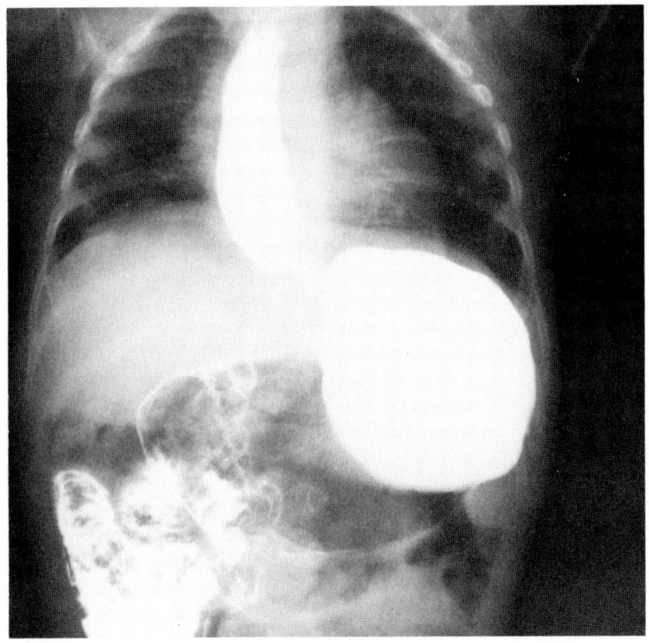

11-2. Massive esophageal reflux resulting from chalasia.

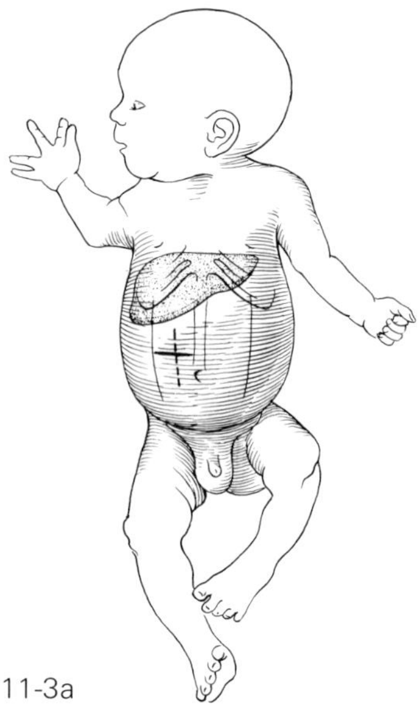

11-3a

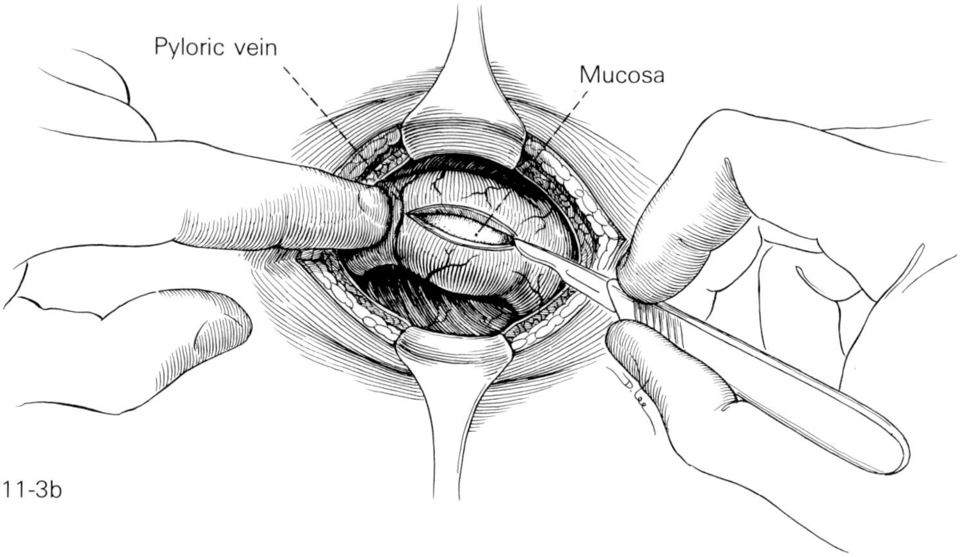

11-3b

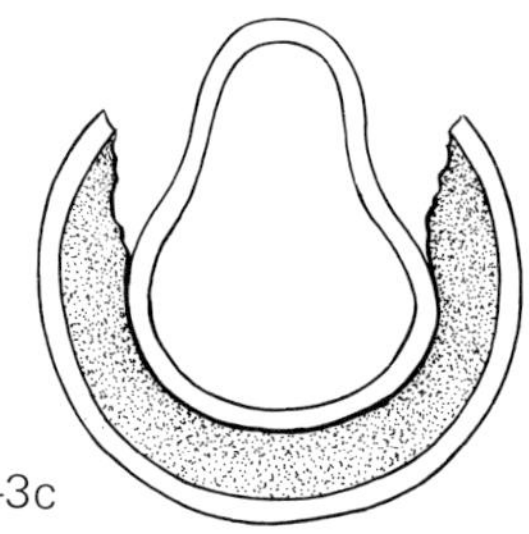

11-3c

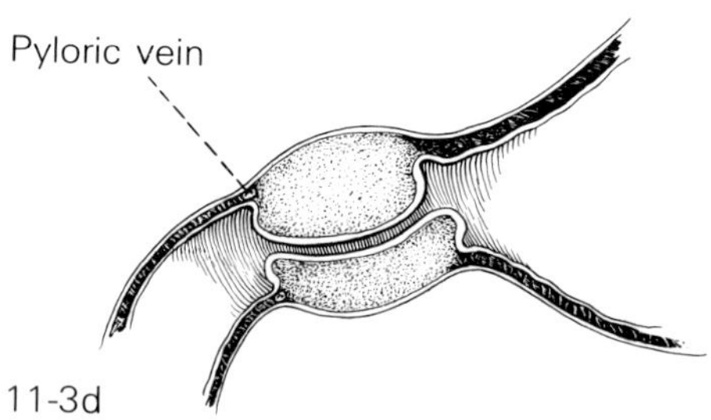

11-3d

ous risk if surgery is done before correction of the metabolic derangement. The child who is seen early in the course of this disease and who wets his diaper while being examined in the doctor's office can usually be operated upon the same day with little or no preoperative preparation. In the more dehydrated patients, however, an intravenous line is placed in position, and fluid correction is undertaken with a solution of 5% dextrose and 0.45 normal saline with 2 to 4 milliequivalents per kilogram of body weight of potassium added. The amount of fluid administered is dependent upon the percentage of dehydration and usually runs between 2,000 and 3,000 cubic centimeters per square meter of body surface area per 24 hours. A nasogastric tube is frequently helpful. It may be placed and left to gravity drainage or inserted every four hours, aspirated, and removed. Patients with severe dehydration may also require plasma (10 cubic centimeters per kilogram of body weight) to bring the child into adequate circulatory balance before surgery.

Operative Technique

The patient is positioned supine. Before induction and intubation, the anesthesiologist passes a large-bore nasogastric tube to be sure that the stomach is completely empty. Transfusion is usually not necessary for this procedure: The operative time is 15 to 30 minutes. A 2-cm transverse incision is made one-third of the way up from the umbilicus to the costal margin directly over the rectus muscle. The skin incision is spread with small vein retractors and a vertical incision is made midway across the rectus fascia (Figure 11-3a). The rectus muscle is separated until the posterior fascia and peritoneum can be seen; they also are incised vertically. At this point it is important that the surgeon not reach for the distal stomach, because the pyloric olive is not pliable and will not move well. Instead, a gentle grasp is taken of the

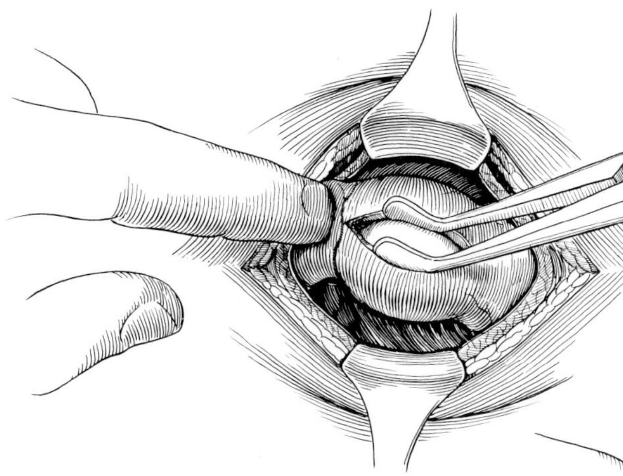

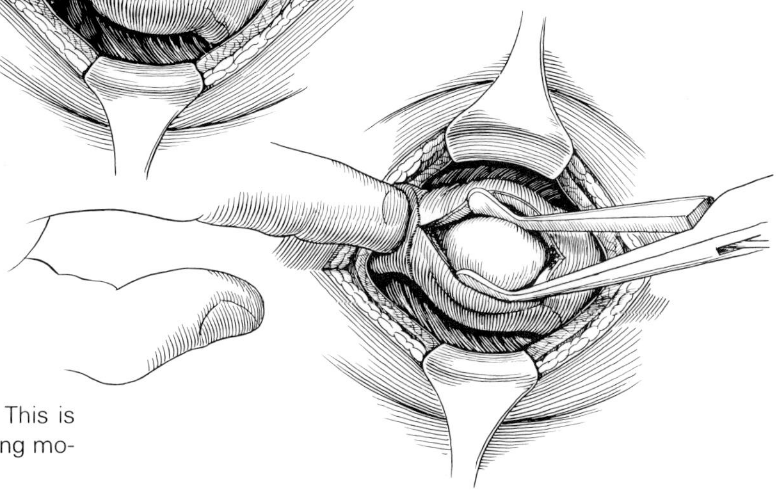

11-3e

midportion of the greater curvature of the stomach. This is brought out into the wound; then, with a gentle rocking motion, the pyloric olive will pop out of the incision.

Now the surgeon places his left index finger against the duodenal wall and invaginates the duodenum into the pyloric olive so that he can readily identify where the duodenum begins and the pylorus ends. The location of the pyloric vein also facilitates this maneuver. Then a scoring incision is made on the serosa of the stomach over the pyloric tumor carried from just proximal to the beginning of the duodenum well onto the stomach wall. Care is taken to make this incision in the relatively avascular plane that is located on the anterior superior aspect of the gastric wall (Figure 11-3b). This incision is then deepened, using the back end of the scalpel. The thick, muscular olive will break under a rocking motion of the scalpel handle. The submucosa of the stomach can then be seen pouting through the pyloric tumor while its fibers are separated (Figure 11-3c). On the gastric side, the pointed end of the hemostat will help break up the fibers. The distal fibers of the olive are left until the end to help avoid entrance into the duodenum, which is very thin-walled and starts abruptly (Figure 11-3d). A Benson pyloric separator is placed with the heels down near the remaining fibers and is gently spread apart until the circular muscles surrounding the duodenum can just be seen (Figure 11-3e). To check that the tumor has been split completely, the surgeon should grasp the pyloric tumor, one hand on each side of the mass, and rock it back and forth. The sides will move independently if the olive has been divided and the obstruction broken (Figure 11-3f). A clean sponge is then placed down at

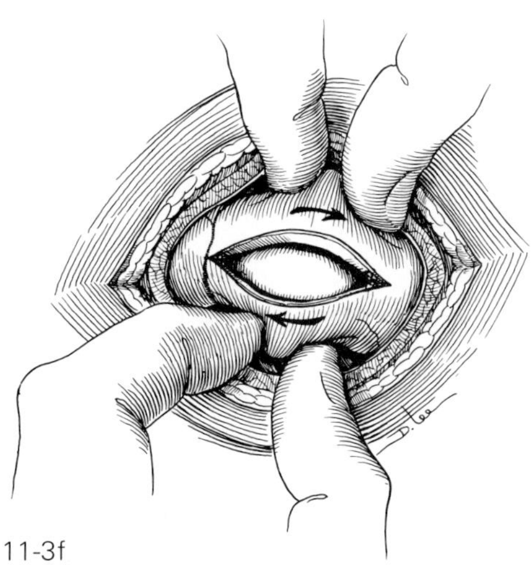

11-3f

the duodenal area. A drop of golden bile is seen if the duodenum has been inadvertently opened. Also, milking the duodenum toward the pylorus will reveal bubbles if the duodenum has been entered. If an opening is detected, a simple suture of 5-0 gastrointestinal silk can be placed to close the defect. This is not a serious complication. It can be tragic, however, if the hole is made and not recognized at the time of surgery. The resultant postoperative duodenal leakage can be fatal.

Frequently venous bleeding is seen in the wall of the pyloric olive after pyloromyotomy. When the stomach is allowed to fall back into the abdomen, however, the venous congestion is decreased and no further treatment for the bleeding is necessary. Posterior fascia and peritoneum are closed with a running 4-0 Dexon suture, and the anterior rectus sheath is closed with an interrupted 4-0 silk. The skin is closed with a subcuticular 5-0 Dexon, and the incision is sealed with collodion.

Postoperative Care

Oral feedings can be started two hours after surgery, at which time 15 cc of dextrose and water is offered to the patient. This is repeated once two hours later. If this is tolerated, the child is switched to half-strength formula at 15 cc every two hours until the following morning, when 30-cc feedings of half-strength formula are started. On afternoon rounds of the first postoperative day, 30 cc of full-strength formula can be tried. The following morning, 60 cc of full-strength formula is offered. By that afternoon the child can be given an *ad lib.* diet and discharged.

In a patient whose duodenum has been inadvertently entered but repaired at surgery, a nasogastric tube is left in place for 24 hours postoperatively and the child is started on broad-spectrum antibiotic coverage and intravenous maintenance. At the end of the 24 hours, if the child is otherwise doing well, he can then be started on the regimen in the preceding paragraph and be discharged four or five days after surgery.

For an infant whose mother desires to breast-feed, the child should be given the same two feedings of dextrose and water and then be started on progressive lengths of nursing. Usually five minutes of nursing will suffice initially, and the time can be gradually raised in five-minute increments.

Occasionally vomiting is seen postoperatively. A single episode can be disregarded. If several episodes of vomiting occur, a nasogastric tube can be placed in the stomach and the stomach irrigated with 30 to 50 cc of half-strength solution of sodium bicarbonate. This helps to alleviate the gastritis, so that the patient can usually be started back on the oral fluid regimen.

Complications

Incomplete pyloromyotomy is a rare complication. Most surgeons believe that leaving several strands of the muscle incompletely divided at the time of surgery probably does not cause recurrent vomiting. Occasionally, however, it becomes obvious that the original vomiting pattern has recurred; if this happens, the surgeon should obtain roentgenographic confirmation of recurrent pyloric obstruction and should plan reoperation. Surprisingly, the peritoneal cavity is usually free of adhesions, and the second procedure can be done without difficulty. Usually the recurrence is the result of incomplete cutting of the muscle at the gastric end. At this time the pyloromyotomy should be done on the opposite side of the pyloric olive.

Most postoperative vomiting is the result of gastritis from the chronic obstruction. This gastritis abates of its own accord and can be helped with instillation of a solution of sodium bicarbonate. Perforation of the duodenum during performance of the procedure should not occur. If it does occur and is recognized at surgery, the perforation presents minimal problems. Wound infections are rarely seen after this operation. With experienced anesthesiologists, the mortality is less than 0.1 percent.

Results

Children are cured by this operation and rarely have any further gastric or duodenal problems afterward.

Spontaneous Perforation of the Stomach

Spontaneous perforation of the stomach in the newborn (SPS) presents as acute abdominal distention with respiratory embarrassment. The lesion was first recognized by Siebold in 1825, yet the cause is still unclear. Ischemia appears to play a role, however, because most of these infants have required cardiorespiratory resuscitation shortly after birth. At the time of the acute episode, the child refuses feedings and becomes lethargic and dusky. Routine chest film reveals massive pneumoperitoneum, and the need for emergency surgery becomes obvious (Figure 11-4). Sometimes it may be difficult to determine whether the pneumoperitoneum is a result of SPS or of necrotizing enterocolitis (NEC). However, patients with SPS usually are term infants who were tolerating oral feedings, while patients with NEC are almost always premature with respiratory distress syndrome (RDS), pneumatosis intestinalis, and hematochezia. Pneumoperitoneum from either disease requires vigorous preoperative preparation and early surgical intervention.

One to two hours of preoperative preparation are needed to counteract the effects of septic shock and to replace in-

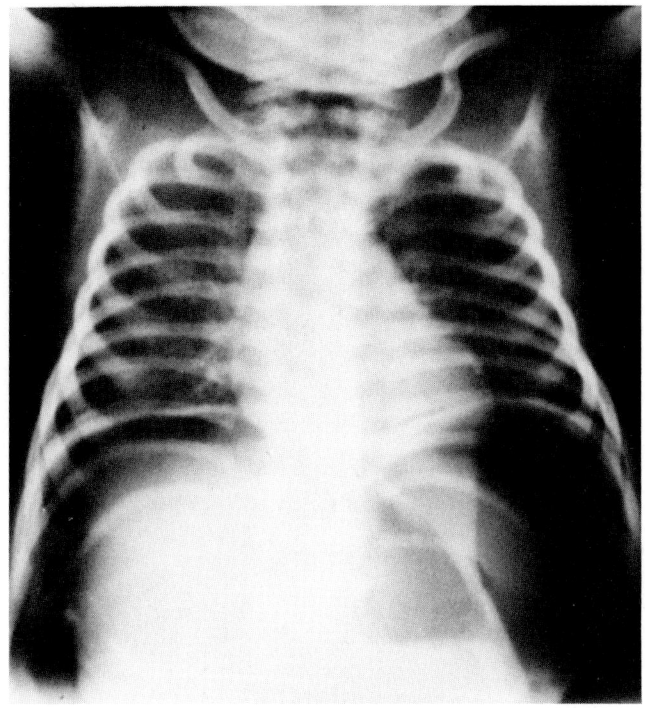

11-4. Massive pneumoperitoneum in a child with spontaneous gastric perforation.

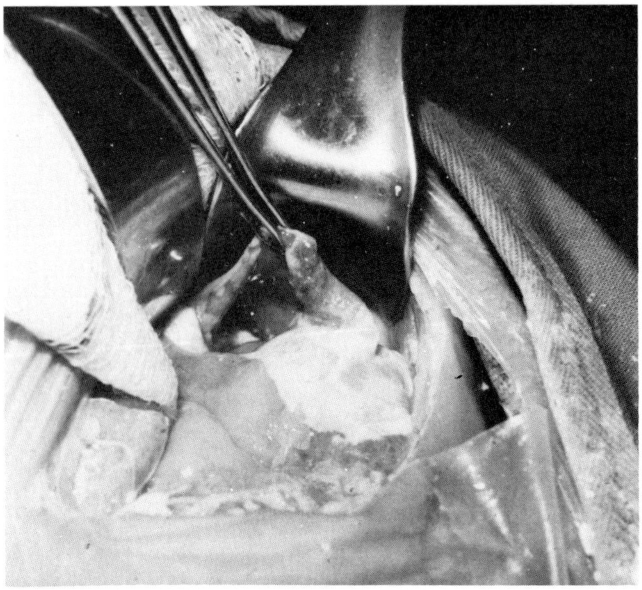

11-5. Forceps shown holding the edge of perforated stomach. Milk curds coat the omentum.

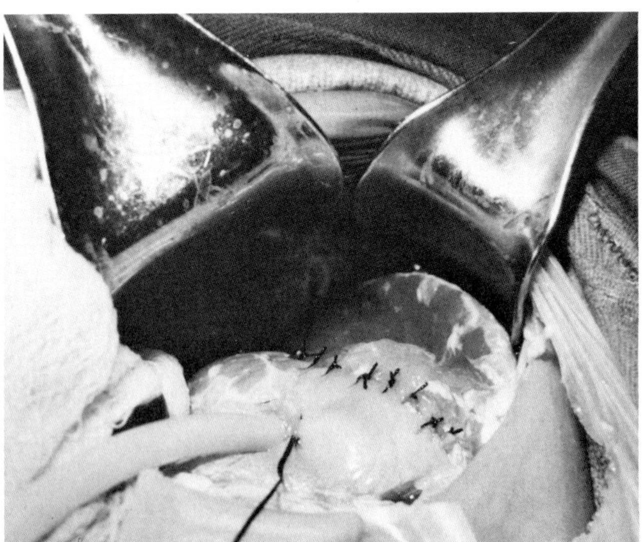

11-6. A gastrostomy in place after the defect has been closed and most of the curd removed.

travascular volume. Ampicillin (150 mg per kg) and gentamicin (2.5 mg per kg) are given; 1 mg of vitamin K and 1 to 2 mg per kg of albumin are administered; and a nasogastric or orogastric tube is inserted. Occasionally diaphragmatic excursion is severely restricted by the free abdominal air, so that needle aspiration of the tense abdomen may be necessary.

Operative Technique

The patient is placed supine on an infant warmer and over a heating blanket. A right-upper-quadrant transverse rectus-cutting incision is used about 1 cm above the level of the umbilicus. This incision may be extended when necessary. A thorough search is made for the source of the perforation. If the small or large bowel is responsible (NEC), resection and exteriorization are necessary (see Chapter 14). On the other hand, if the stomach is the source of perforation, milk and curd will be visibly stuck to much of the bowel. A culture is taken, and the abdomen is irrigated with warm saline solution. Most of the curd can be removed, but some will cake on the bowel and cannot be teased off (Figure 11-5).

The defect in the stomach is often large and may be quite ragged. Nevertheless, the edges must be excised back to viable tissue and the stomach closed in two layers, the mucosa with running 3-0 chromic and the seromuscular layer with interrupted 4-0 silk. A number 14 Malecot gastrostomy tube should be left in the stomach, either in the corner of the defect or through a separate opening (Figure 11-6). The wound is closed in layers.

Postoperative Care

Fluids, electrolytes, colloid, and antibiotics are continued to help treat the peritonitis. The gastrostomy tube is kept on drainage until signs of peristalsis appear and feedings can be tried. The intraoperative cultures may suggest a change in antibiotics.

Complications

These infants usually do amazingly well. Wound infections and intraabdominal abscesses, which are rare, are treated using standard surgical techniques.

Results

Fortunately, most of these babies appear to tolerate this catastrophic episode and fully recover.

Selected References

1. Benson, C. D., and Lloyd, J. R. Infantile Hypertrophic Pyloric Stenosis. In W. T. Mustard, M. M. Ravitch, W. H. Snyder, Jr., et al. (eds.). *Pediatric Surgery*. Chicago: Year Book Medical Publishers, 1969, pp. 818–22.
2. Gross, R. E. *The Surgery of Infancy and Childhood.* Philadelphia: Saunders, 1953, pp. 130–43.
3. Kiesewetter, W. B. Spontaneous rupture of the stomach in the newborn. *Am. J. Dis. Child.* 91:162, 1956.
4. Randolph, J. G. The evolution of an ideal surgical incision for pyloric stenosis. *Arch. Surg.* 93:489–91, 1966.

12

Duodenal Obstruction

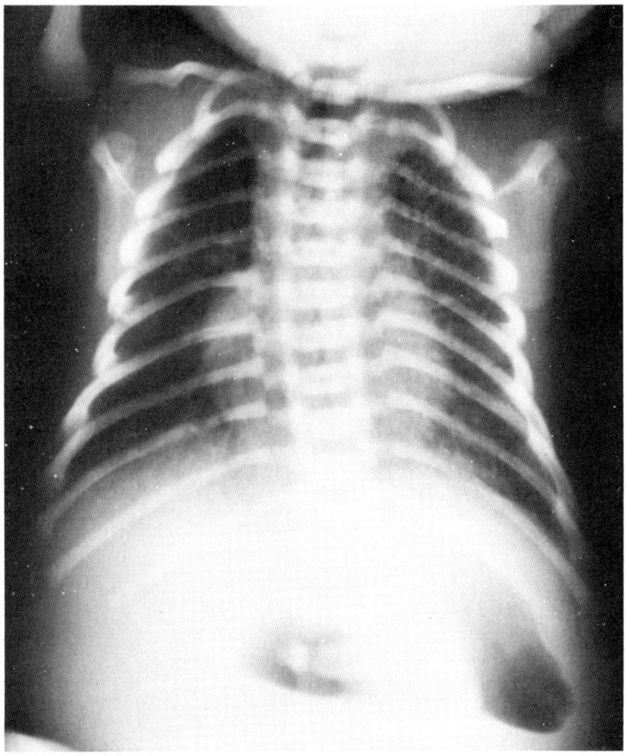

12-1. Typical appearance on a roentgenogram of a double bubble, which can be seen well on both posteroanterior and lateral films in a patient with duodenal obstruction.

Until proved otherwise, bilious vomiting in the newborn is indicative of a mechanical obstruction of the bowel. Certainly in the neonate there are conditions which can cause bilious vomiting that do not require surgery. One must assume, however, that the cause is mechanical until another diagnosis can be established. The common causes of duodenal obstruction in the newborn are duodenal atresia, duodenal stenosis, annular pancreas, and malrotation with obstruction from Ladd's bands. Of these, the commonest causes are duodenal atresia and duodenal stenosis. The incidence of duodenal atresia and stenosis is about one in 5,000 to 10,000 births. There is a high incidence of associated congenital anomalies, especially Down's syndrome, which occurs in about 30 percent of these patients.

Preoperative Evaluation

There is usually a history of maternal polyhydramnios associated with bilious vomiting that occurs shortly after birth. In addition, there is usually failure to pass meconium, although occasionally one can obtain a history of meconium passage. On physical examination, the infant's abdomen usually is minimally distended, because of the high level of intestinal obstruction. The most important diagnostic study to carry out is a plain roentgenogram of the abdomen. In the case of duodenal atresia, one will see a very dilated stomach and duodenum giving the classic appearance of a double bubble with no gas beyond the duodenum (Figure 12-1). In the case of duodenal stenosis, annular pancreas, or malrotation with Ladd's bands, the double bubble is seen, but, in addition, there is often some gas in the distal bowel. The diagnosis of duodenal obstruction can be made from the clinical picture and the radiologic findings, following which definitive therapy can be instituted. In the case of duodenal atresia, duodenal stenosis, and annular pancreas, the infant can be managed overnight with nasogastric decompression and intravenous fluids, and the definitive procedure can be done electively the following morning.

If the obstruction is caused by malrotation, however, then surgery should be carried out as soon as the diagnosis is made in order to prevent development of intestinal gangrene from a midgut volvulus. If a volvulus occurs, the entire small intestine and the proximal large intestine can become necrotic within a very short period of time. Therefore, if one plans to observe a baby with duodenal obstruction overnight, malrotation must be ruled out, which can be done easily, either with a barium enema, which will show the cecum to be in the right upper quadrant or the left upper quadrant of the abdomen (Figure 12-2), or with an upper gastrointestinal series, which will show the absence of a ligament of Treitz (Figure 12-3).

The patient is prepared for surgery by inserting a nasogastric tube and by administering broad-spectrum antibiotics

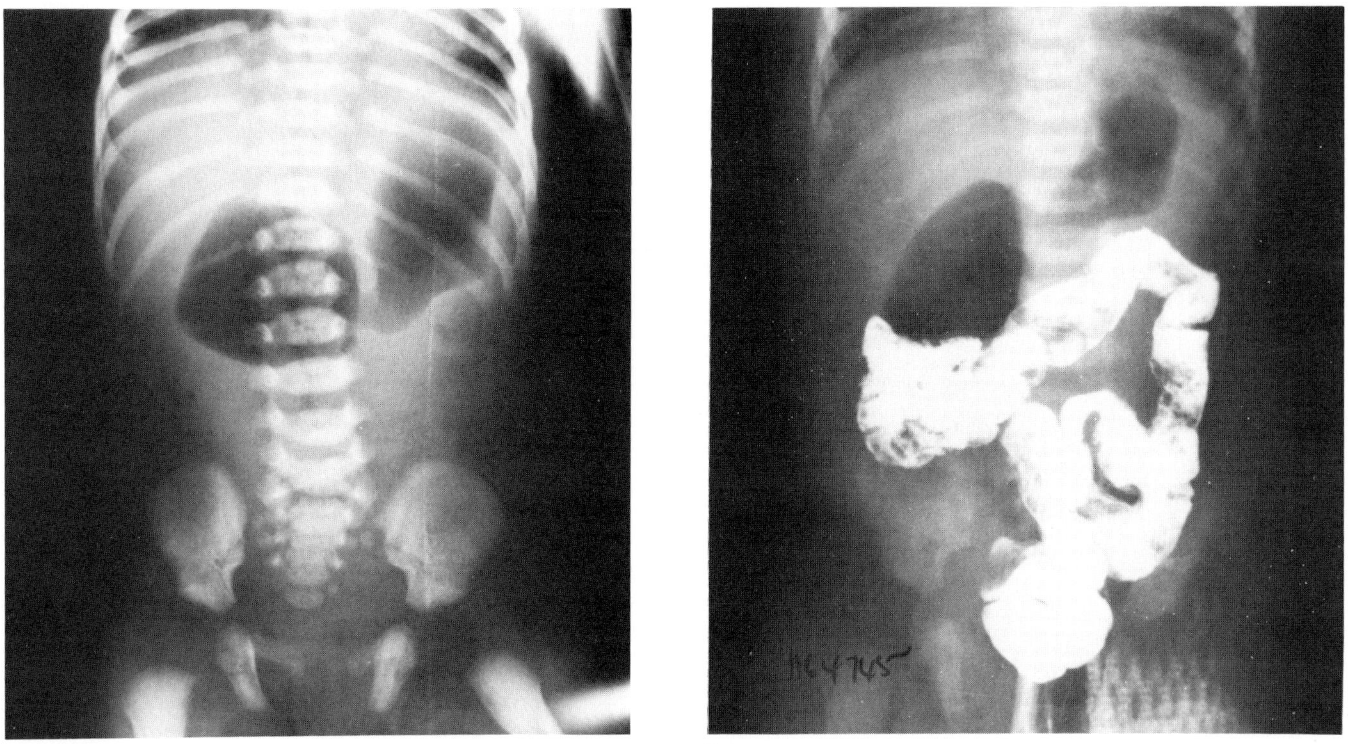

A B

12-2. (A) Double bubble from duodenal obstruction secondary to malrotation. (B) Barium enema showing the cecum in the right upper quadrant in malrotation. Note the double bubble behind the contrast material.

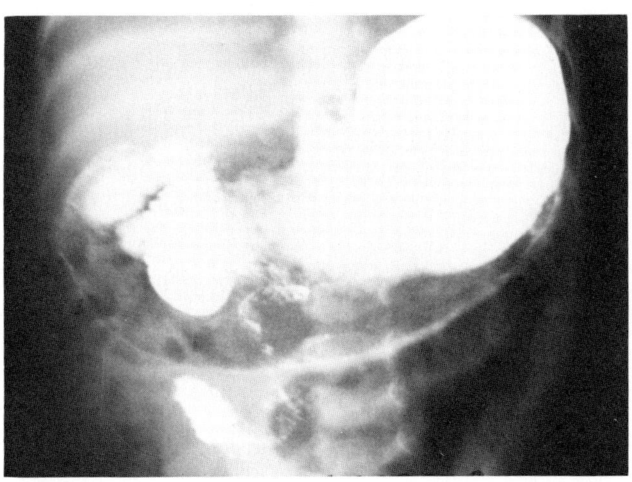

12-3. An upper gastrointestinal series in malrotation showing absence of the ligament of Treitz.

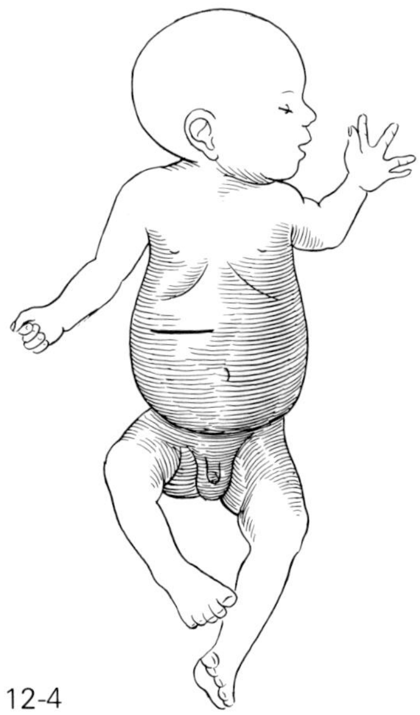

12-4

and vitamin K. Because these infants are usually diagnosed very early in the neonatal period, the amount of fluid lost through vomiting or sequestration into the intestinal lumen is small. Therefore preoperative administration of large volumes of crystalloid or colloid solutions is usually unnecessary.

Operative Technique

In the operating room the patient is placed in the supine position and proper precautions are taken to prevent significant heat loss, as is done with any neonate undergoing major surgery. A proper intravenous line is established, either by a cutdown technique or through a percutaneous catheter. The infant is anesthetized with an endotracheal tube, and the entire abdomen is then prepared and draped. A transverse incision in the right upper quadrant is used; this gives excellent exposure of the entire duodenal area and, in addition, is adequate for a thorough exploration of the rest of the abdomen (Figure 12-4). The rectus muscle is incised with cautery, and the round ligament containing the umbilical vein is preserved. A massively dilated proximal duodenum usually eviscerates through the incision, confirming the diagnosis of duodenal obstruction (Figure 12-5).

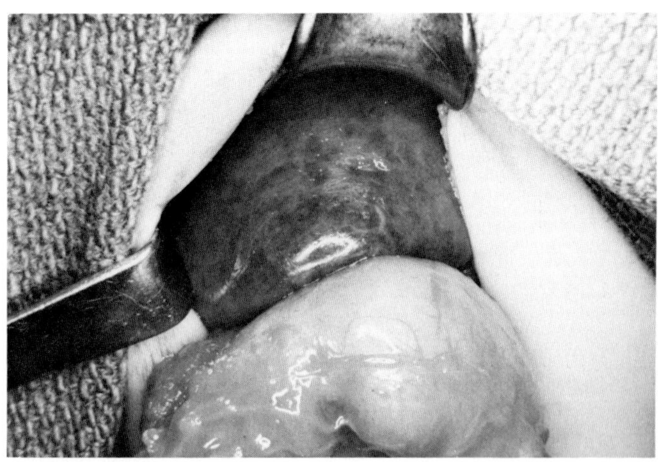

12-5

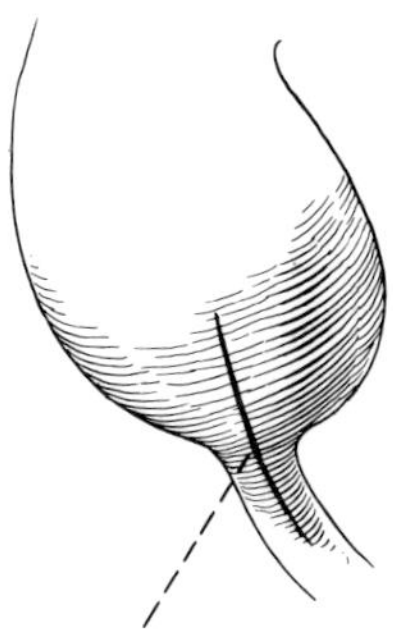

12-6a

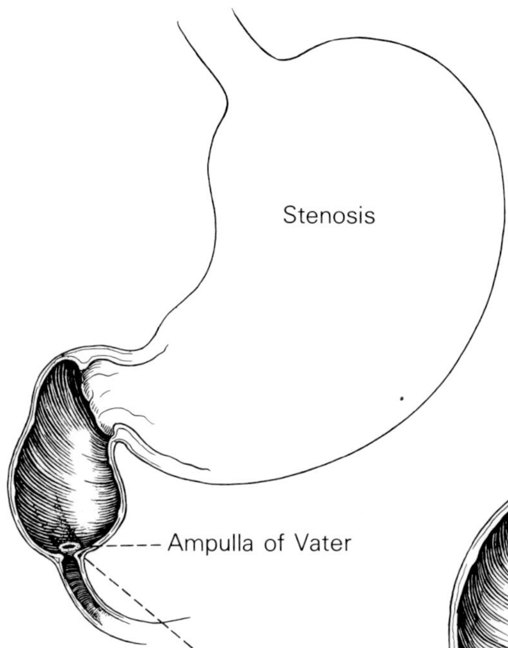

12-6b

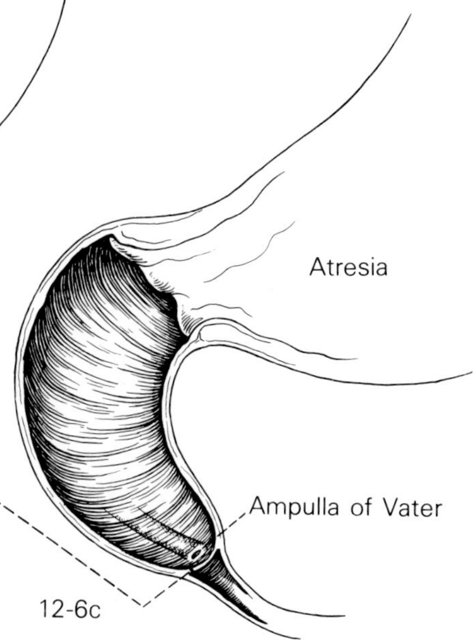

12-6c

At this point, the entire duodenum is inspected to determine the exact cause of the obstruction. Before proceeding with the definitive procedure, the rest of the bowel is inspected for associated atresias. If it appears that one is dealing with a duodenal stenosis or atresia, the proximal dilated duodenum is opened along its antimesenteric border proximal to the area of obstruction to determine the type of stenosis or atresia that is present (Figure 12-6a).

If a diaphragm occluding the intestinal lumen is found, this is excised, taking care to prevent injury to the ampulla of Vater, which often enters at the bottom of the diaphragm (Figure 12-6b and c). After excision of the diaphragm, the duodenotomy can be closed transversely in a Heineke-Mikulicz fashion (Figure 12-6d). If this type of closure is not possible, then a duodenojejunostomy should be done. The duodenojejunostomy is carried out by isolating a proximal loop of jejunum and bringing it, either retrocolic or antecolic, up to the proximal duodenum. The retrocolic approach is preferable. After the proximal jejunum has been brought up to the duodenum, a long side-to-side duodenojejunostomy is carried out using interrupted sutures of 4-0 or 5-0 silk with

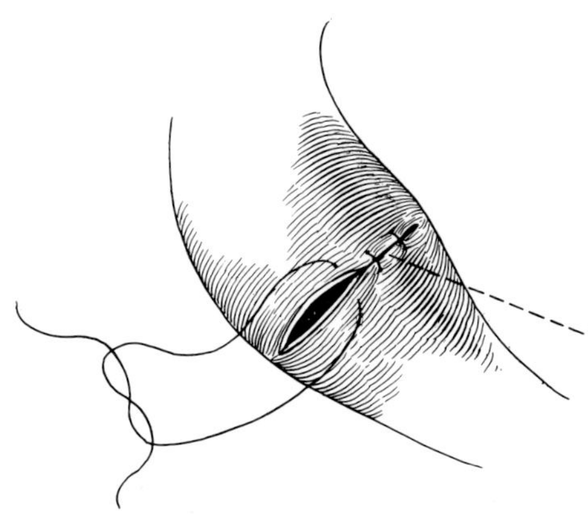

12-6d

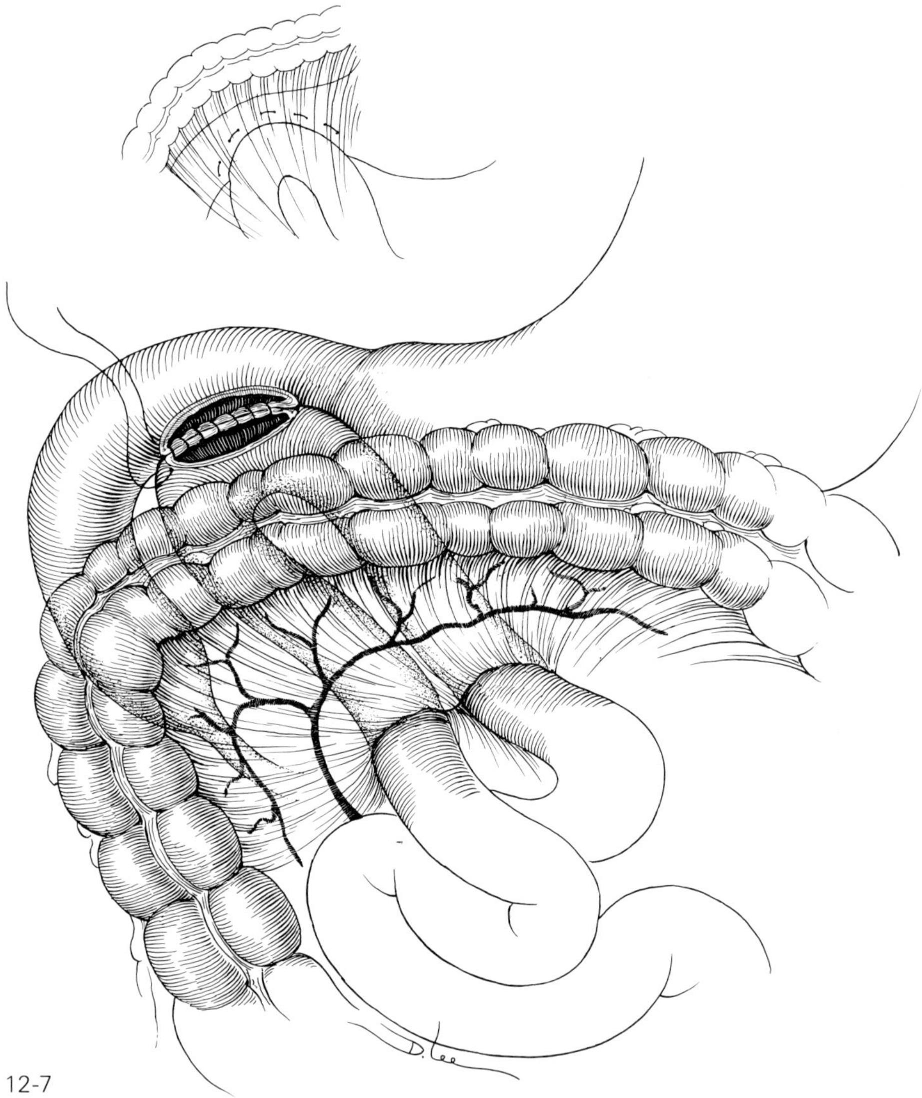

12-7

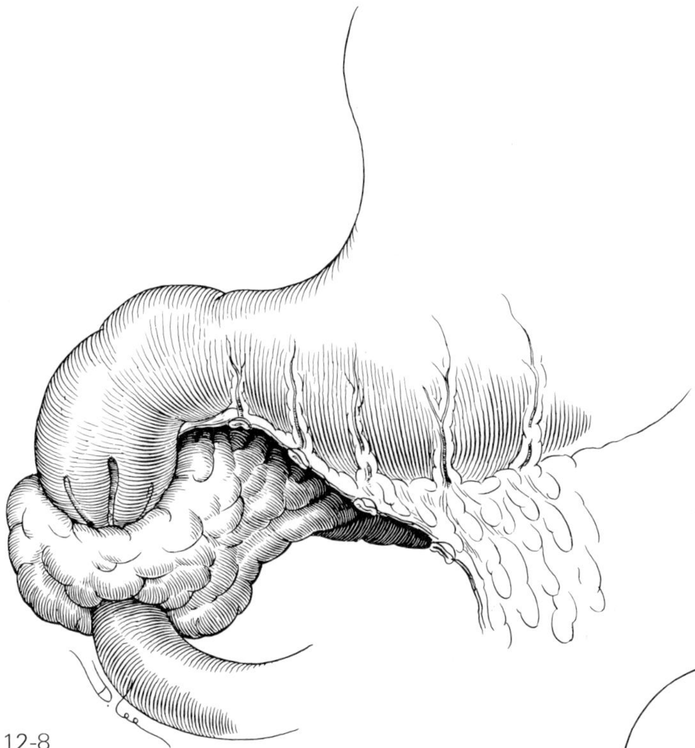

12-8

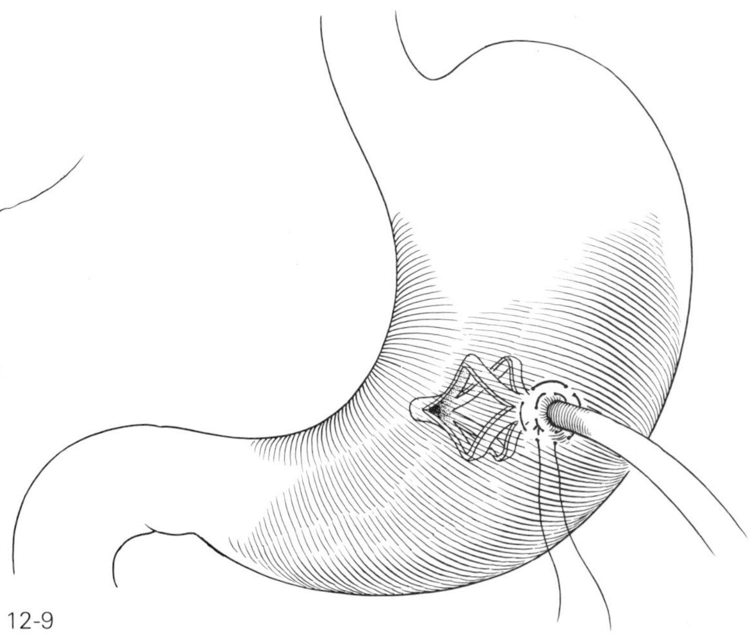

12-9

the knots tied on the inside (Figure 12-7). After the anastomosis has been completed, the jejunal loop is tacked to the surrounding transverse mesocolon with interrupted sutures of 4-0 or 5-0 silk.

In the case of an annular pancreas (Figure 12-8), the preferred procedure is a duodenojejunostomy. One should never perform a gastrojejunostomy to bypass an obstructed duodenum because late complications of stomal ulceration may occur. Occasionally a side-to-side duodenoduodenostomy can be performed, but this is not always technically feasible.

After the duodenoduodenostomy or duodenojejunostomy has been completed, a Stamm gastrostomy is performed in the fundus of the stomach using two pursestring sutures of 4-0 or 5-0 silk and a Malecot catheter (Figure 12-9). The gastrostomy tube is brought out through a separate stab incision medial to the main incision (Figure 12-10). The stomach wall adjacent to the gastrostomy site is tacked to the undersurface of the peritoneum with interrupted sutures of 4-0 silk.

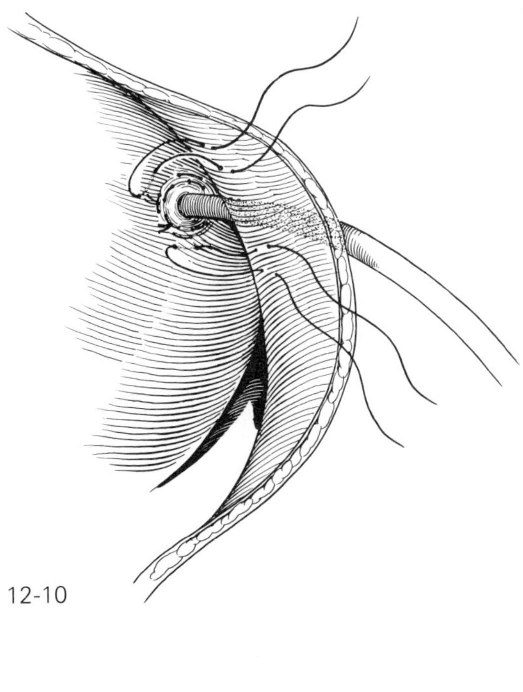

12-10

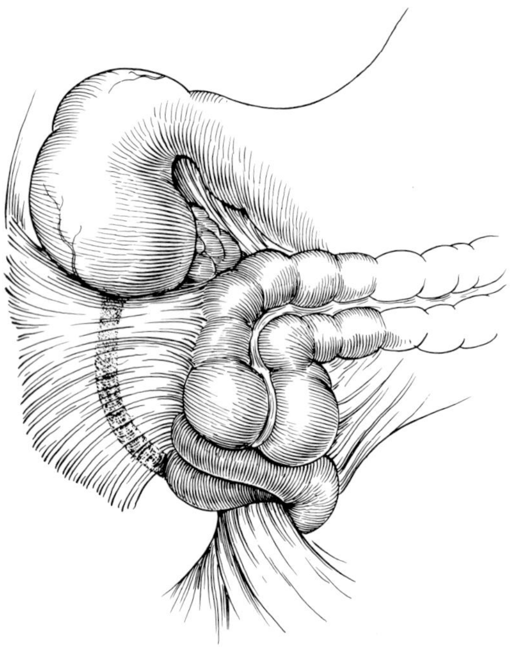

12-11. Typical Ladd's bands, causing duodenal obstruction.

If Ladd's bands (Figure 12-11) are found to be the cause of the duodenal obstruction, then all the bands should be completely lysed (Figure 12-12a). The cecum should then be placed in the left lower quadrant and the small bowel in the right lower quadrant, in order to broaden the mesentery of the small bowel so that a future volvulus becomes unlikely. A small number of cases of duodenal obstruction secondary to Ladd's bands have an associated intrinsic obstruction of the duodenum. One must therefore rule out the presence of this lesion by passing a small Foley catheter through the duodenum by means of a gastrotomy opening (Figure 12-12b). This gastrotomy opening can then be used for the gastrostomy (Figure 12-12c). The abdomen is closed with a running 3-0 chromic suture to the peritoneum and interrupted nonabsorbable sutures to the anterior fascia. The skin can be closed with a running nylon suture.

Postoperative Care

Because of marked distention of the proximal duodenum during intrauterine life, peristalsis in this segment is markedly decreased. Children with duodenal obstruction therefore often experience marked delay in gastric emptying and have great difficulty with feeding postoperatively. It is often two to three weeks before the stomach and duodenum empty adequately to permit the patient to be started on oral or gastrostomy feedings. To prevent the resulting nutritional depletion, one has to resort to other means of nourishing the patient during this critical postoperative period.

In the past, it has been recommended that transduodenal feeding tubes be passed through the gastrostomy site into the duodenum and jejunum distal to the area of anastomosis, a procedure that has often proved very effective in nourishing the patient during the postoperative period. These tubes sometimes become hardened, however, while sitting in the intestinal lumen and they can cause perforation of the bowel. Silastic tubes are less likely to do this than other types of plastic tubing.

In recent years, with increased use of parenteral nutrition, most pediatric surgeons have turned to hyperalimentation of the baby for several weeks postoperatively. Parenteral nutrition can be started on the second or third postoperative day and can be continued until the patient is taking adequate amounts of nourishment orally or by the gastrostomy route.

Broad-spectrum antibiotic coverage is usually continued for about five to seven days postoperatively and then it is stopped unless the clinical course dictates continuance of this therapy. During the postoperative period the patient should be thoroughly evaluated for any associated congenital anomalies. Once the patient is feeding well orally, he can be discharged from the hospital. The gastrostomy tube is usually left in place after the patient has been discharged so that any further difficulties with feeding can be easily managed.

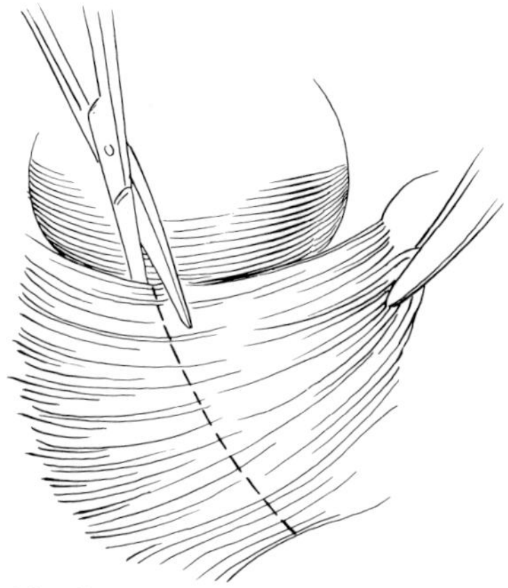

12-12a

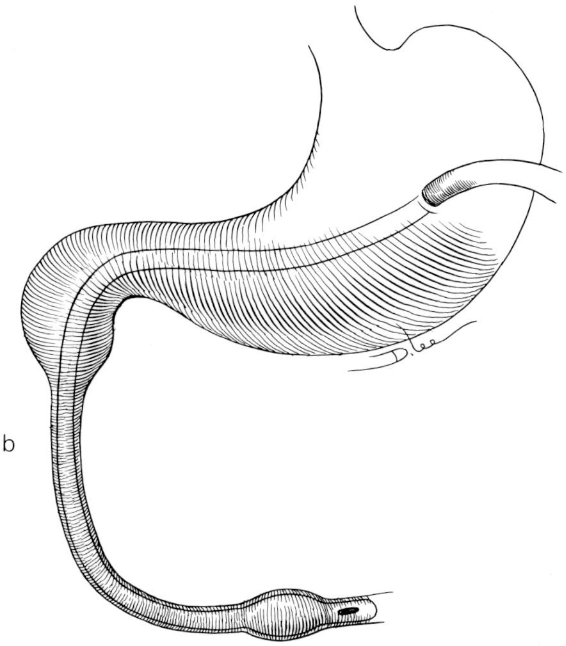

12-12b

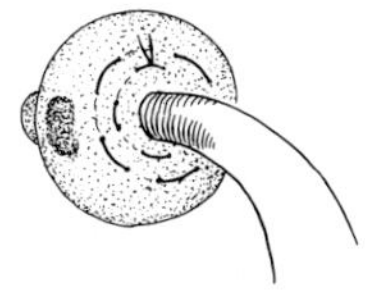

12-12c

Comments

Because a significant percentage of infants with duodenal atresia and stenosis have Down's syndrome, a careful and thorough discussion should be carried out with the parents in regard to the effect of this offspring on the family environment. If the parents want the baby to be treated optimally, then definitive surgery should be performed as soon as the diagnosis has been made.

At one time the preferred surgical approach to duodenal obstruction in the newborn other than that secondary to malrotation with Ladd's bands was to perform a blind duodenojejunostomy without any significant exploration of the area of obstruction in the duodenum. In recent years, however, a more direct approach to the problem has been taken with a thorough exploration of the area of obstruction in the duodenum. This has resulted in the performance of more duodenoduodenostomies. It appears from the clinical experience of most pediatric surgeons that the infants do much better with postoperative feedings following a duodenoduodenostomy than after a duodenojejunostomy. With proper surgical technique and with meticulous postoperative care, including parenteral nutrition, the mortality in this group of patients should be less than 5 percent.

Selected References

1. Brimblecombe, F. S. W., and More, H. D. Duodenal atresia and stenosis. *Ann. Surg.* 172:991, 1970.
2. Fonkalsrud, A. W., deLorimer, A. A., and Hayes, D. M. Congenital atresia and stenosis of the duodenum. *Pediatrics* 42:79, 1969.
3. Longo, M. F., and Lynn, H. B. Congenital duodenal obstruction: Review of twenty-nine cases encountered in a thirty-year period. *Mayo Clin. Proc.* 42:423, 1967.
4. Lynn, H. B. Duodenal Obstruction: Atresia, Stenosis and Annular Pancreas. In W. T. Mustard, M. M. Ravitch, W. H. Snyder, Jr., et al. (eds.). *Pediatric Surgery.* Chicago: Year Book Medical Publishers, 1969.
5. Rickham, P. P., and Johnston, J. H. *Neonatal Surgery.* New York: Appleton-Century-Crofts, 1969.
6. Snyder, W. H., Jr., and Chaffin, L. Malrotation of the Intestine. In W. T. Mustard, M. M. Ravitch, W. H. Snyder, Jr., et al. (eds.). *Pediatric Surgery.* Chicago: Year Book Medical Publishers, 1969.

Intestinal Atresia, Intestinal Stenosis, and Meconium Ileus

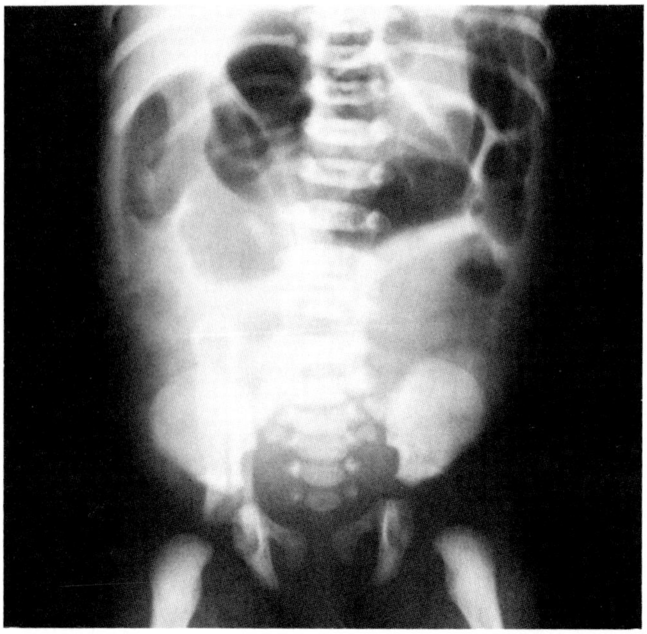

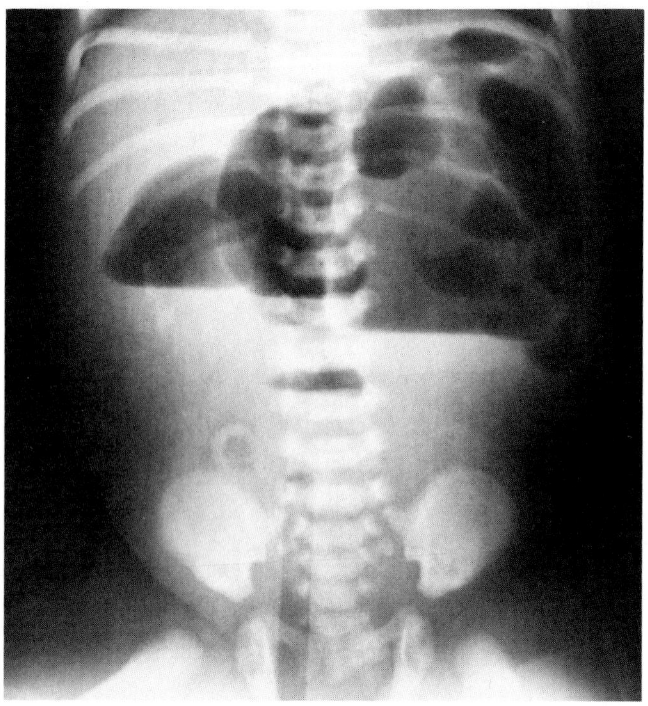

B

13-1. (A) A plain x-ray of the abdomen showing dilated loops of bowel from obstruction secondary to intestinal atresia. (B) The upright film shows air-fluid levels.

The first case of intestinal atresia was reported in 1684 by Goeller. The first successful operation was performed in 1911 by Fockens. In 1947 Potts performed the first resection and primary anastomosis for an intestinal atresia. The incidence of intestinal atresia is between 1 in 1,500 and 1 in 3,000 births.

Although various causative mechanisms have been implicated for bowel atresia, the work by Barnard [1] and Louw [5] clearly demonstrated experimentally that bowel atresia results from a vascular accident occurring in utero. This contrasts with the situation occurring in duodenal atresia, where a failure of revacuolization of the intestinal lumen appears to be the most likely cause of the atresia. The commonest site of atresia is the ileum, followed by the jejunum and the colon; colonic atresia is rare. There is a significant incidence of multiple bowel atresias, so that additional atresias should be looked for during surgery.

Meconium ileus occurs in infants only with cystic fibrosis and is the result of abnormally viscid meconium, which causes obstruction of the intestinal lumen. This can result in a picture of bowel obstruction that is often indistinguishable from intestinal atresia.

Preoperative Evaluation

There is often a history of maternal polyhydramnios, although the incidence of this is lower than in duodenal obstruction. Bilious vomiting with failure to pass meconium usually occurs within the first 24 hours of life; however, if the obstruction is low, as in the colon, the clinical picture may not become obvious until after 24 hours of age. Abdominal distention is almost always present, the degree of distention being related to the level of obstruction in the bowel. Abdominal distention is greater with lower types of obstruction. Often the abdominal skin is tightly stretched and shiny, and large veins can often be seen coursing over the abdominal wall. Severe abdominal distention can lead to a significant compromise of respiratory excursions with subsequent development of respiratory insufficiency.

The most important diagnostic study to carry out is a plain x-ray of the abdomen. In the case of intestinal atresia or stenosis, the x-ray film will usually show dilated loops of bowel with air-fluid levels (Figure 13-1). In meconium ileus, one will also see dilated loops of intestine; air-fluid levels are usually absent, however, and the intestinal lumen has a soap-bubble appearance, which is caused by the mixing of gas and viscid meconium in the bowel (Figure 13-2). If the diagnosis is still in doubt, then a barium enema can be carried out. This will show a microcolon in intestinal atresia, intestinal stenosis, and meconium ileus (Figure 13-3).

If the cause of bowel obstruction is the meconium-plug syndrome, which is seen in babies without cystic fibrosis and is caused by thickened meconium obstructing the colon,

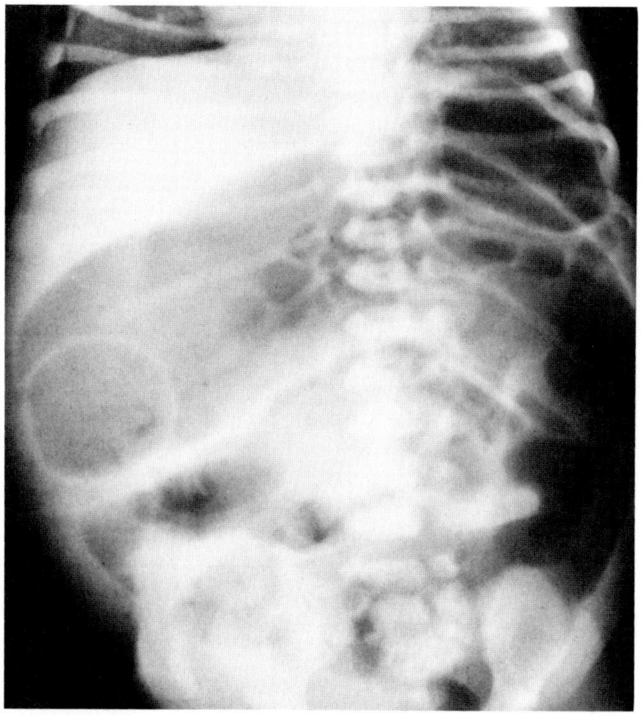

13-2. Intestinal dilatation from meconium ileus. Note the soap-bubble appearance of the luminal contents of the intestine.

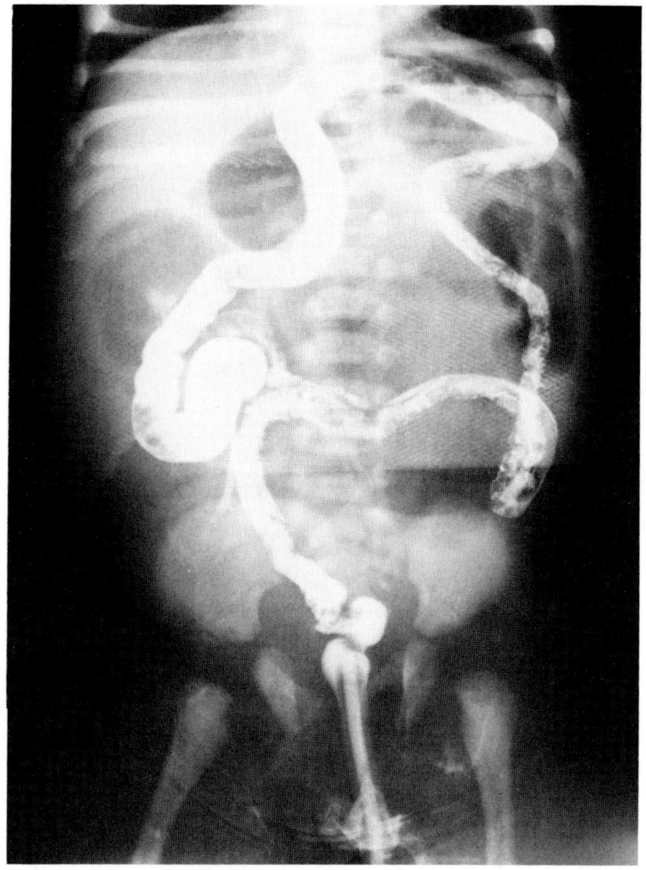

13-3. A typical microcolon is seen on barium enema examination with intestinal atresia.

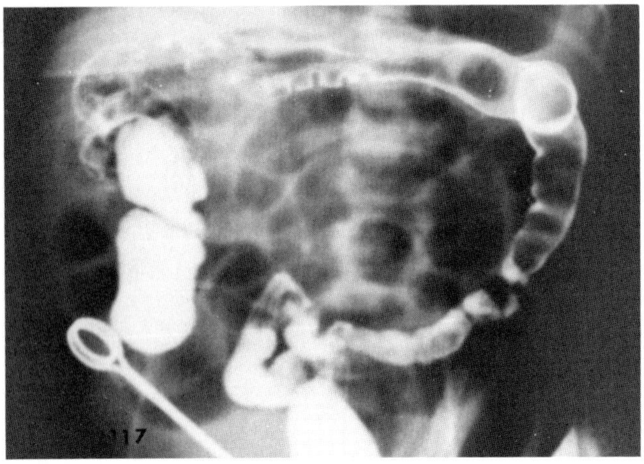

13-4. In the meconium plug syndrome the barium enema demonstrates the large plugs of meconium present in the colon.

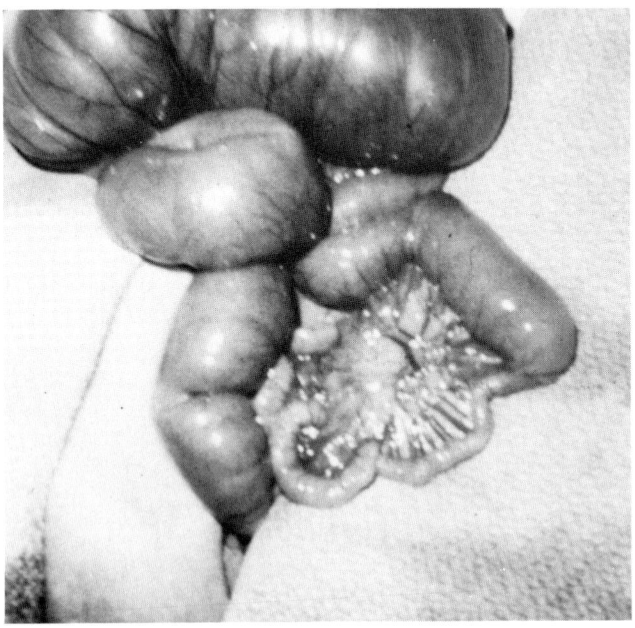

13-5. An operative view showing the entire small intestine eviscerated outside the abdomen. The proximal dilated bowel and distal collapsed bowel are clearly visible.

then the barium enema will demonstrate this syndrome also (Figure 13-4). In the case of the meconium-plug syndrome, the barium enema will usually treat the condition so that no further therapy or surgery is usually needed. If before performing the barium enema examination one strongly suspects meconium ileus, then Gastrografin rather than barium can be used as the contrast material. The Gastrografin will often reflux back into the small intestine and, because of its high detergent properties, will help relieve the obstruction from the viscid meconium. However, because the Gastrografin is very hypertonic, one must have a good intravenous line in the baby before administering it, so that colloid and crystalloid solutions can be given during the procedure. If the Gastrografin enema is unsuccessful in relieving the obstruction, then the infant must be prepared for surgery just as in the case of intestinal atresia or stenosis.

A nasogastric tube is inserted and broad-spectrum antibiotics and vitamin K are administered. If the infant appears dehydrated and hypovolemic, then crystalloid and colloid solutions are administered before the baby is taken to the operating room. The degrees of dehydration and of hypovolemia are related to the level of intestinal obstruction; obstructions lower in the intestinal tract will cause a more significant degree of hypovolemia and dehydration, because of the increased amount of fluid sequestered in the intestinal lumen.

Operative Technique

In the operating room the patient is placed in the supine position and a secure intravenous line is inserted. The abdomen is entered through a transverse incision in the right upper quadrant, and the entire small bowel is eviscerated (Figure 13-5). In intestinal atresia or stenosis, the markedly dilated proximal bowel and the collapsed distal segment are obvious on initial inspection. The presence of associated atresias is determined by injecting saline into the distal collapsed bowel (Figure 13-6a). Next, the dilated bulbous end of the proximal bowel is resected, because postoperatively this portion will not function properly (Figure 13-6a), a phenomenon that was pointed out by Nixon [8]. The distal collapsed bowel is then opened and spatulated along its antimesenteric border for a short distance (Figure 13-6b).

Then an end-to-end or, more precisely, an end-to-back anastomosis is carried out between the proximal and distal bowel. This is done as a one-layer anastomosis using 5-0 or 6-0 silk with the sutures passing through all layers of the bowel and the knots being tied on the inside (Figure 13-6c). The mesenteric defect is closed with interrupted sutures of 5-0 or 6-0 silk (Figure 13-6d).

With the marked improvement in recent years in neonatal anesthesia and in preoperative and postoperative care of neonates, it is rare to have to perform an ileostomy in a baby with intestinal atresia. This becomes necessary only when

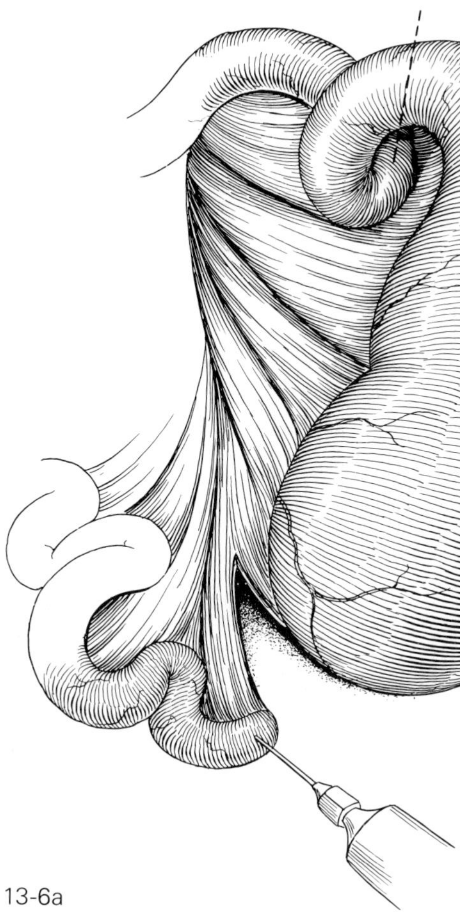

13-6a

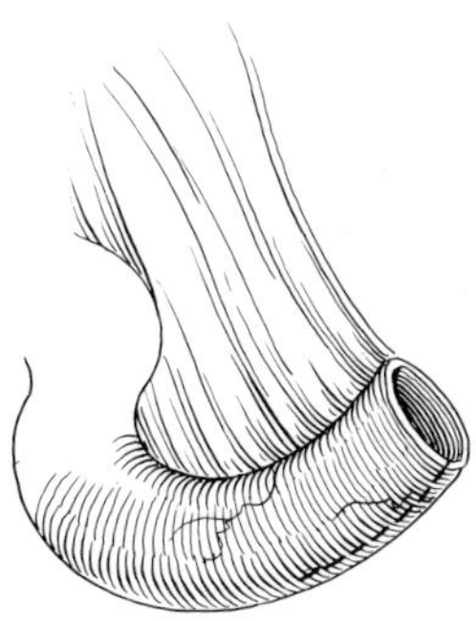

13-6b

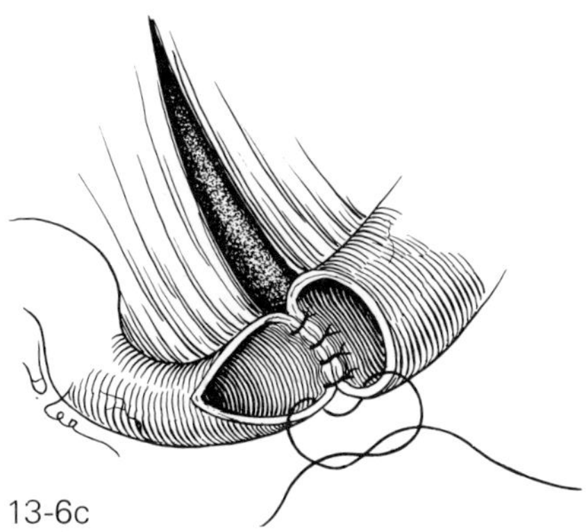

13-6c

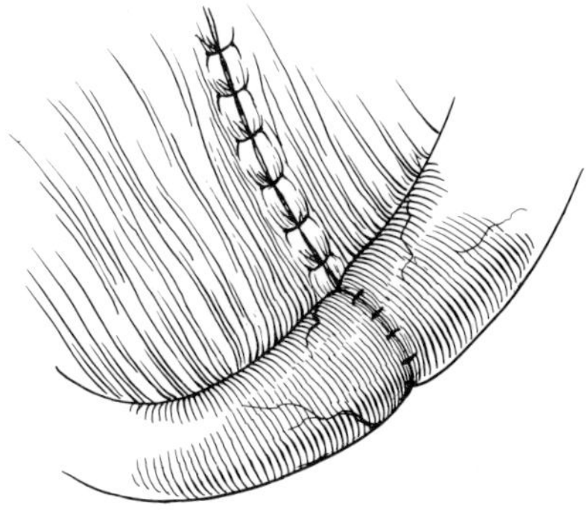

13-6d

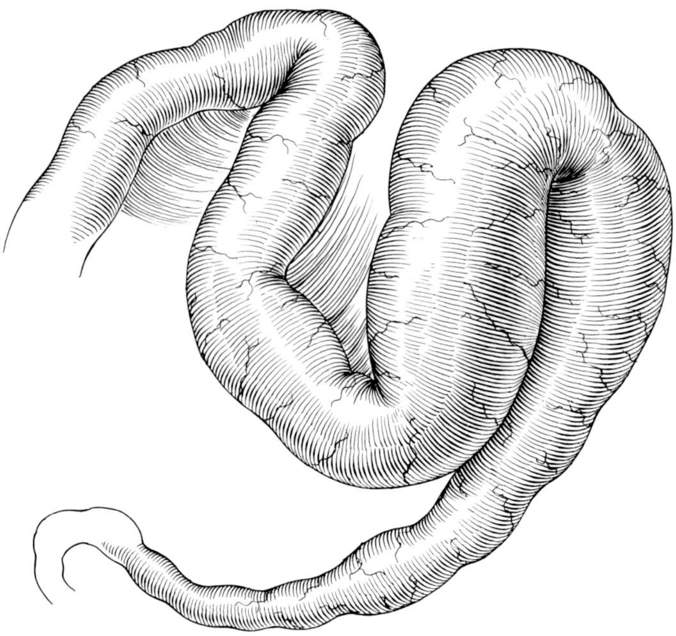

13-7

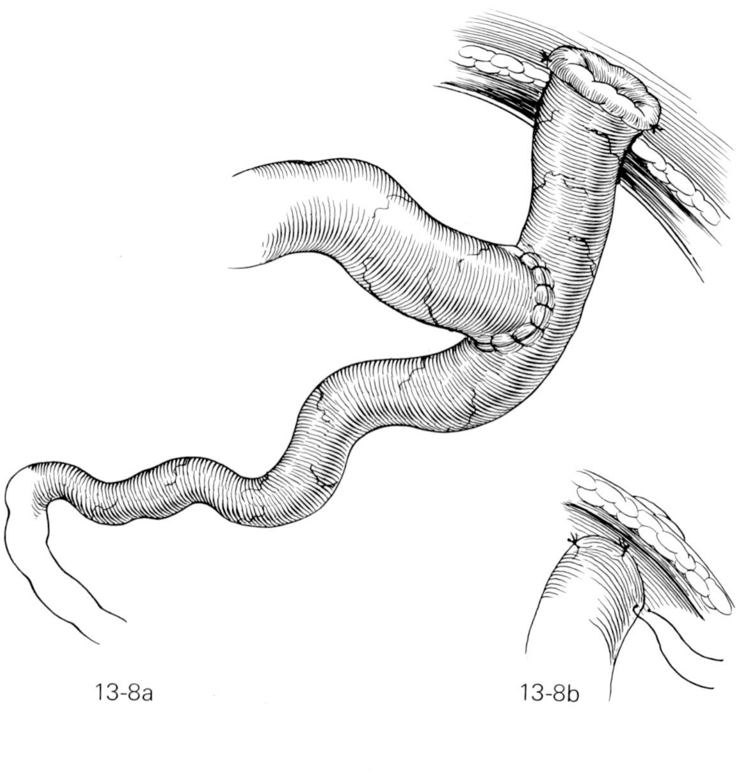

13-8a 13-8b

one is dealing with a meconium or bacterial peritonitis secondary to the atresia, in which case a Bishop-Koop ileostomy is carried out. This will be described in the next paragraph. In meconium ileus the proximal bowel is usually moderately to markedly dilated and is filled with greenish blue meconium. The distal bowel is collapsed but is not as small as that seen in intestinal atresia (Figure 13-7).

Although the Mikulicz ileostomy has been recommended in the past for the management of meconium ileus, we prefer to use the Bishop-Koop ileostomy. This is carried out as an end-to-side enteroenterostomy between the dilated proximal bowel and the collapsed distal bowel (Figure 13-8a). The end of the collapsed distal bowel is then brought out through the incision as an ileostomy (Figure 13-8b). The end-to-side anastomosis is performed with several interrupted sutures or with two running sutures of 5-0 or 6-0 silk. The sutures are placed through all layers of the bowel wall, and the knots are usually tied on the outside (Figure 13-8a). The ileostomy is tacked to the peritoneum and fascia with several interrupted sutures of 5-0 or 6-0 silk (Figure 13-8b). Fistulas can easily result from these tacking sutures so they must be very carefully placed only in the seromuscular layer of the bowel wall.

After the Bishop-Koop ileostomy has been completed in the case of meconium ileus, or after the primary anastomosis has been finished in the case of intestinal atresia or stenosis, a gastrostomy is performed and brought out through a separate stab incision. The techniques for creation of a gastrostomy and for abdominal wall closure are in Chapter 12. If the intestinal atresia is very proximal and it is impossible to resect the dilated bulbous end without coming very close to the ligament of Treitz, then a jejunoplasty can be carried out in which about half of the circumference of the dilated proximal jejunum (Figure 13-9a) is resected along the antimesenteric border, and the opening is closed with a long running suture of 5-0 or 6-0 silk put through all layers of the bowel wall. Following this maneuver, an end-to-end anastomosis is carried out by the technique described above (Figure 13-9b).

Postoperative Care

Most infants will start to pass meconium or feces by the second or third postoperative day following a primary anastomosis for intestinal atresia or stenosis. Infants with high jejunal atresia are often slower to open up and may require a prolonged period of gastrostomy decompression before they can be fed. If the patient cannot begin feedings by the fifth to seventh postoperative day, then one should seriously consider initiating intravenous hyperalimentation. In the case of meconium ileus, the patient will usually be able to tolerate feedings by the third or fourth postoperative day. During the initial phase of feedings one should plan to administer adequate amounts of pancreatic enzymes to the patient by the

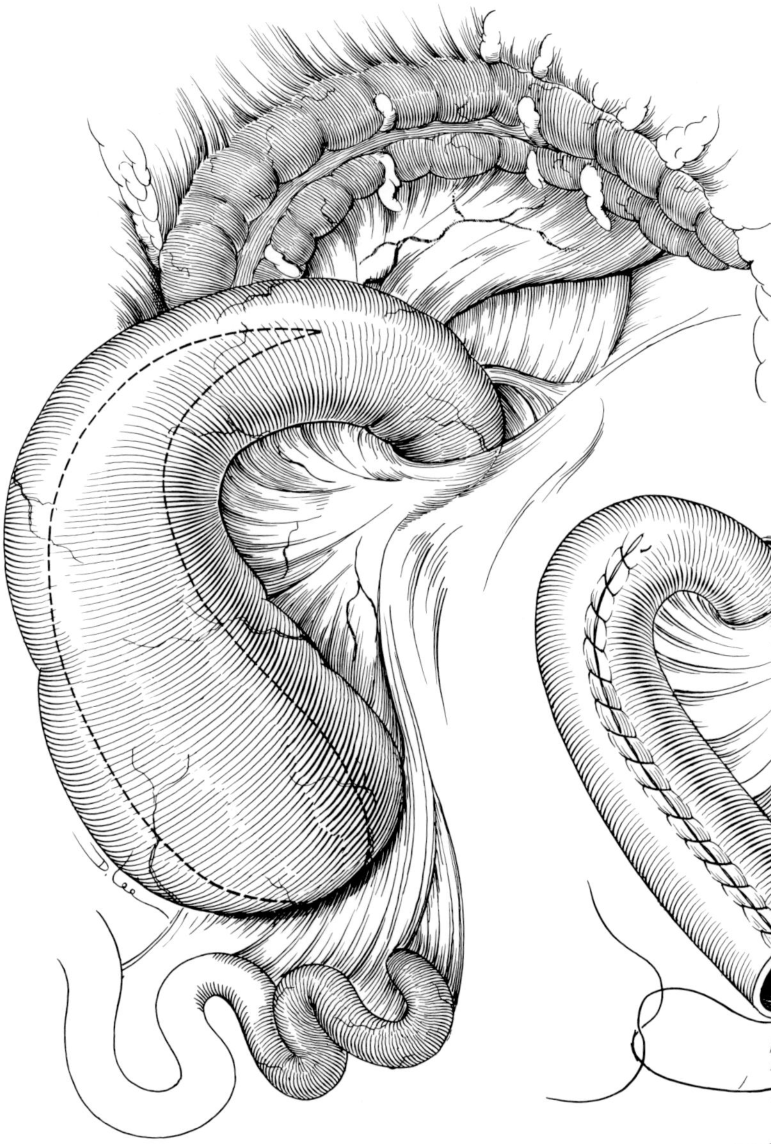

13-9a

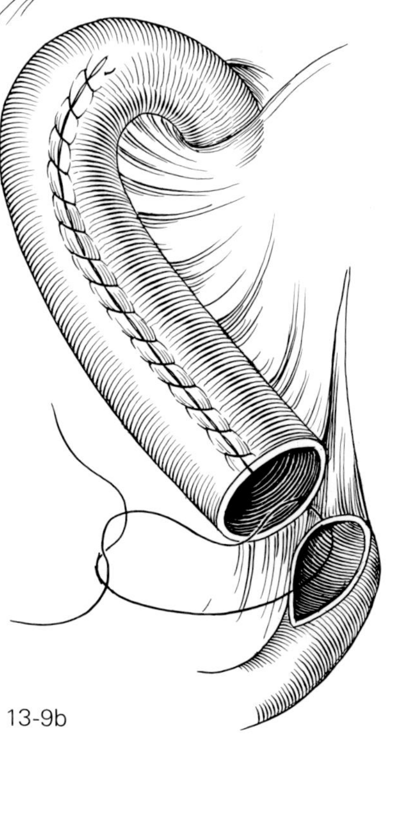

13-9b

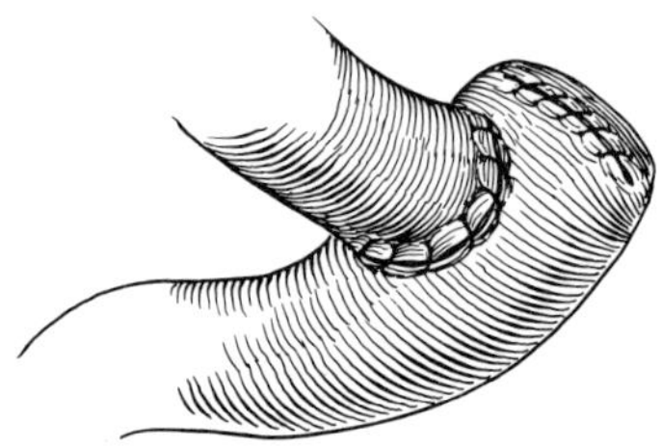

13-10

gastrostomy tube, so that the food will be adequately digested and the fecal stream will flow properly. In addition, during the early postoperative period it is wise to give pancreatic extract enemas through the ileostomy to try to remove all the inspissated meconium present in the bowel distal to the ileostomy.

If during the early postoperative period the ileostomy drainage becomes significant, the ileostomy can be plugged with a small piece of Vaseline gauze so that the fecal stream will pass through the end-to-side anastomosis, and the patient will begin to pass feces per rectum. Once the patient is feeding well and appears to be over the early postoperative period, the ileostomy can be closed by cutting the stoma off flush with the end-to-side anastomosis and oversewing the end (Figure 13-10). This ileostomy closure can be done either extraperitoneally or intraperitoneally; we prefer to do the procedure intraperitoneally. The antibiotic coverage is usually continued for five to seven days. Once the patient is eating and gaining weight, he can be discharged from the hospital with the gastrostomy tube left in place.

Comments

Marked improvement in anesthetic management, fluid and electrolyte administration, and preoperative and postoperative care has changed the approach to intestinal atresia. It is now rare to do an ileostomy in a baby with intestinal atresia who does not have gross peritonitis. Performance of a primary anastomosis in these cases has certainly made postoperative management of these patients much easier by eliminating excessive fluid loss through the ileostomy. In addition, the availability of hyperalimentation has made it much less dangerous to perform a primary anastomosis, which may take a significant period of time to function postoperatively. Use of the Gastrografin enema to relieve the intestinal obstruction from meconium ileus has certainly been a major advance in management of this disease, although a significant number of cases still require surgical decompression.

The meconium-plug syndrome is one that has been recognized only recently. It is important to remember that this syndrome can be easily treated with a rectal examination or a barium enema, and that no further therapy is needed. However, the incidence of Hirschsprung's disease in infants with meconium-plug syndrome is increased and one must be prepared to evaluate these babies for Hirschsprung's disease through further diagnostic tests. Our own feeling is that any infant with a meconium-plug syndrome should have a capsule mucosal biopsy of the rectum to be sure that Hirschsprung's disease is not present.

Selected References

1. Barnard, C. N. The genesis of intestinal atresia. *Surg. Forum* 7:393, 1956.
2. Benson, C. D., and Lloyd, J. R. Atresia and Stenosis of Jejunum and Ileum. In W. T. Mustard, M. M. Ravitch, W. H. Snyder, Jr., et al. (eds.), *Pediatric Surgery*. Chicago: Year Book Medical Publishers, 1969.
3. Bishop, H. C., and Koop, C. E. Management of meconium ileus: Resection, Roux-en-Y anastomosis and ileostomy with pancreatic enzymes. *Ann. Surg.* 145:410, 1957.
4. Dykstra, G., Sieber, W. K., and Kiesewetter, W. B. Intestinal atresia. *Arch. Surg.* 97:175, 1968.
5. Louw, J. R. Congenital intestinal atresia and stenosis in the newborn. *Ann. R. Coll. Surg. Engl.* 25:209, 1959.
6. Louw, J. R. Jejunoileal atresia and stenosis. *J. Pediatr. Surg.* 1:8, 1966.
7. Louw, J. R. Resection and end-to-end anastomosis in the management of atresia and stenosis of the small bowel. *Surgery* 62:940, 1967.
8. Nixon, H. H. Intestinal obstruction in the newborn. *Arch. Dis. Child.* 30:13, 1955.
9. Rickham, P. P., and Johnston, J. H. *Neonatal Surgery*. New York: Appleton-Century-Crofts, 1969.
10. Santulli, T. V. Meconium Ileus. In W. T. Mustard, M. M. Ravitch, W. H. Snyder, Jr., et al. (eds.), *Pediatric Surgery*. Chicago: Yearbook Medical Publishers, 1969.

14

Necrotizing Enterocolitis

Although necrotizing enterocolitis was first discovered in 1891, the first reported series did not appear in the literature until 1967. The disease primarily affects the small, premature infant who has been subjected to some form of stress, such as hypoxia or shock, during the neonatal period. With increased survival of small premature infants in neonatal intensive care units since the early 1970s, the incidence of necrotizing enterocolitis has climbed dramatically. Although the cause of this condition is completely unknown, it appears from clinical and experimental investigations that the disease is secondary to some form of vascular ischemia of the intestinal tract.

Preoperative Evaluation

Onset of symptoms does not usually occur until the fourth to fifth day of life and is rare until after the patient has had initial feedings. The infant is usually a tiny premature weighing less than 1,500 grams, with significant respiratory distress in many cases. Often the patient is on a respirator at the time symptoms appear. The earliest symptom is increasing gastric residuals after gavage feedings, followed shortly thereafter by hematochezia, initially as occult blood and then as gross blood in the stool. During the next 12 to 24 hours the infant develops significant abdominal distention associated with bilious vomiting and failure to pass feces. The entire clinical picture can take anywhere from 4 to 48 hours to emerge completely. Patients who have a rapid development of clinical symptoms usually have a more lethal course.

Once the disease is suspected, roentgenograms of the abdomen should be obtained to look for gaseous distention of the intestine, pneumoperitoneum, pneumatosis intestinalis, and portal venous gas (Figure 14-1). The definitive diagnosis can be made if one sees pneumatosis intestinalis or portal venous gas; about 95 percent of cases will show pneumatosis intestinalis. Roentgenograms should be obtained every 8 to 12 hours in order to detect the early appearance of pneumatosis intestinalis, pneumoperitoneum, or both.

Once the diagnosis has been established, medical therapy—consisting of nasogastric or orogastric decompression of the gastrointestinal tract, intravenous fluids, and intravenous broad-spectrum antibiotics for a minimum of 48 to 72 hours—should be instituted immediately. In 50 percent to 75 percent of the cases, medical therapy is adequate, so that the patients do not develop complete gangrene of the intestine with perforation and peritonitis. The other 25 percent develop full-thickness necrosis of segments of the intestinal tract with resulting peritonitis and gram-negative sepsis. The time lapse from the onset of symptoms until the development of peritonitis can vary from 4 hours to 48 hours; the shorter the time lapse, the more lethal the situation. Diagnosis of peritonitis and bowel perforation in a small

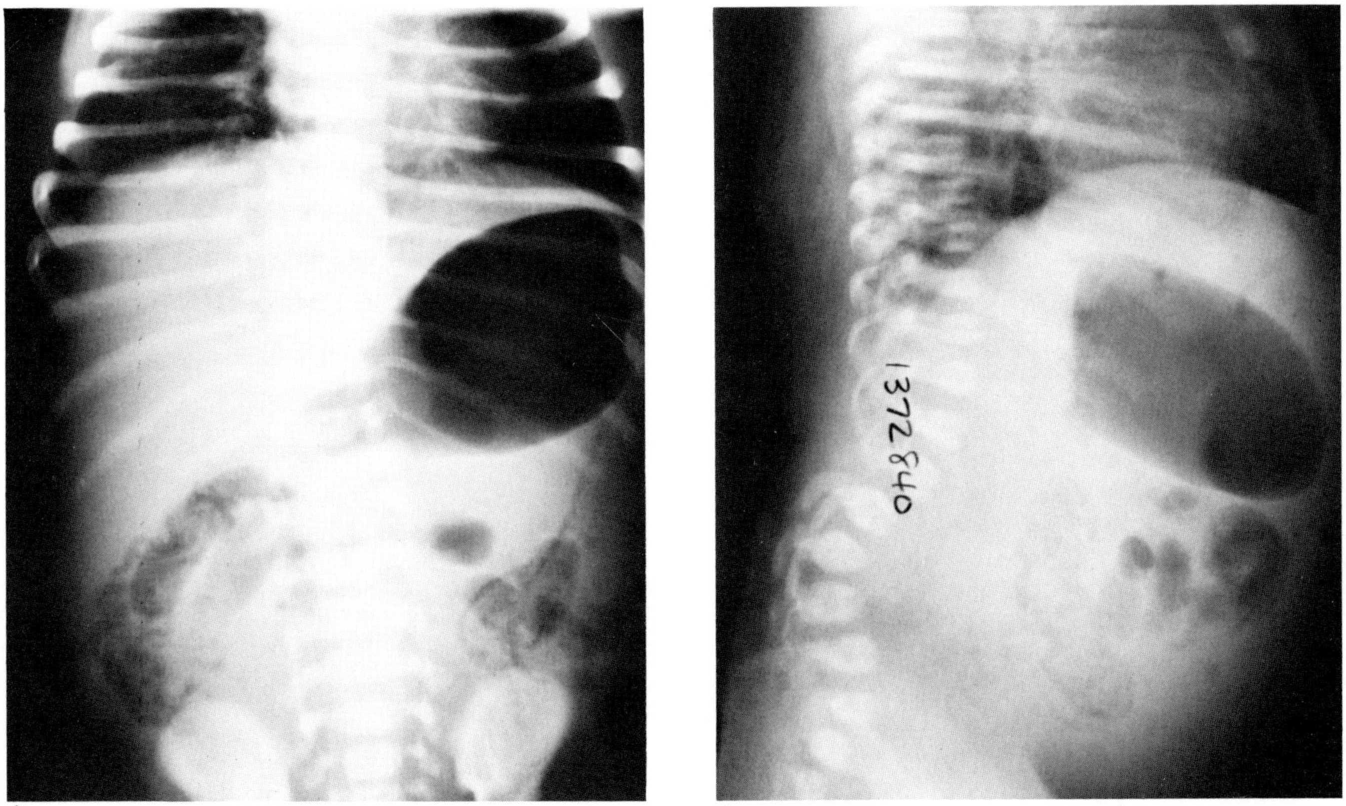

A B

14-1. (A) Posteroanterior and (B) lateral abdominal films demonstrating pneumatosis intestinalis in the region of the ascending colon.

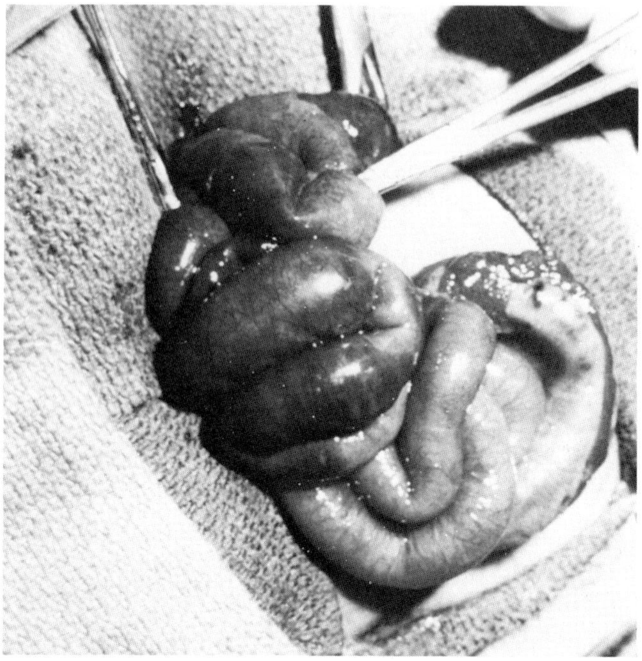

14-2. At operation for necrotizing enterocolitis patchy areas of gangrene can be seen throughout the small intestine.

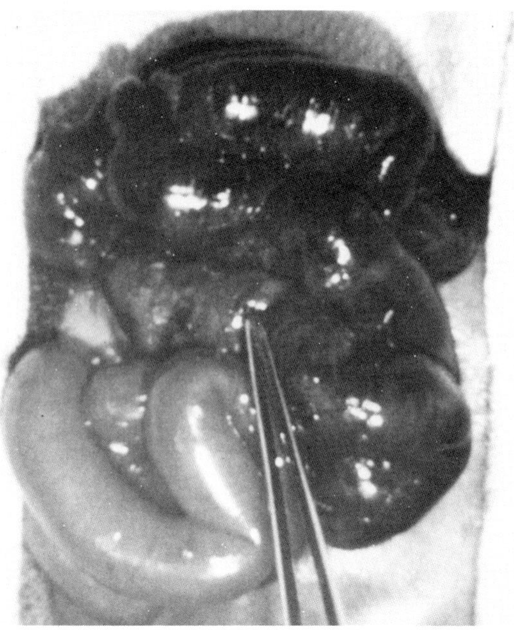

14-3

premature infant is often quite difficult because these babies do not show the classic physical findings of peritonitis. In addition, pneumoperitoneum is seen in only about 25 percent of the cases of bowel perforation secondary to necrotizing enterocolitis. Once the diagnosis of peritonitis has been made, the infant is given colloid solutions intravenously and is taken to the operating room.

Operative Technique

The baby is placed in the supine position on the operating table, and the abdomen is explored through a transverse incision in the right upper quadrant. The small bowel is gently eviscerated after the peritoneal cavity has been opened, and the entire small intestine from the ligament of Treitz to the ileocecal valve is inspected. One must be very careful in handling the bowel because it is extremely friable and can be perforated with only slight palpation. Patchy areas of hemorrhage (Figure 14-2) and gangrene distributed throughout the small and large intestine, often associated with large air cysts (Figure 14-3), are usually noted. The areas most commonly involved are the distal ileum and the right colon, with the left colon being the least often affected.

Once the small bowel has been completely inspected, the entire colon should be carefully visualized so that no areas of colonic gangrene are missed. Occasionally one finds a small localized area of gangrene, usually in the terminal ileum. If 75 percent or more of the small intestine is gangrenous, one should seriously consider performing no resection and merely closing the abdomen. If less than 75 percent of the small intestine is necrotic, then a resection should be carried out. The resection usually involves the distal ileum and the right colon (Figure 14-4). An ileostomy and a colonic mucous fistula are then created by bringing both the stomas out through the incision and tacking them to the medial and lateral corners of the incision (Figure 14-5). The ileostomy and mucous fistula are carefully tacked to the peritoneum and fascia with a few interrupted sutures of 6-0 silk; the sutures are placed only through the seromuscular layer of the bowel wall, to avoid development of subsequent fistulas. Before tacking the stomas to the abdominal wall, a gastrostomy is performed by the technique described in the previous chapters. The gastrostomy tube is then brought out through a separate incision medial to the major incision. The abdominal incision is closed between the two stomas with either interrupted 5-0 silk to the peritoneum or a running 3-0 chromic catgut to the peritoneum. The fascia is closed with interrupted 5-0 silk sutures, and the skin is closed with a running 5-0 nylon suture.

Postoperative Care

These infants are extremely sick postoperatively, with severe sepsis and significant respiratory insufficiency. Most require a ventilator postoperatively, especially those who had hyaline membrane disease or bronchopulmonary dysplasia preoperatively. In addition, the infants who were septic before surgery usually show signs of invasive sepsis postoperatively in the form of disseminated intravascular coagulation. The mortality in this group is extremely high, ranging from 30 percent to 60 percent.

Broad-spectrum antibiotic coverage and gastrostomy tube decompression should be continued for several days postoperatively. Also, these patients usually require intermittent administration of albumin and blood intravenously after surgery.

Once the sepsis is under control and the patient is hemodynamically stable, one can start to feed the baby by the gastrostomy route; most of these patients are too small to feed orally. If a large segment of small bowel has been resected, ileostomy diarrhea, which can lead to significant dehydration, will occur. If severe diarrhea ensues, then one should desist from feeding the patient and institute intravenous hyperalimentation. In many cases no feedings can be given to the patient for the entire period the ileostomy is in place because of the significant fluid loss. This is especially true in those infants in whom more than 50 percent to 60 percent of the small intestine has been resected, in which case the patient should be maintained on hyperalimentation until enough weight has been gained to allow the ileostomy to be closed.

Once the patient's weight has reached 2.27 kilograms (five pounds), either with gastrostomy feedings or with hyperalimentation, the ileostomy can be closed. Before the ileostomy has been closed, a contrast study of the distal bowel through the mucous fistula should be carried out to be sure that there are no strictures present. In the operating room, the ileostomy and mucous fistula are taken down, the edges are trimmed back, and a primary anastomosis is created between these two stomas. The technique for the primary anastomosis is the same as that described in the chapter on intestinal atresia. Two to three days after closure of the ileostomy, the patient can usually be started gradually on oral or gastrostomy feedings. Many patients will manifest the clinical picture of the short-bowel syndrome for many weeks and even months after the ileostomy closure. Even though what appears to be an adequate amount of small intestine has been left in place, this short-bowel syndrome will occur, perhaps because a significant portion of the bowel that was unresected has been altered by the underlying disease process. Infants with symptoms of short-bowel syndrome are very difficult to manage: They require multiple formula changes for several weeks to months postopera-

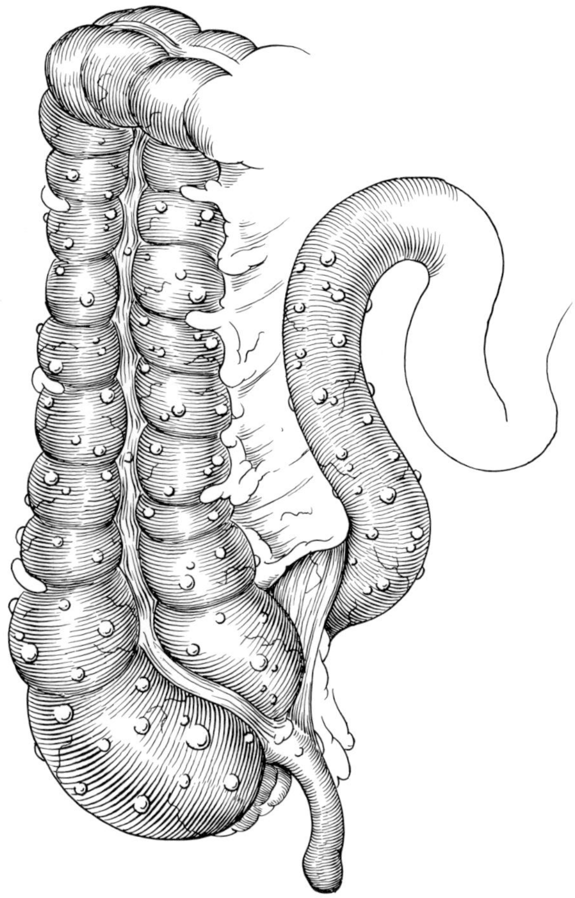

14-4. The distal ileum and proximal colon are necrotic, with multiple air cysts throughout. These are the areas that are resected.

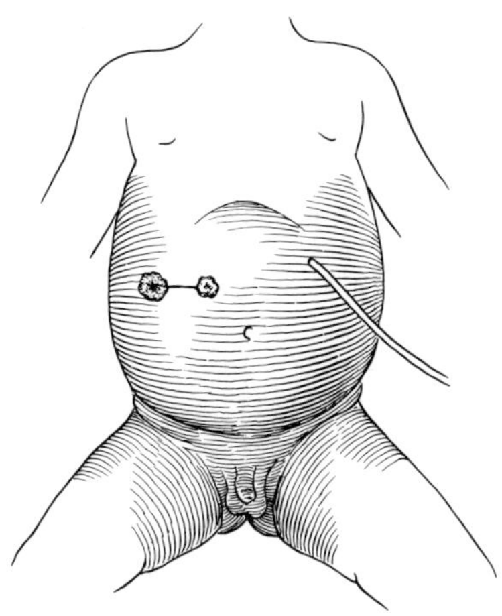

14-5

tively, to decrease the diarrhea and to improve the caloric and protein intake. Intermittent periods of hyperalimentation are often required while formula changes are being carried out.

Comments

Necrotizing enterocolitis is a disease that normally does not require surgical intervention. The pediatric surgeon becomes involved in the management of this condition only when evidence of complete necrosis of the bowel wall or bowel perforation is present. Because of the diffuse distribution of the disease, surgical therapy is at best a reasonable compromise. As neonatologists and pediatricians are learning to recognize this entity earlier and are instituting medical therapy immediately, the number of infants coming to surgery has significantly decreased. In addition, as neonatologists and pediatric surgeons become more adept at recognizing the early signs of peritonitis in the neonate, infants are being operated upon for peritonitis much earlier than in the past, with subsequent marked improvement in the salvage rate. Many babies with necrotizing enterocolitis are also plagued by the presence of a patent ductus arteriosus with significant left-to-right shunting through this defect. The left-to-right shunting through the ductus may contribute to the mesenteric vascular insufficiency that is present in necrotizing enterocolitis. Also, the marked left-to-right shunt can lead to significant congestive heart failure in these infants, which compounds the postoperative management problems. Because of the significant congestive heart failure that often results, many of these babies have to undergo an emergency ligation of the patent ductus arteriosus in the early postoperative period.

Selected References

1. Dudgeon, D. L., Coran, A. G., Lauppe, F. A., et al. Surgical management of acute necrotizing enterocolitis in infants. *J. Pediatr. Surg.* 8:607, 1973.
2. Santulli, T. V., Schullinger, J. N., Heird, W. C., et al. Acute necrotizing enterocolitis in infancy. *Pediatrics* 55:376, 1975.
3. Stevenson, J. K., Oliver, T. K., Jr., Graham, C. B., et al. Aggressive treatment of neonatal necrotizing enterocolitis, 38 patients with 25 survivors. *J. Pediatr. Surg.* 6:28, 1971.
4. Touloukian, R. J., Berdon, W. E., Amoury, R. A., and Santulli, T. V. Surgical experience with necrotizing enterocolitis in the infant. *J. Pediatr. Surg.* 2:389, 1967.
5. Touloukian, R. J., Rosch, J. M., and Spencer, R. The pathogenesis of ischemic gastroenterocolitis of the neonate. *J. Pediatr. Surg.* 7:194, 1972.
6. Wilson, F. E., and Woolley, M. M. Primary necrotizing enterocolitis in infants. *Arch. Surg.* 99:563, 1969.

15

Hirschsprung's Disease

Hirschsprung's disease, which is congenital absence of ganglion cells in the distal colon and rectum, is rapidly becoming one of the commonest causes of intestinal obstruction in the neonatal period. In fact, in many of the major neonatal centers, Hirschsprung's disease as a cause of bowel obstruction in the newborn is more common than intestinal atresias and stenoses. The aganglionic segment of bowel maintains an unremitting state of severe spasm, which leads to intestinal obstruction in the infant and chronic constipation in the child.

Preoperative Evaluation

Most newborn infants with the symptoms of Hirschsprung's disease are full-term babies, although occasionally one sees a premature with the classic findings. The commonest clinical finding in the neonatal period is failure to pass meconium during the first 24 to 48 hours of life. Any newborn who fails to pass meconium during the first 48 hours of life should be highly suspect of having Hirschsprung's disease and should be evaluated further to rule in or out this diagnosis. Not uncommonly, the neonate may present a full-blown picture of intestinal obstruction with bilious vomiting (Figure 15-1). Occasionally superimposing enterocolitis may develop—a grave complication of Hirschsprung's disease in the neonate. This is associated with a significant morbidity and mortality in the newborn period. On physical examination, the infant's abdomen is often found to be moderately to markedly distended, depending on the degree of obstruction. Rectal examination usually shows normal findings; however, after removal of one's finger from the infant's rectum, there is often an explosive passage of meconium or feces.

Although examination by barium enema in the older infant and child is usually diagnostic of Hirschsprung's disease, showing a narrowed rectosigmoid with dilated colon above it, this is usually not the case in the neonatal period. The best clue to the radiologic diagnosis of Hirschsprung's disease in the newborn is the presence of barium on a plain film of the abdomen taken 24 hours after the initial examination (Figures 15-2, 15-3). This retention of barium is highly suggestive of Hirschsprung's disease, although it is not diagnostic. Further studies have to be carried out to make a definitive diagnosis in the newborn.

Classically, the next diagnostic step taken after a barium enema that makes one suspicious is to perform a full-thickness rectal biopsy under general anesthesia to look for the presence of ganglion cells in the myenteric plexus of the rectum. Frozen sections are obtained during anesthesia. If no ganglion cells are present, the surgeon then proceeds to a colostomy. Although this is certainly an acceptable approach to the management of this condition, rectal biopsy is not always a technically easy procedure to perform in the small neonate. During the past few years we have taken a different

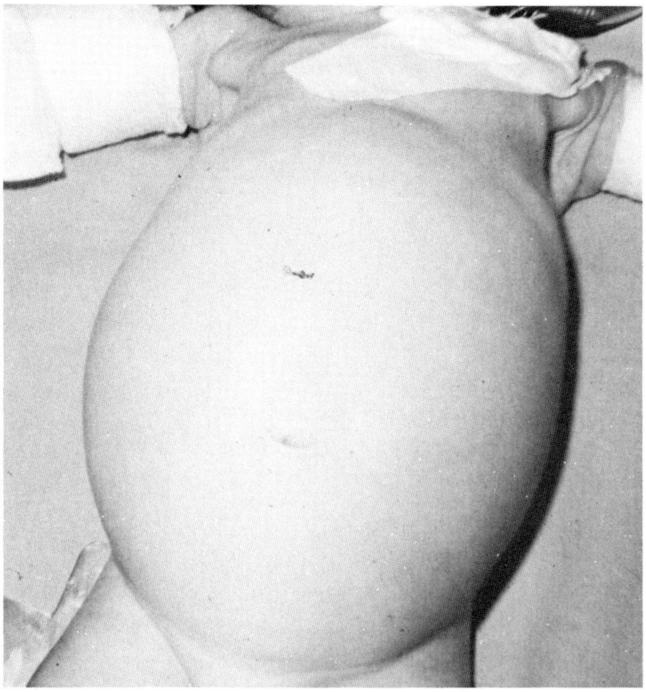

15-1. Marked abdominal distention from Hirschsprung's disease.

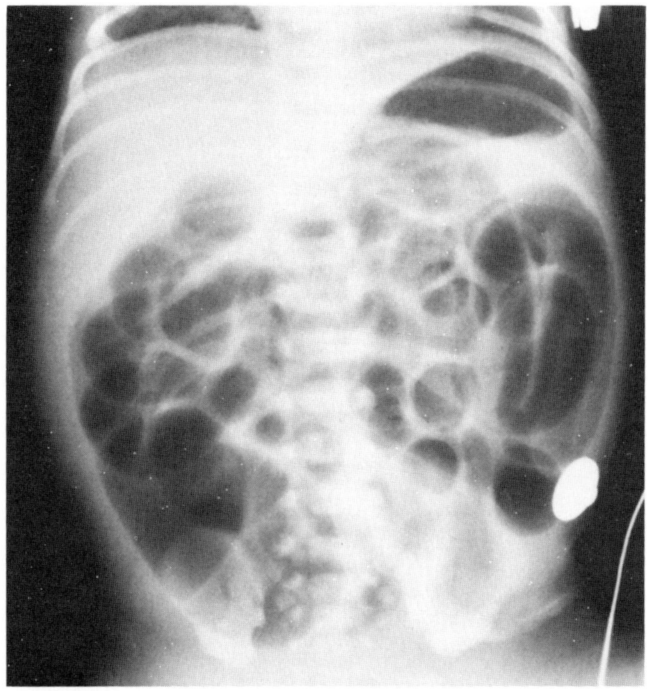

15-2. Plain roentgenogram of the abdomen of an infant with bowel obstruction from Hirschsprung's disease.

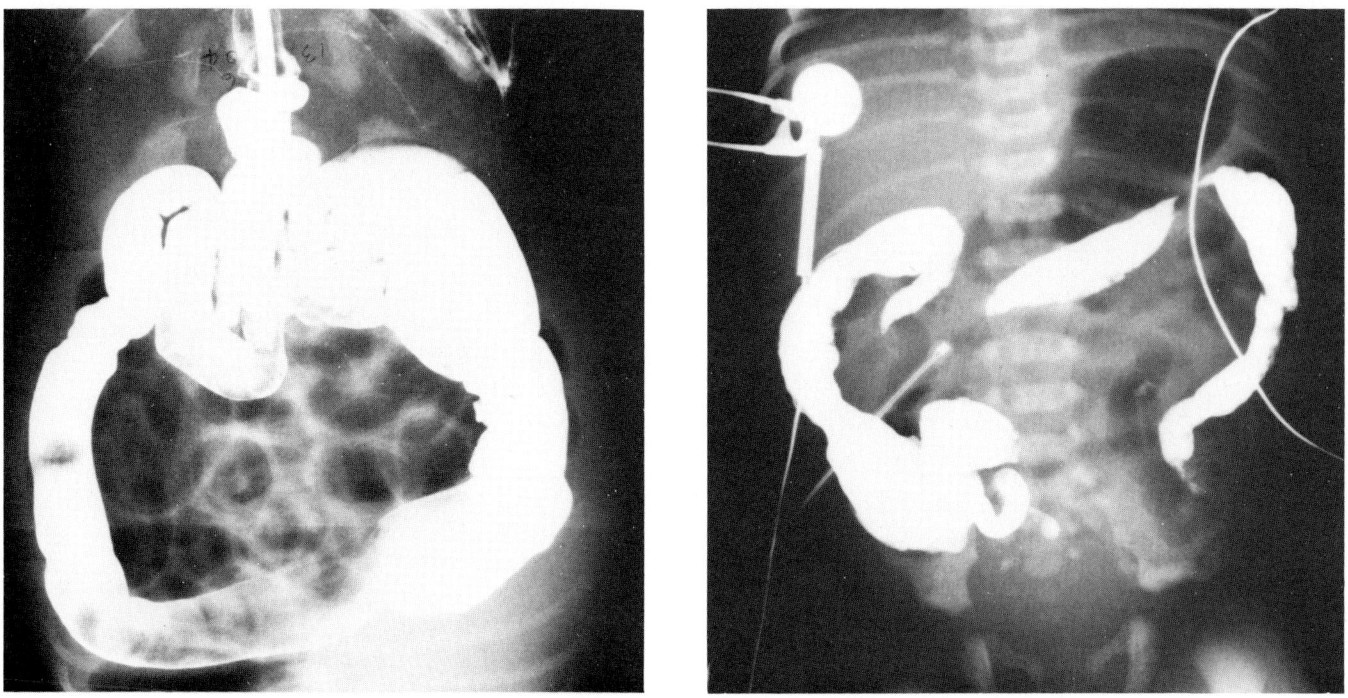

A

B

15-3. (A) Barium enema that shows normal findings in a newborn with Hirschsprung's disease. (B) A 24-hour film showing barium retention.

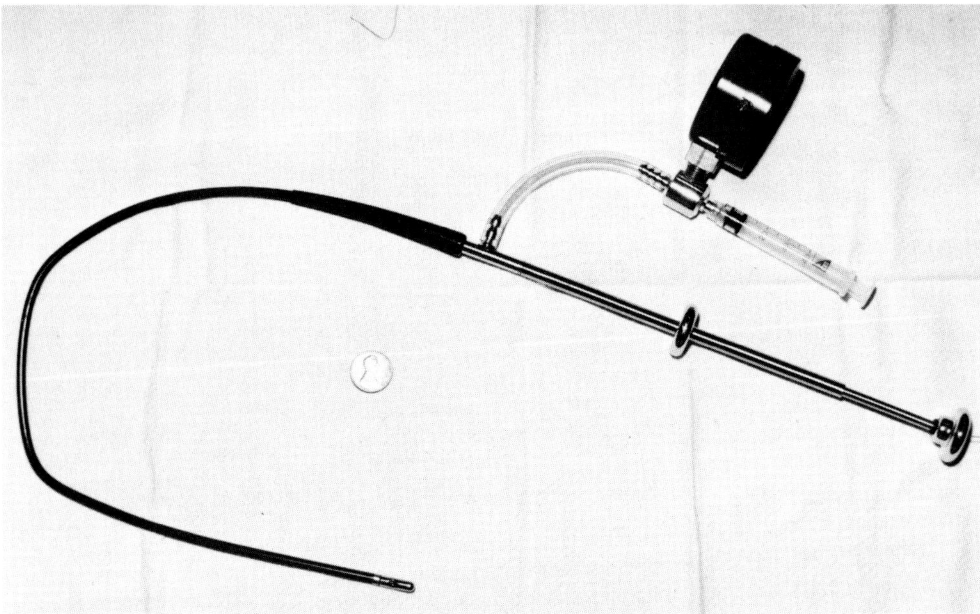

15-4. Biopsy capsule kit (manufactured by Quinton Instruments, Inc., Seattle, Washington). The capsule is inserted into the rectum a distance of 2 cm. Suction is obtained with a syringe.

approach to this problem by using a biopsy capsule kit that will obtain a piece of mucosa and submucosa from the rectum without the necessity of administering any anesthesia; in fact, the procedure can be entirely done at the bedside (Figure 15-4). An experienced pathologist can then determine whether or not ganglion cells are present in the submucosal or Meissner's plexus. Although the absence of ganglion cells in the submucosal plexus is not as definitively diagnostic of Hirschsprung's disease as is the absence of ganglion cells in the myenteric (intermuscular) plexus, it does allow one to proceed with definitive management of the patient in the neonatal period. The other great advantage of not performing a full-thickness rectal biopsy in the patient is that the definitive pull-through procedure carried out at a later date is made much easier by the absence of scarring in the low rectum of the infant.

Once the diagnosis has been established, the infant is prepared for surgery by inserting a nasogastric tube and administering broad-spectrum antibiotics and vitamin K. If there is clinical or hemodynamic evidence of significant third-space loss of fluid into the gastrointestinal tract or the peritoneal cavity, then appropriate volumes of crystalloid or colloid solutions are given intravenously before taking the newborn to the operating room.

Operative Technique

In the operating room the infant is placed in the supine position, and precautions are taken to prevent significant heat loss (Figure 15-5a), either by wrapping the infant's arms and legs with sheet wadding or by placing an overhead heater above the operating table. A nasogastric tube is already in place, and a proper intravenous line is established, either by a cutdown technique or through a percutaneous catheter. The infant is anesthetized with an endotracheal tube, and the entire abdomen is prepared and then draped.

Many surgeons advocate performing a blind transverse colostomy in normally ganglionated bowel during the neonatal period and determining the exact level of aganglionic intestine at the time of the definitive pull-through. We prefer to determine the exact level of aganglionic bowel during the initial operation and to perform a colostomy just above this area. This usually means that (except in the case of long-segment or total colonic Hirschsprung's disease), one is performing a sigmoid colostomy, which is much easier to manage during the first year of life. The entire procedure can be carried out through a small incision in the left lower quadrant, rather than by performing a formal large laparotomy (Figure 15-5a). We use a small oblique incision in the left lower quadrant in which the oblique muscles are split just as is done in a classic McBurney approach on the right for acute appendicitis (Figure 15-5b).

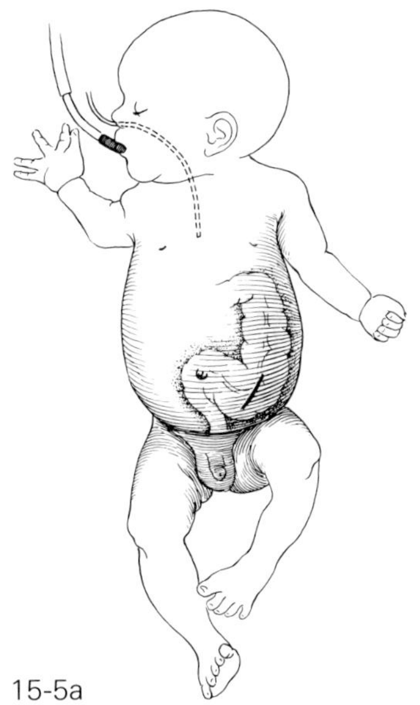

15-5a

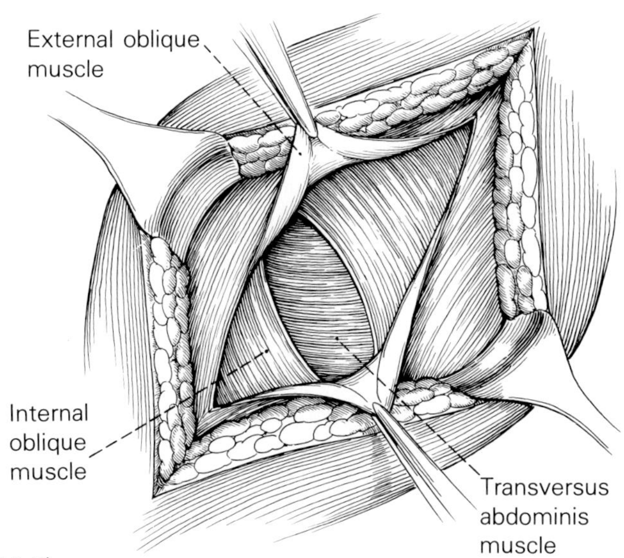

15-5b

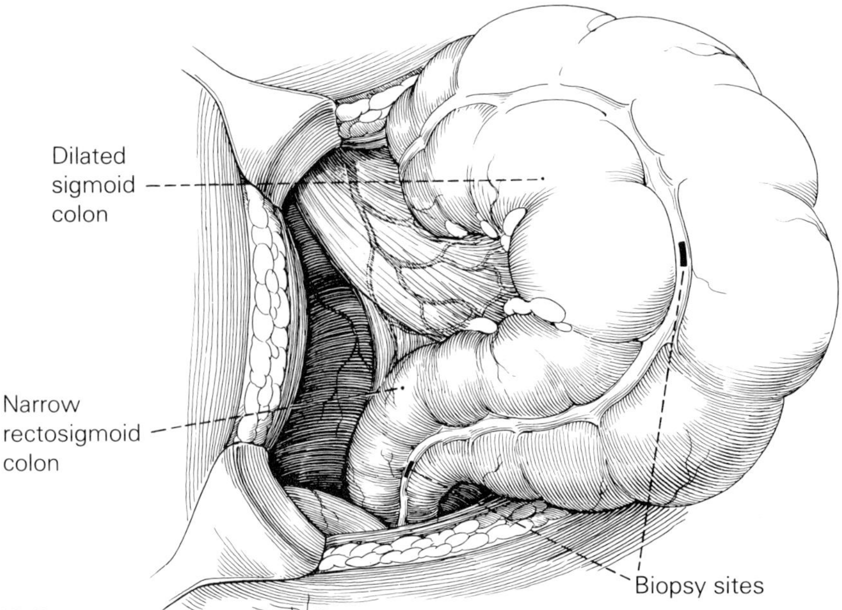

15-5c

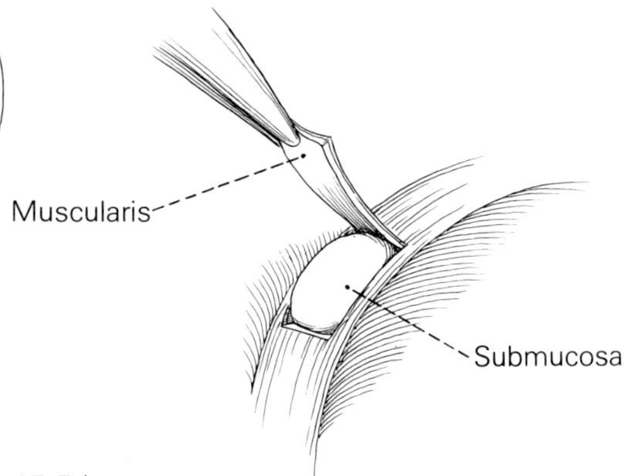

15-5d

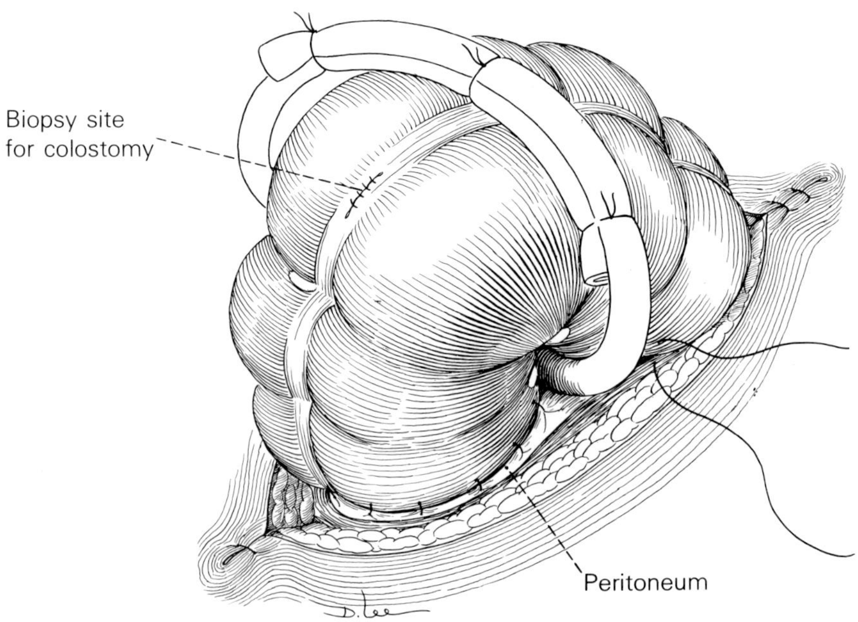

15-5e

This small incision gives one adequate exposure for determining the level of aganglionic bowel and for performing the colostomy. If one notes a significant disparity between the distal and proximal sigmoid colon, indicating a transition zone (Figure 15-5c), then an extramucosal muscle biopsy is taken from the narrowed segment to determine if ganglion cells are present. A similar biopsy is taken from the most distal dilated portion (Figure 15-5d). The report on the frozen section will usually indicate that there are no ganglion cells in the narrowed distal segment and that there are ganglion cells in the proximal dilated sigmoid colon. The colostomy is then performed in the most distal portion of the dilated sigmoid colon, where ganglion cells have been proved to be present by frozen section (Figure 15-5e). We prefer to use a colostomy of the loop type rather than a divided one because it is just as effective and easier to perform. The selected segment of sigmoid colon is exteriorized and is carefully tacked to the peritoneum with interrupted sutures of 4-0 or 5-0 silk placed through only the serosa and muscularis of the bowel wall. A small opening is then made in the middle of the sigmoid mesentery just next to the bowel wall. A small segment of a 16 French rubber catheter is brought through the opening and tied to itself to act as a rod. A few additional tacking sutures of 4-0 or 5-0 silk are placed between the muscle layers of the abdominal wall and the seromuscular layer of the colon. These sutures are not as critical as the peritoneal sutures, which must be placed carefully in all colostomies performed in infants to prevent evisceration. Usually the loop of colon fills the entire incision and no additional closure is required; however, if some of the muscle is still left open it can be closed with interrupted sutures of 3-0 chromic catgut. Any skin that is left open can be closed with interrupted sutures of 5-0 nylon. If the infant is in a stable condition and is not markedly obstructed, the colostomy can be opened the next morning on the ward by simply making an incision of 1 to 1½ centimeters along a taenia; this can be done with cautery or by crushing the area to be incised with a hemostat before cutting it. If the infant is quite sick and has a severe degree of intestinal obstruction, then it is preferable to open the colostomy in the operating room once the skin has been closed. Although this increases the risk of a wound infection, the risk is certainly acceptable in an unstable infant during this operative procedure.

Postoperative Care

For the first one to two postoperative days the infant is maintained on intravenous fluids until there is evidence that the colostomy is working. Once the colostomy is functioning, the infant is gradually started on oral feedings. The broad-spectrum antibiotic coverage is usually continued for three to five postoperative days. Once the infant is eating and stooling normally, he can be discharged home. The colostomy is easily cared for by the mother merely by placing the diaper a little higher on the infant's abdomen. Some surgeons prefer to use a colostomy bag, which is certainly acceptable. The fecal output of a sigmoid colostomy in an infant is really no different from that of a normal infant passing feces per rectum; therefore skin irritation and other problems related to a colostomy are really minimal with this type of colonic diversion in a newborn. The catheter can be removed in the office on the tenth postoperative day.

Comments

A small minority of pediatric surgeons prefer to manage neonates with Hirschsprung's disease without a colostomy by performing daily rectal irrigations with moderately small volumes of warm saline. They feel that this technique can relieve the infant of the acute intestinal obstruction and can prepare him for a definitive pull-through procedure. The pull-through procedure is then performed during the newborn period. Most surgeons feel, however, that the risk of perforation of the colon with saline irrigations is significant and that the results of definitive pull-through procedures performed during the neonatal period are less satisfactory than those obtained when the procedure is carried out at one year of age.

Selected References

1. Ehrenpreis, T. Megacolon in the newborn. *Acta Chir. Scand.* 94(Suppl.):112,1946.
2. Pilling, G. P., and Cresson, S. L. Hirschsprung's Disease. In W. T. Mustard, M. M. Ravitch, W. H. Snyder, Jr., et al. (eds.), *Pediatric Surgery.* Chicago: Year Book Medical Publishers, 1969.
3. Rickham, P. P., and Johnston, J. H. *Neonatal Surgery.* New York: Appleton-Century-Crofts, 1969.
4. Swenson, O., and Bill, A. H., Jr. Resection of rectum and rectosigmoid with preservation of the sphincter for benign spastic lesions producing megacolon. *Surgery* 24:212, 1948.
5. Swenson, O., Fisher, J. H., and McMahon, H. E. Rectal biopsy as aid in the diagnosis of Hirschsprung's disease. *N. Engl. J. Med.* 253:632, 1955.

16

Imperforate Anus

Imperforate anus was well recognized in ancient times by Greek, Roman, and Arab physicians. Because the diagnosis can usually be made by simple inspection, it is not surprising that this condition was recognized early in medical history. The incidence is approximately 1 in every 3,000 to 4,000 live births. The condition is somewhat more common in males than in females, but there is no racial predisposition.

There are many different classifications in the literature used to describe imperforate anus; however, a sound understanding of the anomaly and its treatment can be gained by placing infants with imperforate anus in four major categories: high and low and male and female (Figure 16-1). In general, most males have high lesions while most females have low ones. A high imperforate anus exists when the terminal end of the rectum lies at or above the levator sling (pubococcygeal and puborectalis muscles). A low imperforate anus is one in which the rectum has traversed this sling but has not terminated at the normal site of the anus. High lesions in males are almost always associated with a rectourethral fistula. Since the levator sling is the major structure responsible for fecal continence, patients with low lesions have a good chance for normal rectal control after careful surgery. In infants with high lesions, meticulous surgery should also result in good bowel control, but the results in general are somewhat poorer, and the morbidity is slightly higher than in patients with low anomalies. In most pediatric surgical centers, a sigmoid colostomy is performed in the newborn period for high lesions. When the baby reaches 9 to 11 kilograms in weight (20 or 25 pounds) a formal pull-through procedure is performed because the sling mechanism is easier to locate and less prone to iatrogenic injury. On the other hand, babies with low lesions, usually have excellent results if primary perineal surgery is done during the first few days or weeks of life.

For proper classification of a newborn with imperforate anus, the surgeon first assesses the sex, which is usually obvious. If examination of the perineum reveals a fistulous opening, the child almost surely has a low lesion. No visible opening usually means that a high lesion is present, but occasionally the opening of a low lesion is very small or hidden in the vagina or the median raphe of the scrotum. For this reason, we prefer to watch these infants for 12 to 24 hours because a small speck of meconium may appear on the perineum and point the way to the fistula. (Note: It is safer to do an occasional colostomy on a child with a low lesion than to try a perineal exploration in a newborn with a high lesion.)

If after 24 hours no fistulous opening on the perineum is seen, then a high lesion should be suspected. The surgeon should seek confirmation and then proceed with a colostomy because these infants obviously will develop symptoms of intestinal obstruction.

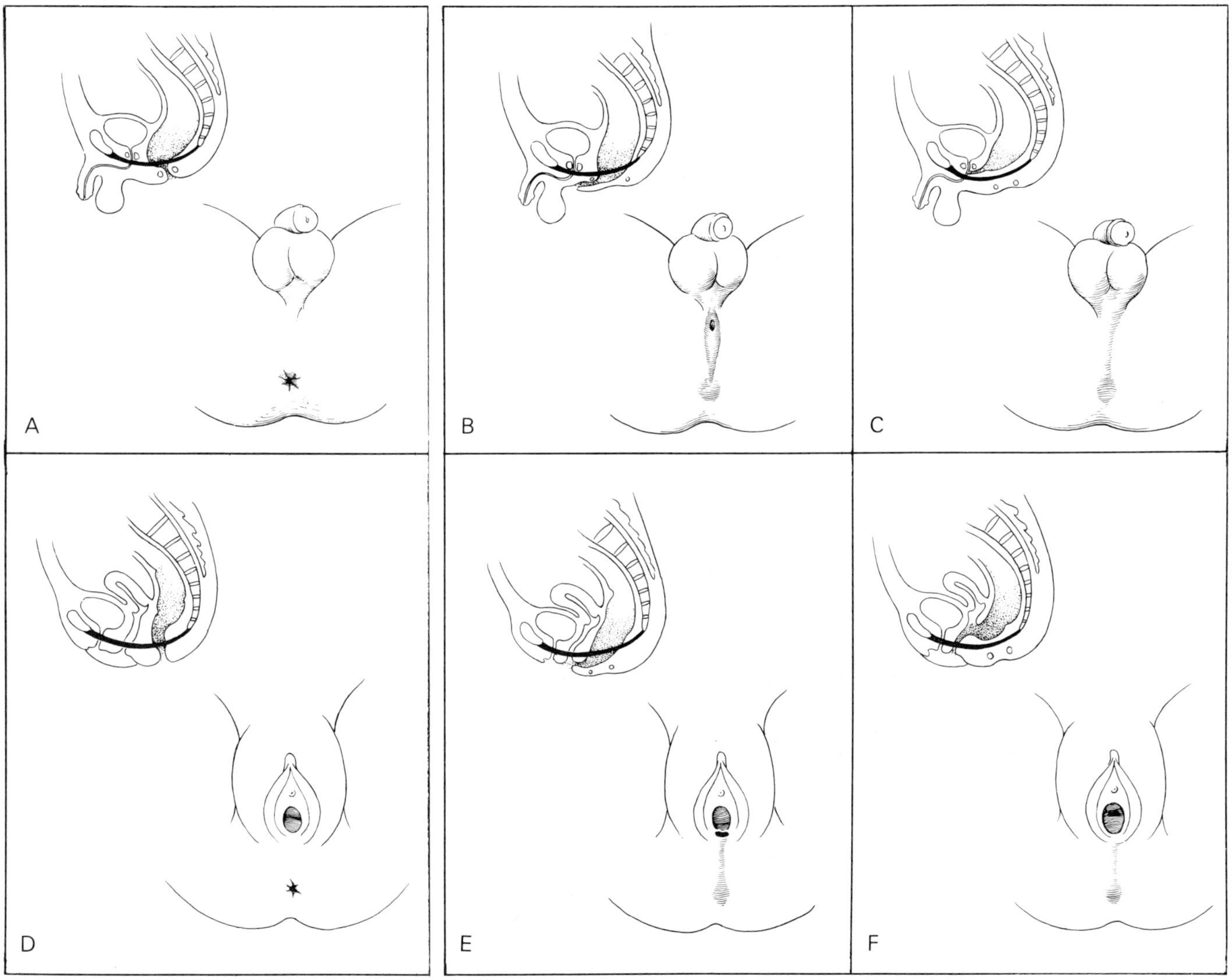

16-1. (A) Normal male. (B) Male with low imperforate lesion and anterior subcutaneous fistula. (C) Male with high lesion. Rectum ends in the posterior urethra. (D) Normal female. (E) Female with low imperforate anus and fistula at vaginal fourchette. (F) Female with high lesion. Rectum ends in the upper vagina.

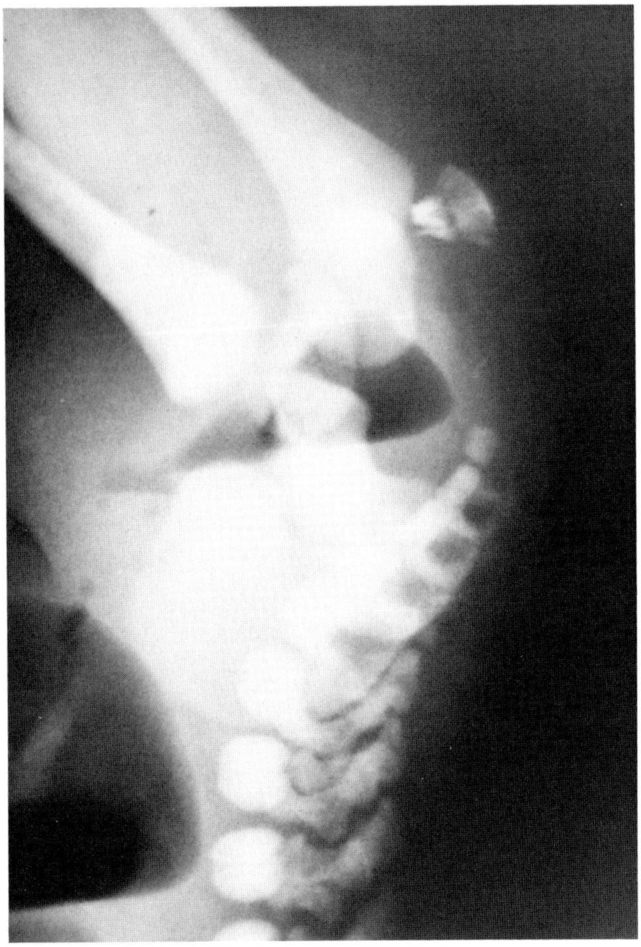

A

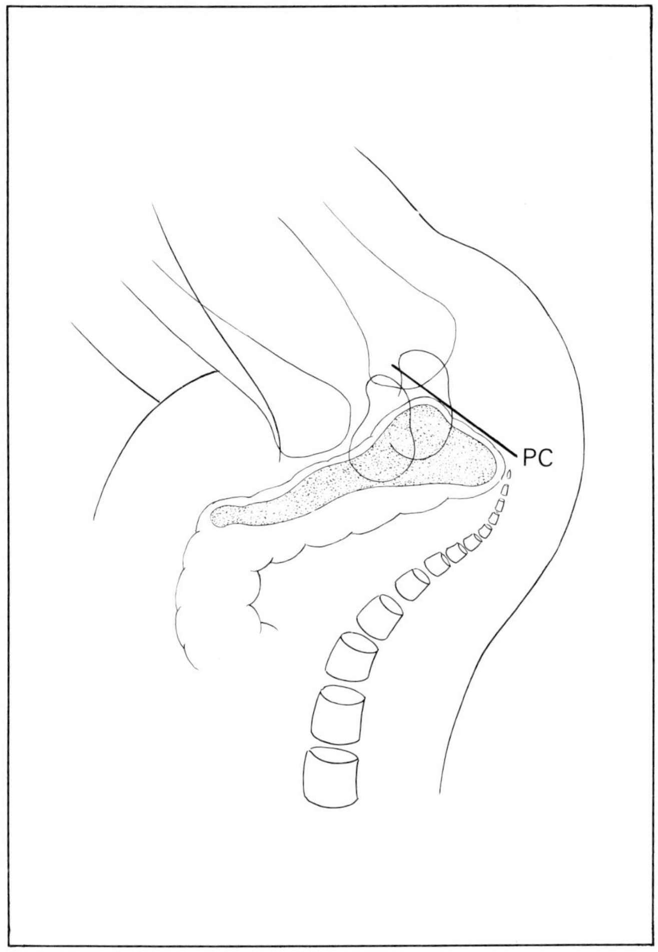

B

16-2. (A) Lateral upside-down x-ray film of male with the air column ending at the pubococcygeal (PC) line, indicating that the rectum has not gone through the levator sling. (B) The PC line drawn to show position of levator sling.

Males with High Imperforate Anus

In a male infant who at 24 hours has had no evidence of a fistulous communication to the perineum, an upside-down lateral abdominal x-ray film is taken. By 24 hours of age, intestinal air should reach the most distal portion of the colon. This air column can be related to the levator sling. Since the sling runs from the pubis to the coccyx, a line can be drawn on the x-ray plate and the relationship of the levator sling to the level of the air column can be assessed (Figure 16-2). If the column of air is well beyond the pubococcygeal (PC) line, a low lesion with a fistula exists and a perineal anoplasty can be performed. In a baby with a high imperforate anus, the air column has not traversed the PC line and a sigmoid colostomy should be carried out. A loop colostomy is satisfactory and can be performed in the manner described in Chapter 15. Formal pull-through procedures (usually sacroperineal) in these males are performed at approximately 12 months of age. An intravenous pyelogram (IVP) is obtained before discharge to search for urinary and spinal anomalies.

Two specific complications are seen in the interim between colostomy and pull-through. Because the distal end of the colon usually ends in the posterior urethra or bladder (fewer than 10 percent of males with a high lesion have no urinary fistula), these boys may have urinary reflux into this segment of colon with resultant hyperchloremia and acidosis. This can be treated by the addition of small amounts of sodium bicarbonate solution to the baby's formula. In a similar fashion, the mucous and bacterial contents of the distal colon can enter the bladder and cause occasional urinary tract infection. Antibiotics can be used for acute infection. Fortunately, chronic urinary tract infection is rare in this situation.

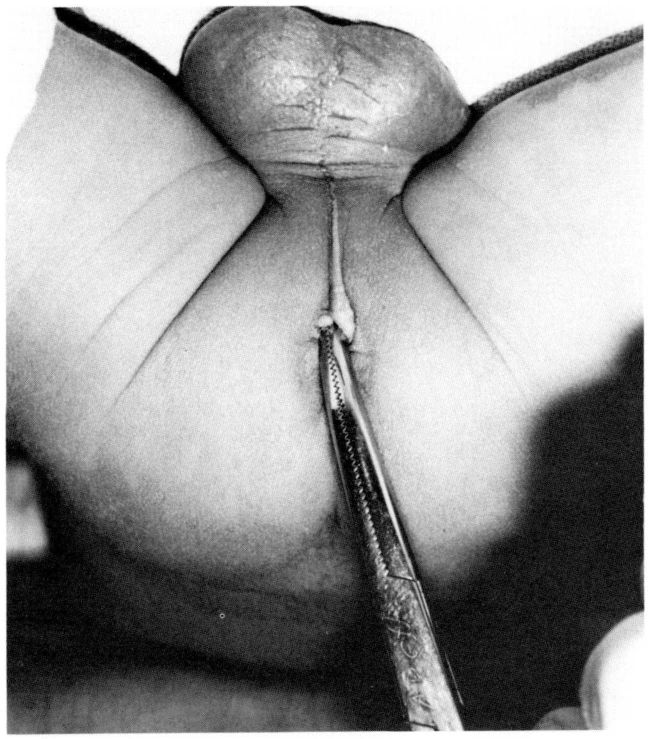

16-3. Male with low imperforate anus and thickened median raphe.

Males with Low Lesions

A visible fistula in a male almost always means that the colon has traversed the levator sling. The opening is usually small and is often anterior to the normal location (Figure 16-3). The area of the so-called fistula is gently probed with a hemostat or a needle and syringe. When meconium is encountered this opening is carefully enlarged. Simple anal dilatation may cure minor lesions, but perineal anoplasty may be needed to correct the problem in more significant low lesions.

Perineal Anoplasty or Cutback in a Male

After the induction of general anesthesia, the infant is positioned on skis at the end of the table. The site of the new anus is determined by locating the anal wink of the external sphincter and marking it on the skin (Figure 16-4a). A clamp is placed in the fistula and pointed posteriorly (Figure 16-4b). An incision is then made over the clamp, opening the anus all the way back through the anterior fibers of the external

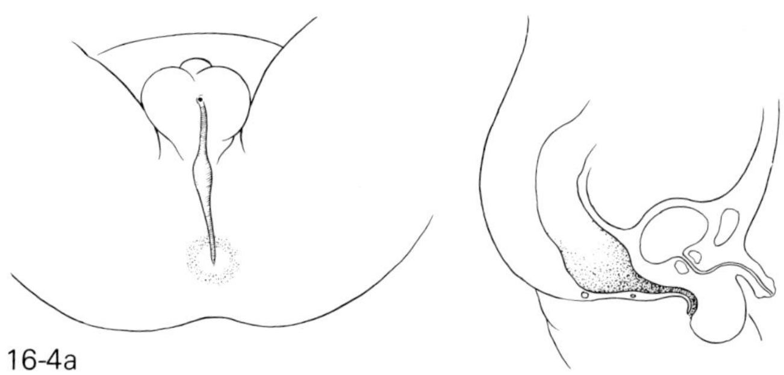

16-4a

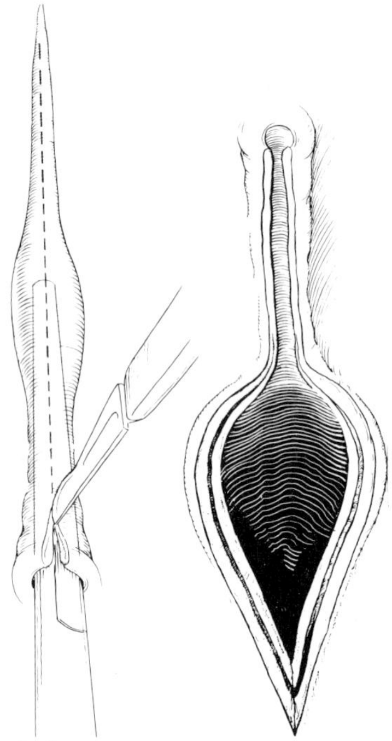

16-4b

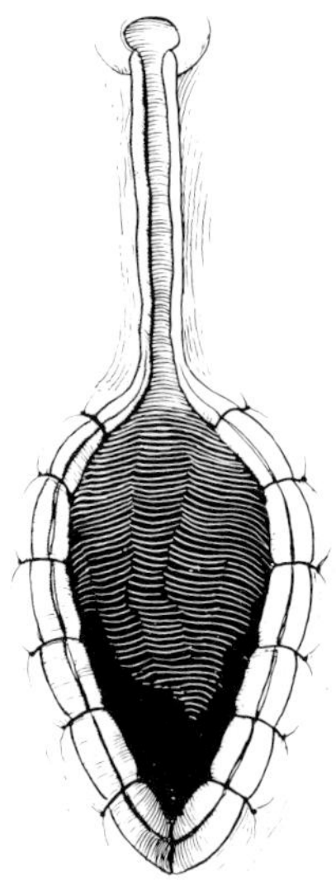

16-4c

sphincter to the previously marked site. The mucous membrane and skin are freed and then approximated with interrupted stitches of 4-0 or 5-0 Dexon (Figure 16-4c). At this point, a finger or Hegar dilator placed into the anus will release a moderate amount of meconium. In an occasional male infant, the fistula may extend all the way up the median raphe. A small metal probe is placed in this tract and an incision is made over it to filet it open. Then a routine cutback anoplasty is performed. After 10 days gentle dilatations are begun, first with the fifth finger or with Hegar dilators. Gradually over the next few weeks the index finger or larger Hegar dilators are used until the anus appears supple and soft. This may take two to three months, but mothers can learn to do this on a daily basis. These male infants should have an excellent result, with normal bowel control, when they are older.

A common complication seen after this type of repair is stricture of the anastomosis; this is both prevented and treated by appropriate dilatations.

Females with Low Imperforate Anus

Most females have low lesions; the terminal end of the rectum is visible somewhere anterior to the normal site. The fistula can be just anterior to the anus, in the vaginal fourchette, or in the distal vagina. Fistulas that lie on the perineum just anterior to the anus can be cured with a cutback procedure identical to that done for males with low lesions. The more anterior fistulous openings require a formal procedure; however, these openings are large enough for the infants to stool through. For this reason, surgery can be postponed until the child is a month or more of age, at which time a formal Potts transfer procedure is carried out.

Potts Transfer Anoplasty

The child is placed in the lithotomy position with the legs on skis, a Foley catheter is inserted into the bladder, and the perineum is prepared with Betadine and draped appropriately (Figure 16-5a). Either with the child awake or before she is paralyzed, the wink of the external sphincter is found so that the location for the new anus can be marked. A circumferential incision is then made directly around the end of the fistula (Figure 16-5b). With stay sutures on the end of the fistula, the bowel is dissected free from surrounding structures. Small lateral extensions of the incision are frequently needed to allow access to this area.

The anterior rectal wall is in close apposition to the posterior vagina. For this reason, the surgeon should be extremely careful while dissecting the anterior wall of the rectum, because inadvertent injury to the vagina or the rectum can result postoperatively in a rectovaginal fistula. The dissection should be carried up proximally until sufficient length of colon has been freed to allow creation of the anoplasty without

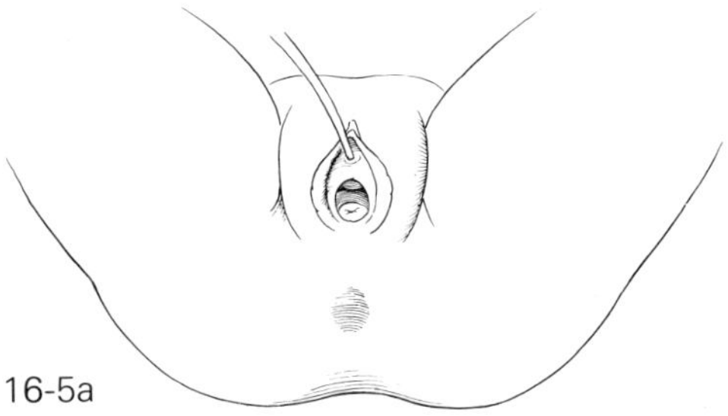

16-5a

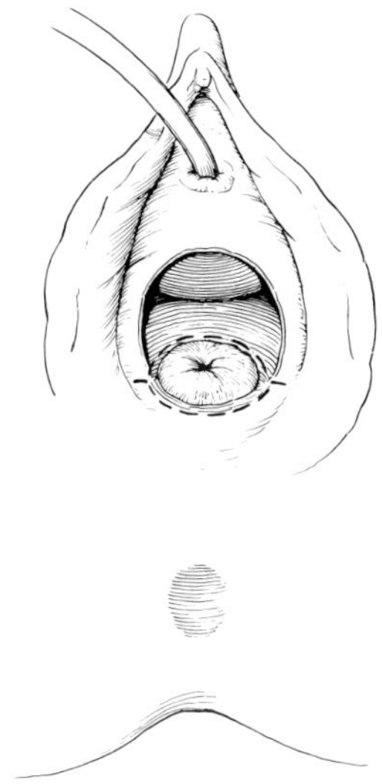

16-5b

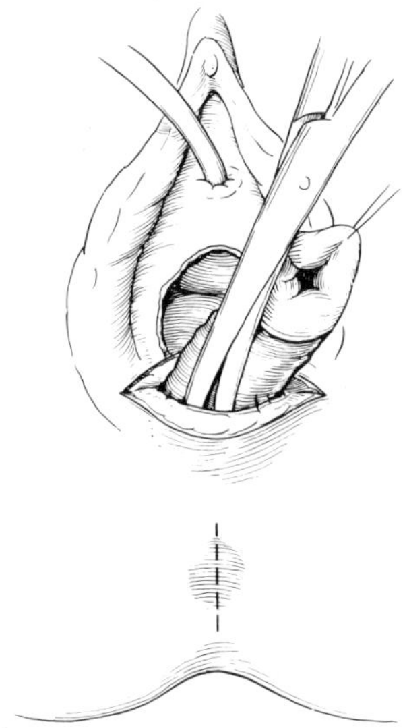

16-5c

tension (Figure 16-5c). The dissection has usually been carried out adequately when the levator muscles are visualized. Almost invariably, the restriction in length is from the anterior part of the rectal dissection. When sufficient length has been obtained, a single vertical incision of 10 to 15 millimeters is made, centered over the area of the planned new anus; with gentle dissection the circular fibers of the external sphincter are visualized. A blunt clamp is then placed through the center of this area, the stay sutures on the end of the rectum are grasped, and the rectum is pulled through the subcutaneous tissue to emerge at the new location (Figure 16-5d). The area between the two incisions will become the new perineal body as the child grows, so great care should be taken to be certain that this skin remains viable. The external sphincter is sutured to the serosa of the rectum with interrupted stitches of 4-0 silk. A new anus is then constructed by using interrupted stitches of 4-0 Dexon going through the entire wall of the rectum and then the skin. The anterior incision is then closed in layers with interrupted 4-0 Dexon suture (Figure 16-5e). A drain is not normally left in place. When the procedure is finished, the anal opening is calibrated with Hegar dilators. A small amount of antibiotic ointment can be left on the incision but no other dressing is applied.

The Foley catheter is removed at 48 hours. A large notice should be placed on the patient's bed to avoid rectal temperatures or any other trauma to this area. Stools should be gently wiped away with a damp cloth. At ten days the new anal opening is calibrated with the fifth finger or with number 8 to 10 Hegar dilators, and the child is discharged. Three weeks after surgery the child is seen in the office, and the mother is instructed about daily dilatations. The dilatations are continued until the anus is large enough and supple enough so that the risk of further stricturing is unlikely.

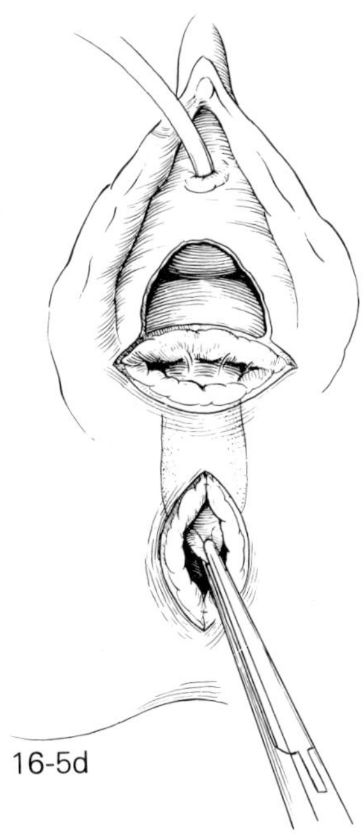

16-5d

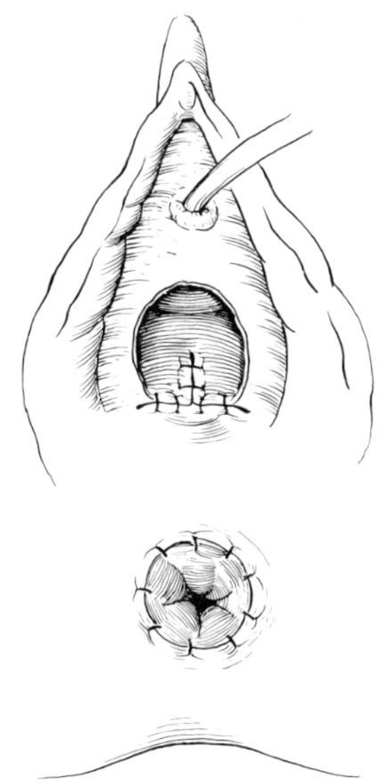

16-5e

Postoperative Complications

Stenosis of the anastomosis is frequently seen and is best prevented and treated by careful dilatations.

Deep wound infections and rectovaginal fistulas are infrequently seen following this type of surgery. If either oc-

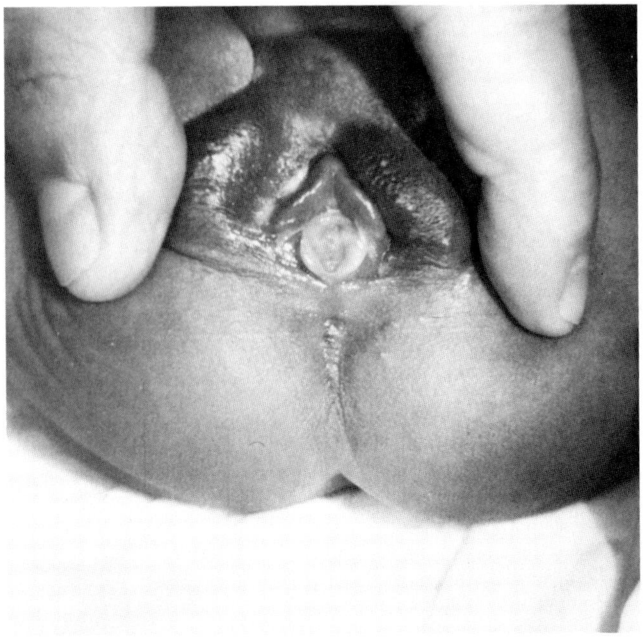

16-6. Female with low imperforate anus discovered by separating the labia.

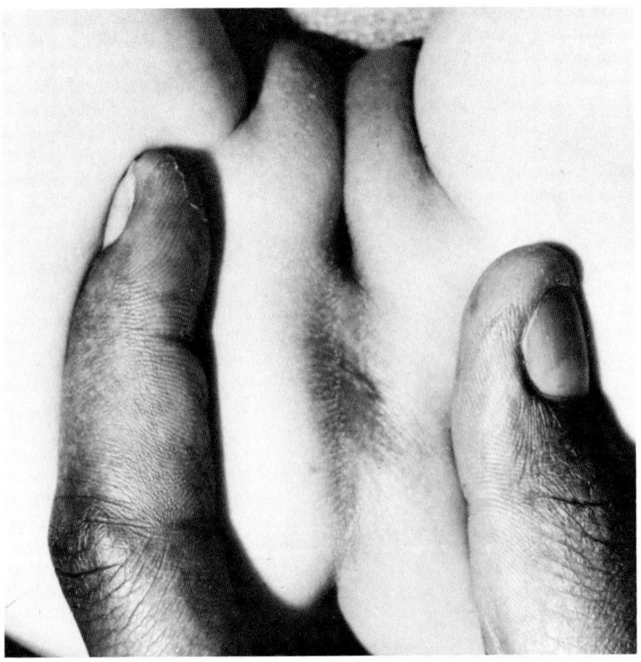

16-7. Female with high imperforate lesion.

curs, careful observation may be the only treatment necessary. Occasionally, a rectovaginal fistula may require a colostomy to allow spontaneous closure. Chronic urinary tract infections are not usually seen in females after this type of surgery.

Females with High Imperforate Anus

If, at 24 hours, careful inspection of the perineum and gentle spreading of the labia fail to demonstrate a low fistulous tract (Figure 16-6), a lateral upside-down abdominal film is taken to assess the end of the air column in relation to the PC line. High lesions are uncommon in females (Figure 16-7), so that examination under anesthesia may be necessary to demonstrate the fistulous opening in the proximal part of the vagina. If a high anomaly is confirmed, a sigmoid loop colostomy as described in Chapter 15 should be performed. Six to 12 months later a sacroperineal pull-through can be done safely. Again, an intravenous pyelogram and roentgenograms of the spine should be obtained before discharge because anomalies in these areas are common in females with high lesions. Urinary fistulas are rare in these infants; thus hyperchloremic acidosis and urinary tract infections are very uncommon.

Associated Anomalies in All Types of Imperforate Anus

Reported incidence of associated anomalies in patients with imperforate anus varies between 25 percent and 75 percent. The most common anomalies are in the urinary tract and the spine. Congenital heart disease and intestinal atresias are also encountered.

Of special note is the high association of esophageal atresia and imperforate anus. In these patients, a colostomy and gastrostomy are done on the first day of life, followed by repair of the esophagus in a few days. The pull-through procedure is carried out when the child is older.

Females with high imperforate anus frequently have genital abnormalities, such as vaginal atresia, vaginal septum, bicornuate uterus, and ambiguous genitalia.

Complications after Anal Surgery

Infants often develop perineal excoriation following surgery for imperforate anus. Local hygiene, use of bland ointments, and gentle removal of stool from the perineum help to eliminate and treat this problem.

Separation of the recto-cutaneous suture line with retraction of the bowel is obviously a serious and potentially life-threatening complication, which requires immediate surgical intervention. If the breakdown is only anterior, as is usually the case, reanastomosis can occasionally be undertaken. A more serious separation should be treated with a proximal colostomy and reanastomosis distally. In both males and females alternate incisions have been tried to relieve suture-

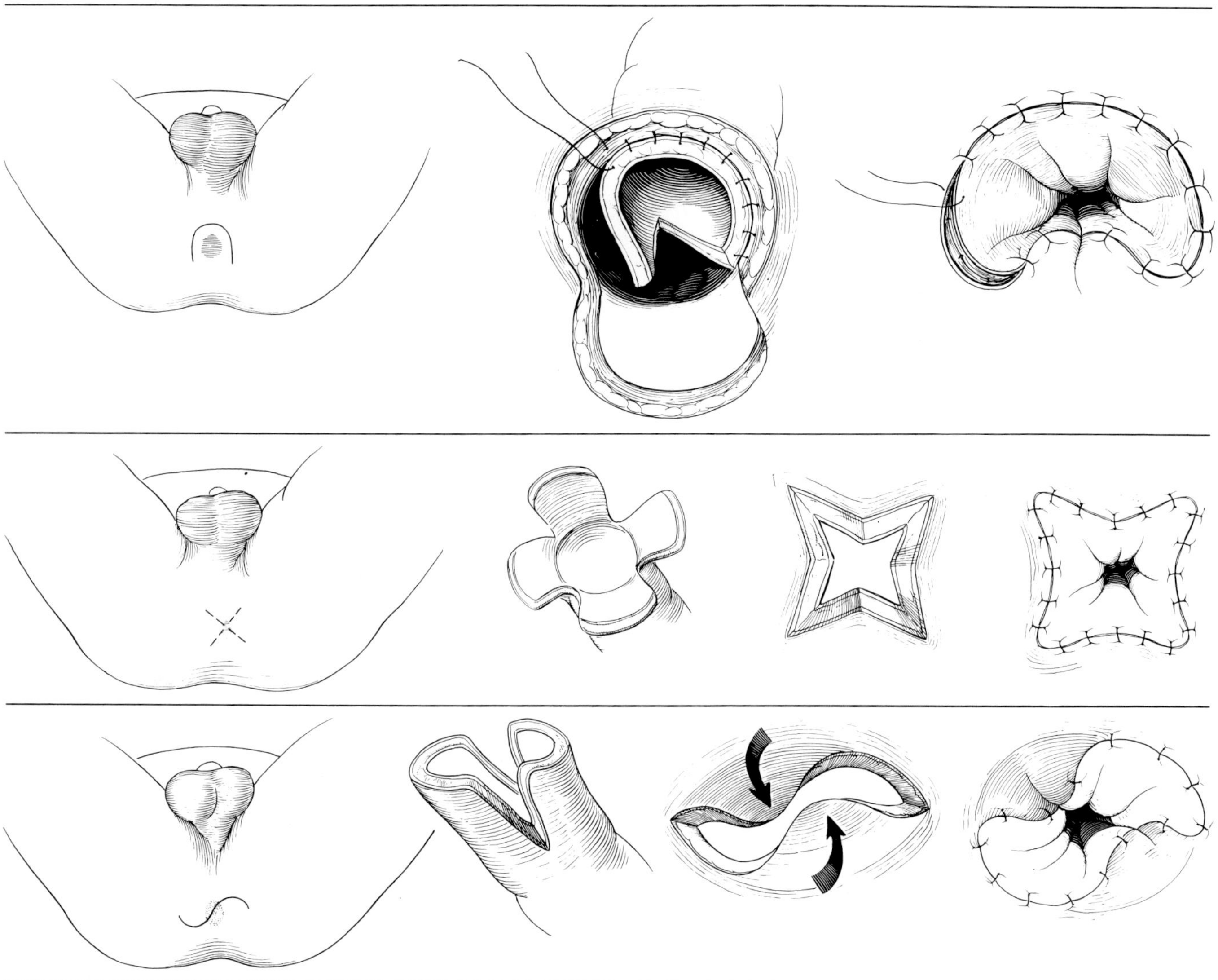

16-8. Three alternative incisions and closures for construction of the anus.

line tension and create a more normal mucocutaneous junction (Figure 16-8). We still prefer the simple vertical incision in Figure 16-5c.

Injury to the urethra, especially in males, can occur if the child does not have a Foley catheter in place. Careful intraoperative attention to this area should prevent such a complication. Urinary retention or incontinence occurs occasionally but it is usually due to a primary neurologic deficit associated with spinal abnormalities rather than to the surgery.

Postoperative fistulas between the rectum and urethra or vagina do occur but are uncommon. Careful surgical technique is the best way to avoid this complication, but treatment may require a backup colostomy and a second surgical procedure.

Permanent fecal incontinence is uncommon in children with low lesions because the rectum has traversed the levator sling, which is the main muscle of continence.

Results and Prognosis

Of children with low anomalies, 85 percent to 90 percent should have normal or near-normal continence. On the other hand, only 50 percent to 65 percent of children with high anomalies will be continent at all times. The remaining patients in both groups will have constipation with or without occasional soiling, particularly during periods of gastroenteritis. Permanent end sigmoid colostomy is rarely necessary except for severe, uncontrollable fecal incontinence.

Selected References

1. Santulli, T. V., Schullinger, J. N., Kiesewetter, W. B., et al. Imperforate anus: A survey from the members of the surgical section of the American Academy of Pediatrics. *J. Pediatr. Surg.* 6:484, 1971.
2. Stephens, F. D., and Smith, E. D. *Anorectal Malformations in Children.* Chicago: Year Book Medical Publishers, 1971.
3. Taylor, I., Duthie, H. L., and Zachary, R. B. Anal continence following surgery for imperforate anus. *J. Pediatr. Surg.* 8:497, 1973.
4. Wiener, E. S., and Kiesewetter, W. B. Urologic abnormalities associated with imperforate anus. *J. Pediatr. Surg.* 8:151, 1973.

17

Omphalocele, Gastroschisis, and Other Anomalies of the Abdominal Wall

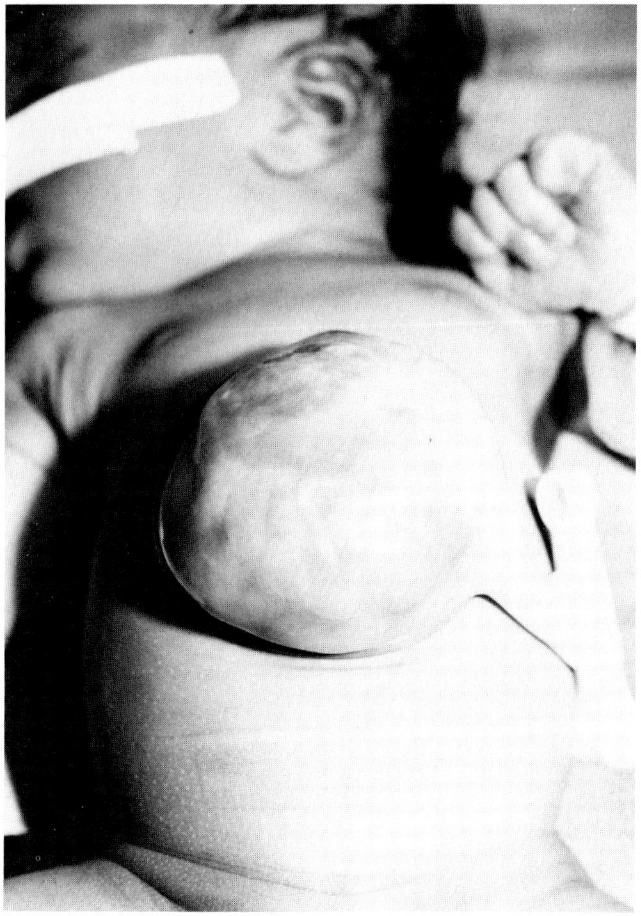

17-1. Medium-sized omphalocele. Umbilical cord is on sac.

Omphalocele

An omphalocele is a herniation of the abdominal viscera into the base of the umbilical cord. It appears as a spherical membranous sac with the umbilical cord inserted on the end of the sac (Figure 17-1). The size of the defect can vary from 2 cm up to the entire breadth of the anterior abdominal wall. The smaller sacs may contain only one or two loops of bowel. In the larger sacs, however, liver, spleen, and much or all of the intestinal tract may be encountered. The diagnosis of omphalocele is usually obvious on gross inspection, so that no studies need be done for confirmation.

Preoperative Preparation

A sterile towel soaked in warm normal saline solution is placed around the sac to protect it. The child is placed in an infant warmer and an intravenous line is started, preferably in the upper extremity. Preoperatively the child is begun on broad-spectrum antibiotics and vitamin K. Type and crossmatch of blood is performed, and a nasogastric tube is placed into the stomach. Loss of colloid occurs across the membranous sac, so that albumin (one gram per kilogram of body weight) is administered.

Operative Technique

General endotracheal anesthesia is used. We prefer balanced anesthesia with muscle relaxants because use of nitrous oxide can increase the amount of gas in the intestine and make it more difficult to reduce the contents back into the abdomen.

The patient is placed in the supine position and the abdomen, umbilical cord, and sac are prepared with Betadine. In those patients in whom the defect is small, the sac can be excised and the intestines returned to the abdomen (Figure 17-2). In this situation the abdominal cavity is closed in layers with 3-0 silk sutures, much as an umbilical hernia is repaired (Figure 17-3). An attempt is made to make the scar look like an umbilicus.

Unfortunately, most omphaloceles are medium to large in size, and the intestines do not fit back into the abdominal cavity without undue pressure on the vena cava (which obstructs venous return) and on the diaphragm (which results in respiratory compromise). Manual stretching of the lateral muscles and fascia of the abdominal cavity occasionally may provide sufficient additional space to allow primary closure.

When primary closure is not feasible, the sac is excised, and the umbilical arteries and vein are ligated (Figure 17-4). Ladd's bands are cut to prevent any potential duodenal obstruction. A standard Stamm gastrostomy (see Chapter 12) is performed and brought out through a separate stab

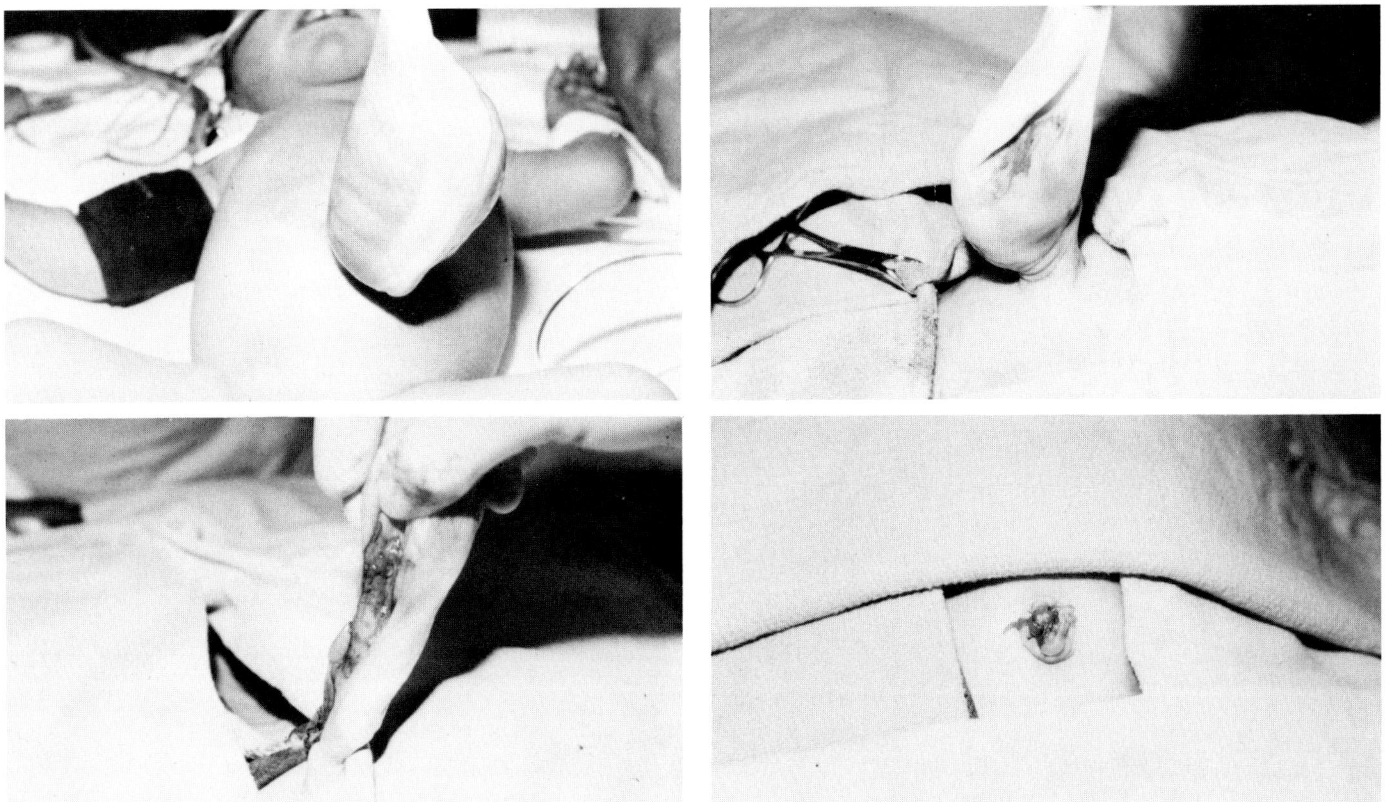

17-2. Sequential views of primary closure of small omphalocele.

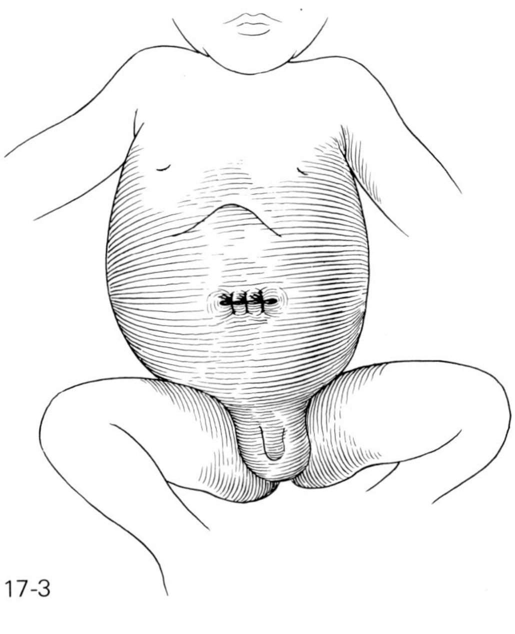

17-3

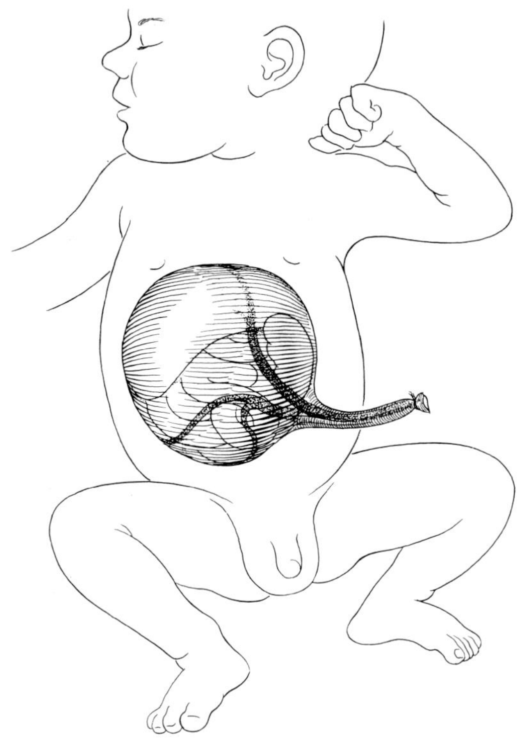

17-4. Large omphalocele with the umbilical vein visible superiorly and the two arteries seen inferiorly. Liver, bowel, and spleen are visible within the sac.

incision in the left upper quadrant. Then a silo of reinforced Silastic mesh (Dow-Corning number 501-3) is created. The mesh is placed next to the edge of the defect, and a running-locking suture of 2-0 Polydek is started at the superior margin and continued all the way around the defect, thus creating a funnel. The suture is placed through all layers of the abdominal wall, including skin and peritoneum (Figure 17-5a). The open end of the mesh is then closed with the same running-suture material (Figure 17-5b). This creates a tall, cylinder-shaped silo. Beginning at the top, the silo is then gently manipulated downward toward the abdomen with a milking motion. Intraabdominal pressure is increased only slightly, so as to have a minimal effect on venous return and diaphragmatic movement. An umbilical tape is then tied around the silo to create a complete pouch. To prevent infection at the junction of the skin and the mesh, the child's abdomen and the silo are wrapped with a Kerlex gauze that has been dipped in Betadine solution. The child is returned to the neonatal intensive care ward in an incubator in which the top of the silo is supported to prevent it from falling to one side (Figure 17-5c).

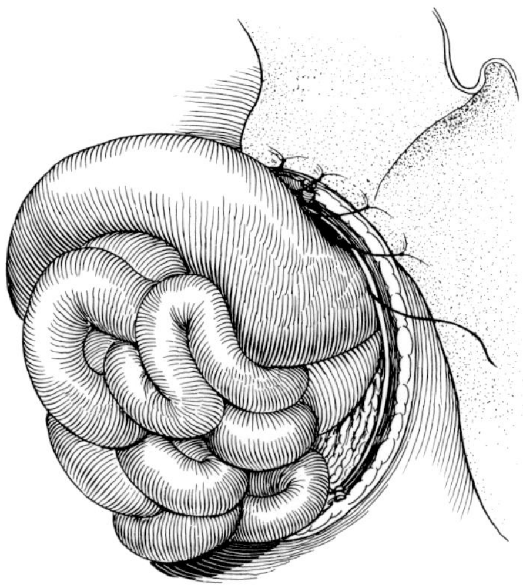

17-5a

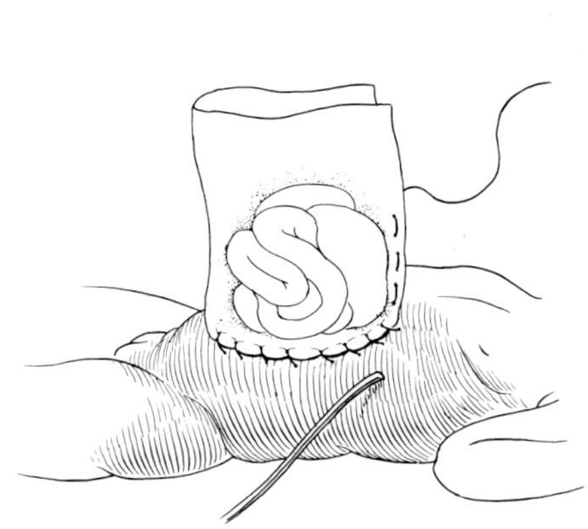

17-5b

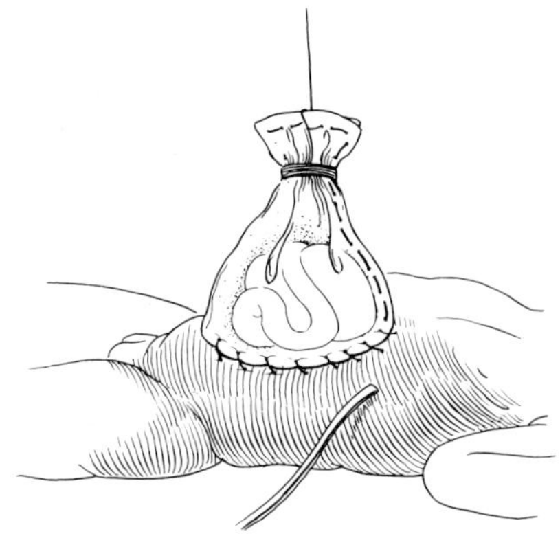

17-5c

Postoperative Care

Fluids are given intravenously according to the infant's needs. The day after surgery, peripheral hyperalimentation is begun to promote positive nitrogen balance while the silo is in place. Antibiotics are continued until three days after the silo has been removed. Once each day, in the child's warmer or isolette, the surgeon gently compresses the silo farther down toward the abdomen and ties a new umbilical tape at each new level (Figure 17-6). Within five to ten days the abdomen will have enlarged enough to accept the intestinal contents, and the lowest umbilical tape will be flush with the anterior abdominal wall. The sequence rarely takes longer than seven days. In fact, by 10 to 12 days the sutures begin to pull out of the skin and fascia, so that every effort should be made to reduce the contents back into the abdomen as quickly as possible. Betadine solution is dripped on the silo continually during this period.

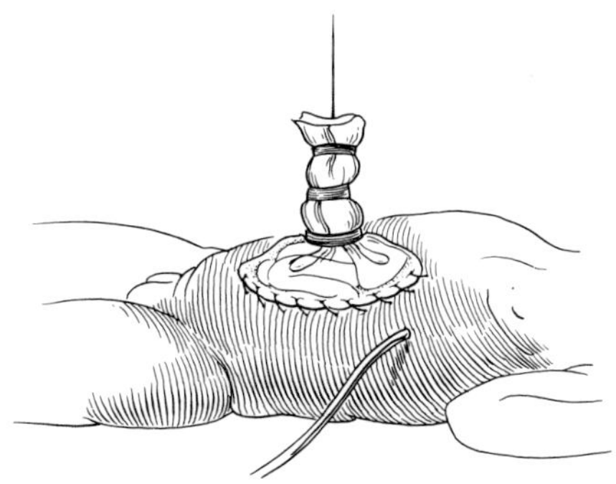

17-6

Once the viscera have been reduced into the abdominal cavity, the child is taken back to the operating room, and the silo is removed. Again, nitrous oxide is not used as an anesthetic. An appendectomy may be performed to avoid appendicitis in future years in a colon that is abnormally rotated. The appendectomy is not done at the original operation because of the presence of a foreign body, the silo. The fascia is freed from the skin all the way around the defect and is then closed with interrupted simple sutures of 2-0 and 3-0

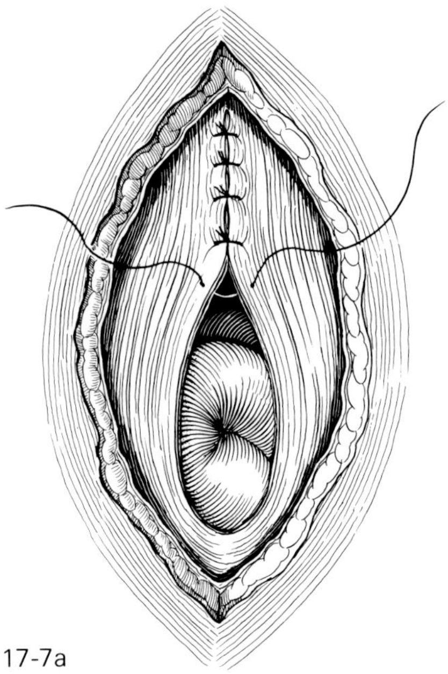

17-7a

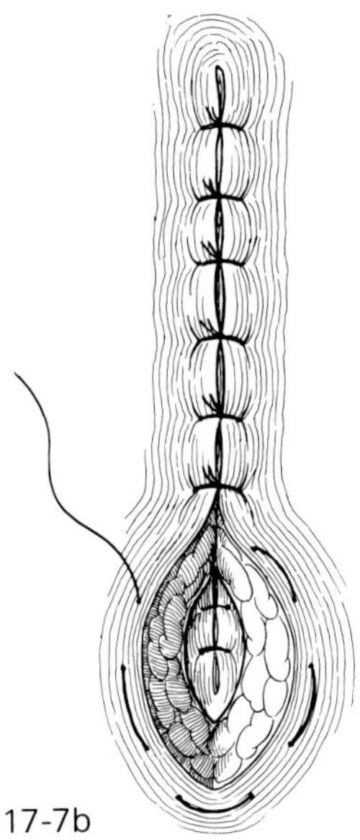

17-7b

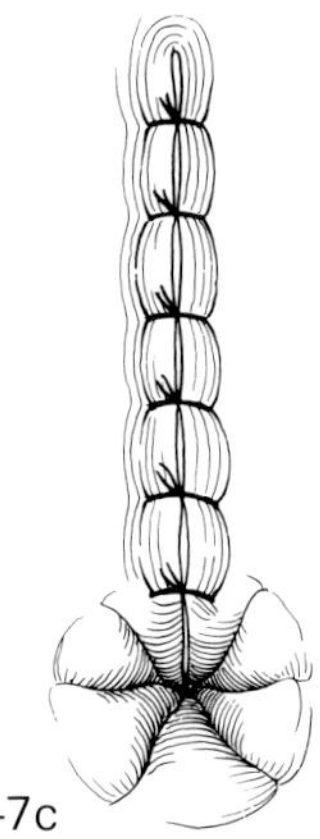

17-7c

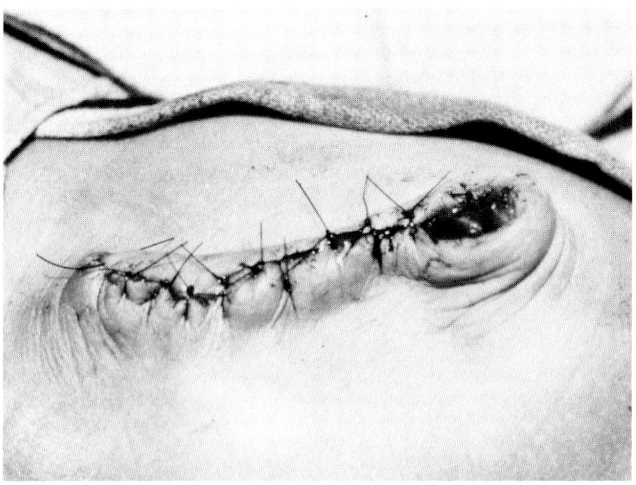

17-8. Skin closed in infant with omphalocele. The inferior aspect is closed with a pursestring to create the impression of an umbilicus.

silk or Tefdek (Figure 17-7a). The skin is closed with interrupted 4-0 silk (Figure 17-7b). For cosmetic reasons, an attempt is made to create a new umbilicus. This is easily done by using a pursestring suture to close the inferior 2 cm of the incision (Figure 17-7c). The puckered appearance is not perfect but usually is satisfactory (Figure 17-8).

Postoperatively, the child is gradually advanced on oral feedings and is discharged after a search for associated anomalies has been completed.

Conservative Treatment

Occasionally an intact omphalocoele is so large as to preclude any type of primary or secondary closure, or a child may be seen with severe associated congenital anomalies that make immediate surgery impractical. In this situation it is possible to paint the sac with 2% tincture of Mercurochrome every four hours. With this regimen the sac will become crusted and hard and will slowly shrink down and close. At a later date a ventral herniorrhaphy will be necessary. This method should not be used except in extreme cases.

Ruptured Omphalocele

An antepartum or postpartum rupture of an omphalocele will be associated with all the problems that have previously been discussed under unruptured omphalocele. In addition, these infants will have the intestinal problems seen with gastroschisis and should be handled in the same way as patients with gastroschisis.

Complications

Compromise of the venous return from the lower extremities is best treated by avoiding primary closure in larger lesions (Figure 17-9). If primary closure has already been carried out and the patient has obvious severe venous stasis in the lower extremities, the child should be returned to the operating room, the fascia opened, and a silo inserted.

Atelectasis, especially in the lower lobes, is common after repair of large omphaloceles. Meticulous pulmonary toilet, occasionally with an endotracheal tube in place, may be needed to clear the atelectasis. In severe cases, again, consideration should be given to reducing abdominal pressure by placement of a silo if a primary closure has been performed.

The Silastic pouch can pull away from the skin before the extraabdominal contents have been returned into the abdomen. The wound separation requires reoperation and reformation of the silo.

Sepsis has been a frequent complication of silo insertion. The addition of the continuous Betadine drip to the pouch has reduced the infection rate significantly.

Incarceration or strangulation of the bowel in the pouch by the edges of the defect can occur. This is best avoided by careful suturing of the original silo. If incarceration or strangulation of the bowel is encountered, secondary repair of the silo with appropriate intestinal surgery is indicated. Intestinal resections and anastomoses or ileostomies can be performed in combination with primary closure or silo insertion.

Midgut volvulus has been reported in patients with repaired omphaloceles and is related to malrotation. This should not occur if a Ladd's procedure is done at the original operation, but volvulus must always be considered in the postoperative patient who develops signs of intestinal obstruction.

An important late complication is the development of a ventral hernia (Figure 17-10). Whether large or small, these hernias should not be repaired until the child is at least two years old. Reoperation is usually difficult and hazardous because the abdominal viscera are adherent to the underside of the skin. Rarely is prosthetic material necessary to repair the defect.

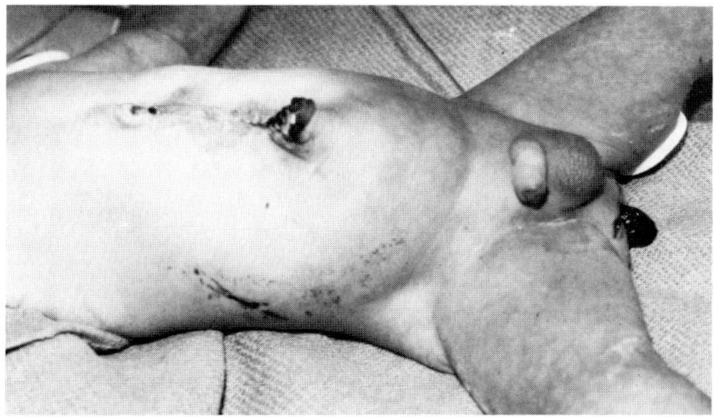

17-9. Infant with omphalocele closed primarily under too much tension with subsequent venous stasis.

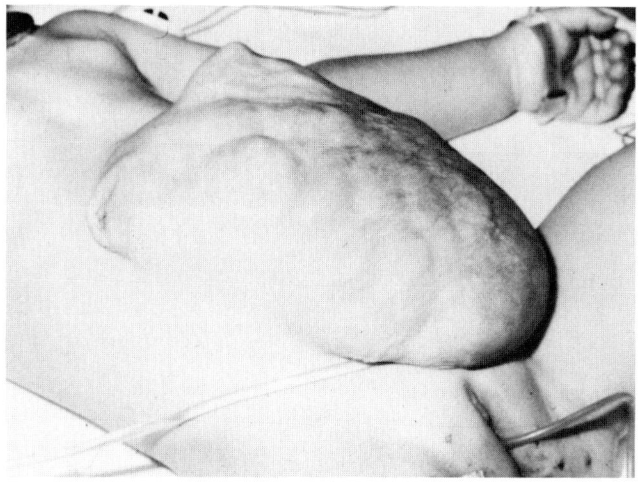

17-10. Large ventral hernia that occurred after treatment of an omphalocele by a skin closure only.

Results

In children without associated anomalies, the overall results should be excellent.

Table 17-1. Differentiation between omphalocele and gastroschisis

Factor	Omphalocele	Gastroschisis
Defect size	2–15 cm	2–3 cm
Sac	Always (may rupture)	Never
Umbilicus	End of sac	Left of defect
Contents	Bowel, liver, or both	Bowel
Quality of bowel	Normal	Edematous
Nonrotation	Yes	Yes
Alimentation	Normal	Delayed
Associated anomalies	Approximately 50%	Uncommon

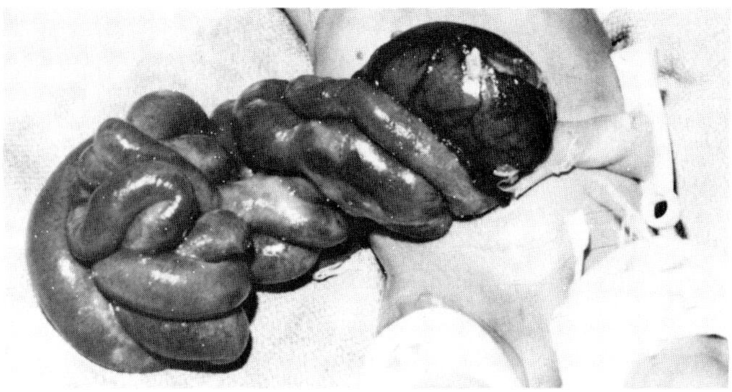

17-11. Newborn with gastroschisis.

Gastroschisis

Gastroschisis can usually be clinically differentiated from a ruptured omphalocele. However, the operative management of both is similar. In general, the clinical differentiation between omphalocele and gastroschisis is useful; Table 17-1 lists a number of categories that help make the distinction. An omphalocele is a hernia of the intestinal contents into the base of the umbilical cord, while gastroschisis is a defect of the abdominal wall to the right of the midline that allows bowel to escape from the abdomen in utero. In gastroschisis a normal umbilical cord is always present, and the bowel is not protected by a sac; as a result, the bowel becomes irritated by its contact with the amniotic fluid. This bathing with amniotic fluid results in significant intestinal-wall inflammation and fibrosis, with resultant decrease in the peristaltic and absorptive capabilities of the bowel during the postoperative period (Figure 17-11).

Patients with gastroschisis have a low incidence of associated congenital anomalies when compared to babies with omphalocele. Therefore, although infants with gastroschisis have a more prolonged immediate postoperative course because of poor bowel function, their late survival rate is better than that of babies with omphalocele.

The diagnosis of gastroschisis is simple. Usually it is made by the obstetrician or pediatrician immediately after birth.

Preoperative Preparation

The patient should have an adequate intravenous line placed in an upper extremity. The infant is started on broad-spectrum antibiotic coverage and is given vitamin K; a sterile towel soaked with warm normal saline solution is placed around the intestines. Great care must be taken to keep the child warm, because heat loss from the exposed intestine can be very rapid. In addition, there is considerable loss of protein and electrolytes from the bowel wall; therefore albumin is administered intravenously at the rate of 1 to 2 g per kilogram of body weight during the hour that the patient is being prepared for surgery.

Surgery is done on an infant warmer with the patient in the supine position (Figure 17-12). The patient is only painted

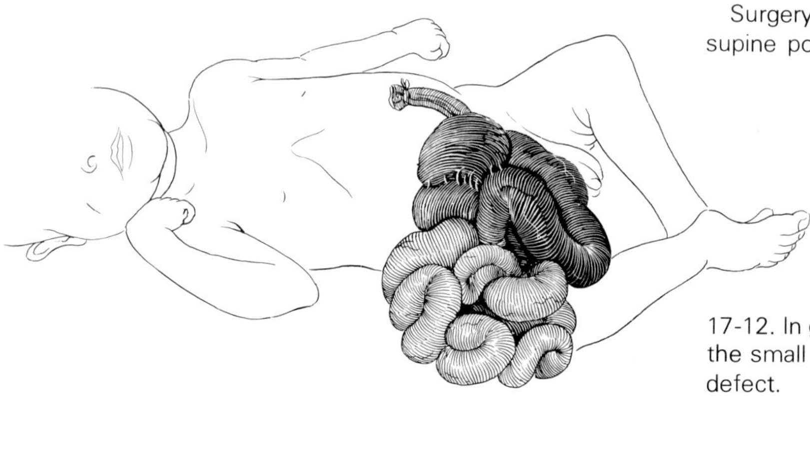

17-12. In gastroschisis only the bowel protrudes through the small defect. The umbilicus is to the left of the infant's defect.

with Betadine, because a regular preparation will cause excessive heat loss from evaporation. As in patients with omphalocele, nitrous oxide should be avoided as part of the anesthetic regimen. Our choice for anesthesia is a balanced technique with muscle relaxation.

The abdominal defect is always small. To allow adequate exposure, it is enlarged superiorly in the midline approximately one inch (Figure 17-13). If the amount of bowel outside the abdomen is not excessive, the intestine may be placed back into the abdomen after gentle stretching of the abdominal wall, and primary closure may be achieved. In these patients a midline fascial closure with 2-0 or 3-0 Tefdek and a skin closure of 4-0 silk is possible. Children who can be treated thus usually have a benign postoperative course with relatively rapid return of bowel function.

Unfortunately, the amount of thickened, edematous bowel is often too great to allow primary closure, and the patient must be treated with a silo similar to that created for the large omphalocele, described in the first portion of this chapter. The exposed bowel may appear foreshortened, atretic, or even necrotic, but true necrosis is rarely the case. In fact, no intestinal surgery should be undertaken because it is hazardous, bloody, and usually not necessary. Instead, a Stamm gastrostomy with a number 12 or 14 Malecot catheter should be performed (see Chapter 12) and brought out through a stab wound in the left upper quadrant. Then a number 501-3 Dacron reinforced Silastic sheet should be sewn completely around the defect using a 2-0 Polydek suture with a running-locking stitch (Figure 17-14). The side of the silo is then sewn in a similar fashion and the top is tied off with umbilical tape, as has been previously described for omphalocele. A Kerlex roll soaked with Betadine is wrapped around the silo. The umbilical vessels are ligated close to the skin.

Postoperative Course

Delayed function of the intestinal tract is the rule in patients with gastroschisis. Hyperalimentation is therefore almost always necessary. We use peripheral hyperalimentation to eliminate the need for a central venous catheter. The gastrostomy tube is left to gravity drainage. Each day the Silastic chimney is compressed downward, and a new umbilical tape is tied on it to keep pressure on the abdominal contents. The silo is supported from the top of the isolette or infant warmer to prevent kinking.

In gastroschisis the silo can usually be reduced much more quickly than in omphalocele. One of the reasons for this is that the edematous fluid in the intestinal wall rapidly returns to the circulation by gravity. As a result, the actual volume of the extracoelomic contents is reduced. It is important to achieve rapid reduction of the silo because the sutures holding the silo to the abdominal wall will not last longer than 10

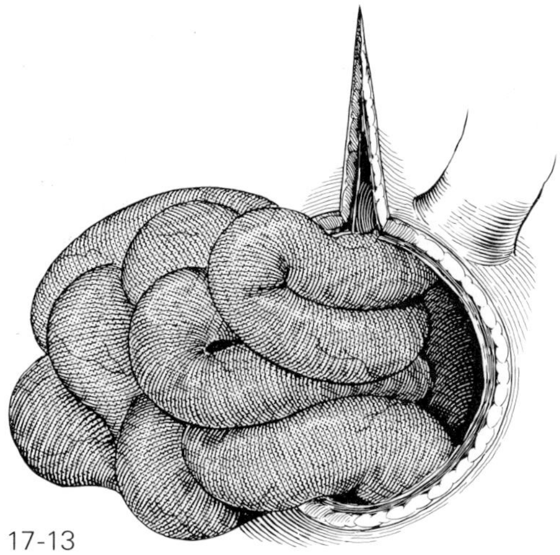

17-13

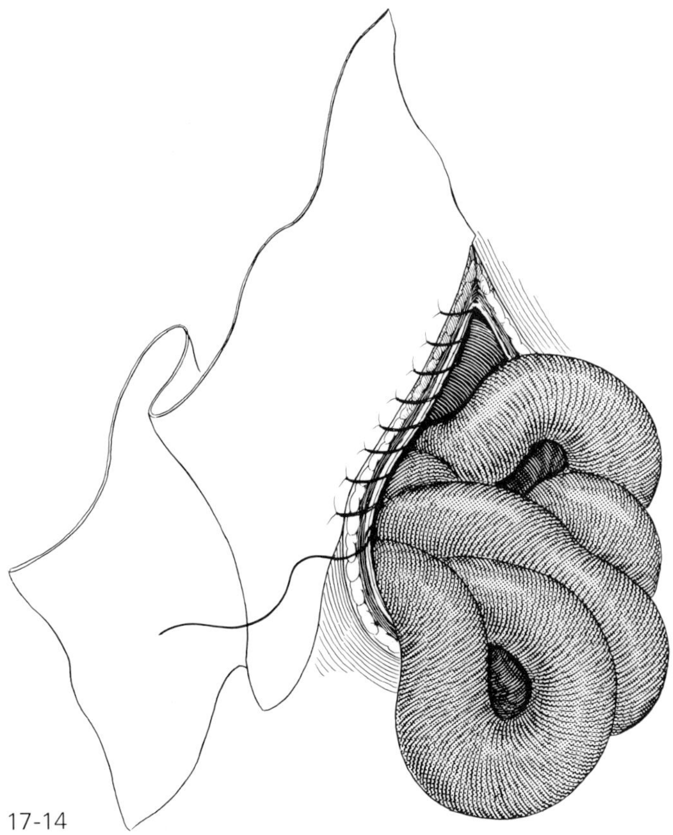

17-14

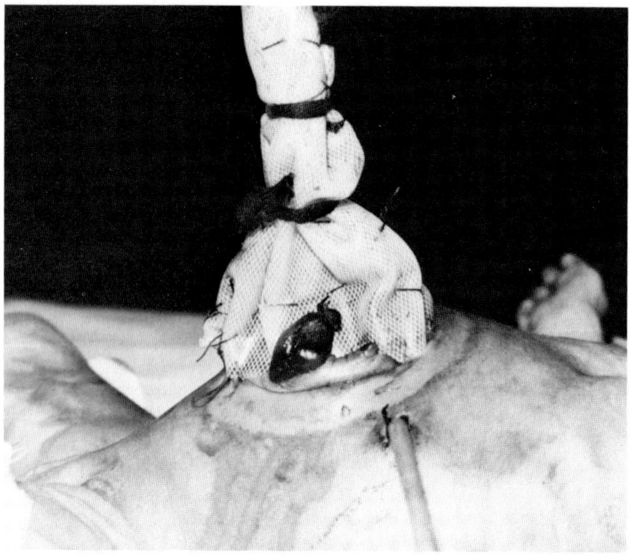

17-15. Infant with gastroschisis. Silon has been completely reduced and the baby is ready for delayed primary closure.

to 12 days. In gastroschisis the reduction is accomplished within four to six days, at which time the patient is taken back to the operating room and the sheeting is excised (Figure 17-15).

In gastroschisis the large number of intestinal adhesions significantly reduce the likelihood of postoperative volvulus. Appendectomy is not routinely undertaken because of the edema and inflammation of the intestinal wall. The fascia and the skin are separated, the midline fascia is closed with 2-0 or 3-0 Tefdek, and the skin is closed with 4-0 silk.

After the final operation intestinal motility slowly returns, usually within three weeks. Peripheral hyperalimentation is continued until oral nutrition is adequate. If an associated bowel atresia (incidence of 15 percent) is suspected, this should not be repaired until about three weeks after the final operation. At that time the intestines are much easier to resect and anastomose.

Complications

All the postoperative problems encountered in omphalocele patients are also seen in gastroschisis. In addition, decreased intestinal motility and enterocutaneous fistulas contribute to the morbidity and mortality of infants with gastroschisis. Hyperalimentation is helpful in each of these complications and is continued until normal intestinal function returns. Occasionally the fistulas require resection and anastomosis.

Results

Poor postoperative intestinal function and enterocutaneous fistulas resulted in a mortality approaching 95 percent before institution of Silastic pouches and hyperalimentation. The addition of these modalities has reversed the mortality figures, so that now most of these infants can be expected to survive and lead a normal life.

Other Abnormalities of the Abdominal Wall

Umbilical Hernias

This defect is asymptomatic and more than 90 percent undergo spontaneous closure during the first two years of life. Surgical treatment of this defect should therefore be delayed until well beyond infancy.

Omphalomesenteric Remnants

Persistence of parts of the omphalomesenteric duct is uncommon, but a number of variations can be encountered. Figure 17-16 depicts six of the possible presentations. These may be cystic, may bleed, may cause volvulus, or may drain stool or mucus. Each can be explored through a transverse infraumbilical incision, through which the umbilical end is excised and the intraabdominal portion is reconstructed as necessary.

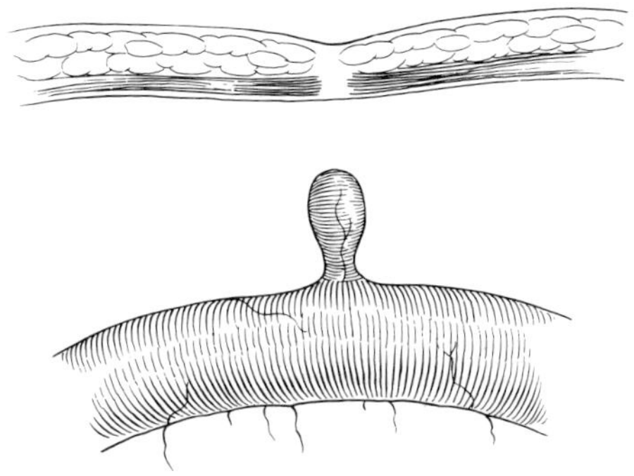

17-16a. Meckel's diverticulum.

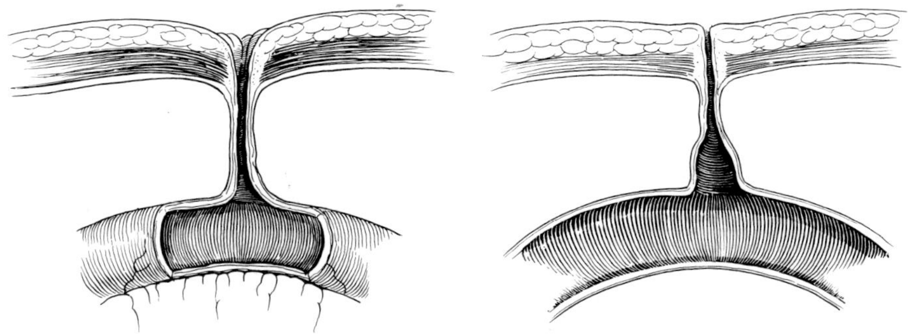

17-16b, c. Patent omphalomesenteric ducts.

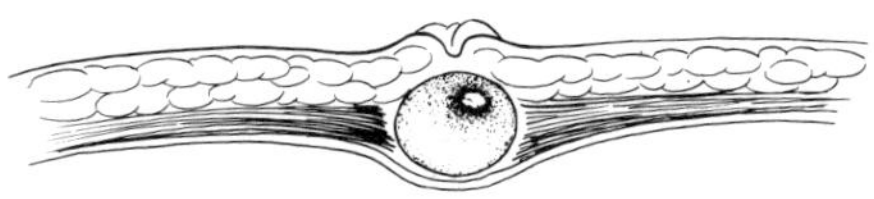

17-16d. Omphalomesenteric duct cyst.

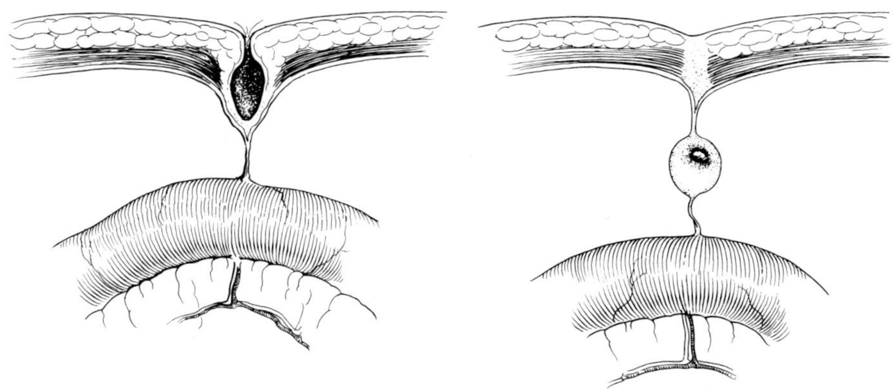

17-16e, f. Omphalomesenteric duct cyst with vitelline duct remnant.

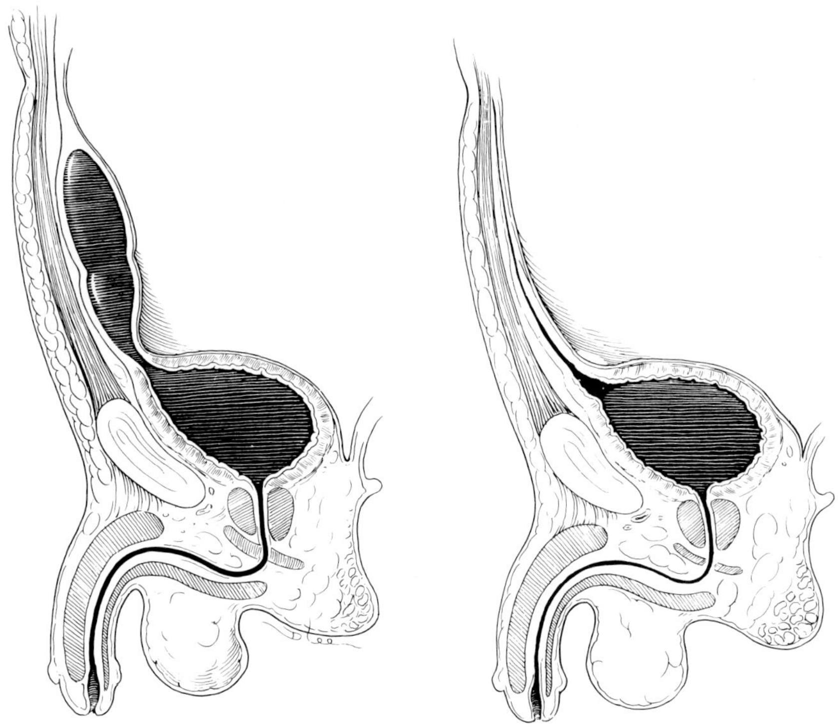

17-17. Small and large urachal remnants may be open at the umbilicus.

Urachal Remnants

A so-called wet umbilicus is suggestive of a patent urachus (Figure 17-17). An intravenous pyelogram may be obtained for preoperative evaluation. The patient is explored through a transverse infraumbilical incision. The urachal remnant, which is extraperitoneal, is excised, and the dome of the bladder is closed in two layers with 3-0 chromic catgut.

Exstrophy of the Bladder

Exstrophy of the bladder is a result of failure of the bladder to turn in and fuse. The bladder mucosa is exposed, and the ureteral orifices are visible. Early surgical intervention in these infants is unnecessary. The infants usually do well at home with no initial therapy. When they weigh 10 kilograms (20 pounds) or more, a turn-in procedure or a urinary diversion can be considered.

Exstrophy of the Cloaca

Exstrophy of the cloaca is one of the most complex and serious congenital anomalies. Infants who have exstrophy of the cloaca are usually premature. The anomaly consists of exstrophy of the bladder, omphalocele, imperforate anus, agenesis of the colon, decreased small bowel length, and vesicointestinal fistula (Figure 17-18). More than half of the patients also have myelomeningoceles (and subsequent hydrocephalus). Initial sex determination is often difficult, so that chromosomal studies are necessary. Anomalies of the upper urinary tract and orthopedic anomalies are frequently present.

The diagnosis is apparent at birth. From the outset, a multispecialty approach is needed. The family should be made aware of the long-term prognosis, especially in the infants with myelomeningocele.

At surgery, the omphalocele sac is excised, and the umbilical arteries and vein are ligated. The intestine is traced distally to its end in the middle of the exstrophied bladder. The end is transected, and an ileostomy is created in the right lower quadrant. There may be a small remnant of right colon connected to the bladder; this can be left in place for future use in reconstructing bowel or bladder. A gastrostomy is created, and the defect of the abdominal wall is closed in a single or double layer with 2-0 or 3-0 Tefdek and 4-0 silk. At the end of the first operation the child is left with exstrophy of the bladder and a permanent ileostomy (Figure 17-19). Reconstruction of the urinary system is undertaken in 12 to 24 months.

Postoperative problems are frequent. Voluminous fluid loss from the ileostomy is common and accurate measurement of intake and output is essential. Urine output is difficult to quantitate but measurements of specific gravity are helpful in assessing the state of hydration.

The problems of omphalocele closure and short-gut syndrome may add to the nutritional problems. Proper sex assessment usually requires chromosomal studies.

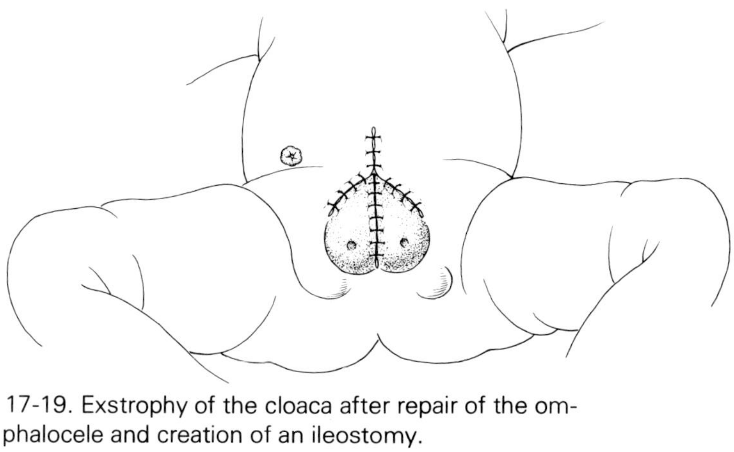

17-19. Exstrophy of the cloaca after repair of the omphalocele and creation of an ileostomy.

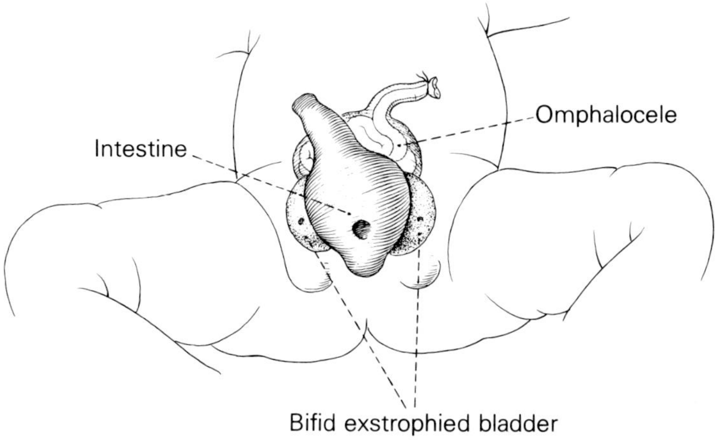

17-18. Exstrophy of the cloaca. The omphalocele and the vesicointestinal fistula in the center of the exstrophied bladder are visible.

Selected References

1. Allen, R. R., and Wrenn, E. L., Jr. Silon as a sac in the treatment of omphalocele and gastroschisis. *J. Pediatr. Surg.* 4:3, 1969.
2. Bill, A. H. In W. T. Mustard, M. M. Ravitch, W. H. Snyder, Jr., et al. (eds.), *Pediatric Surgery.* Chicago: Year Book Medical Publishers, 1969.
3. Binnington, H. B., Keating, J. P., and Ternberg, J. L. Gastroschisis. *Arch. Surg.* 108:455, 1974.
4. Cordero, L., et al. Staged repair of gastroschisis with Silastic sheeting. *Surgery* 65:676, 1969.
5. Croom, R. D., III, and Thomas, C. G., Jr. Repair of gastroschisis. *Surg. Gynecol. Obstetr.* 132:689, 1971.
6. Girvan, D. P., Webster, D. M., and Shandling, D. The treatment of omphalocele and gastroschisis. *Surg. Gynecol. Obstetr.* 139(2):222–4, 1974.
7. Hollabaugh, R. S., and Boles, E. T., Jr. The management of gastroschisis. *J. Pediatr. Surg.* 8:263, 1973.
8. Lewis, J. E., Jr., Kraeger, R. R., and Danis, R. K. Gastroschisis: Ten-year review. *Arch. Surg.* 92:218, 1973.
9. Schuster, S. R. A new method for the staged repair of large omphalocele. *Surg. Gynecol. Obstetr.* 125:837, 1967.
10. Wesselhoeft, C. W., Porter, A., and Deluca, F. G. The treatment of omphalocele and gastroschisis. *Ann. Chir. Infant.* 13:237, 1972.
11. Zwiren, G. T., and Patterson, J. H. Exstrophy of the cloaca: Report of a case treated surgically. *Pediatrics* 35:687, 1965.

18

Abdominal Masses

Abdominal masses are surprisingly common in the newborn. Although many masses are asymptomatic, others may affect the function of the urinary system or result in intestinal obstruction. It is often possible to make a correct preoperative diagnosis in infants with abdominal masses after a careful physical examination and a few selected laboratory or radiologic procedures.

Differential Diagnosis

A proper physical examination of an infant requires much patience on the part of the surgeon. The child should be quiet; a pacifier or bottle may help. Flexing the patient's thighs at the hips with the left hand while gently palpating with the right is frequently helpful to the right-handed surgeon. Removal of gastric fluid and air with a nasogastric tube may also aid in the examination. Rectal examination is useful in the small infant; a bimanual examination is possible with the finger in the rectum. If at all possible, the surgeon's index finger should be used in the rectum, because it allows for better proprioception than does the fifth finger.

Chest roentgenogram, along with flat and upright views of the abdomen, are occasionally diagnostic, but frequently further x-ray studies are needed. An intravenous pyelogram done through an ankle vein is the single most useful radiologic procedure. With the foot as an injection site, an early film provides an inferior vena cavagram, while subsequent films delineate the kidneys and collecting system. A voiding film or film taken after voiding is obtained to evaluate the bladder neck, urethra, and ureteral reflux. Retrograde pyelography is rarely possible or necessary in the newborn. Upper and lower gastrointestinal series can also be helpful in a number of circumstances. It is particularly helpful if the surgeon is present during the fluoroscopic studies to assist the radiologist in interpreting the study and correlating it with the physical findings. Arteriograms and radionuclear scans may also help to define certain problems.

Abdominal masses in the neonate fall into five general categories:

- URINARY TRACT
  - Midline
    - Distended bladder
    - Horseshoe kidney
    - Urachal remnants
  - Bilateral flank
    - Hydroureter and hydronephrosis
      - Ureteropelvic junction obstruction
      - Posterior urethral valves
      - Prune-belly syndrome
      - Ureteroceles
    - Polycystic disease
  - Unilateral flank
    - Multicystic disease
    - Ureteropelvic junction obstruction
    - Wilms' tumor
    - Renal vein thrombosis
- GASTROINTESTINAL TRACT
  - Duplications
  - Mesenteric cysts
- GENITAL TRACT
  - Hydrocolpos
  - Ovarian cysts
  - Intersex
- HEPATOBILIARY SYSTEM
  - Hepatoma
  - Hepatoblastoma
  - Hepatic cyst
  - Choledochal cyst
  - Vascular abnormalities
    - Hemangioma
    - Hemangioendothelioma
    - Arteriovenous malformation
- OTHER
  - Adrenal hematoma
  - Splenic hematoma
  - Splenic cyst
  - Anterior myelomeningocoele
  - Neuroblastoma
  - Sacrococcygeal teratoma

Each of these conditions will be discussed in detail in this chapter. Occasionally a true exploratory laparotomy is necessary to diagnose and to treat an abdominal mass.

Exploratory Laparotomy

The preoperative preparations depend on the suspected diagnosis but in general follow the guidelines set up in Chapters 1 and 2. The intravenous line should be placed in an upper extremity so that, if excessive bleeding is encountered, blood can be administered above the lesion.

For the laparotomy, a transverse incision in the right or left upper quadrant is made 1 cm above the umbilicus. The rectus is transected with the cautery. The peritoneum is entered carefully under direct vision. All the abdominal contents of a neonate can be thoroughly inspected and operated upon through this incision. The intestines are eviscerated and covered with a warm moist pad. An orderly, stepwise approach is taken in order to inspect everything. Warm wet sponges are used, and the surgeon must be very gentle in order to avoid injury to the delicate organs of a newborn. In certain ways, the exploration of a newborn's abdomen must be differentiated from the exploratory laparotomy in an adult. There is essentially no fat in the omentum of a neonate, and the thin, filmy structure tears easily. The spleen is very mobile but also quite friable. Thus the spleen also must be handled with great care. When the bowel is examined it must be kept warm and moist and handled cautiously, because the serosa tears readily. Moreover, loss of heat or protein, or both, occurs rapidly.

When closing the abdomen of a neonate, the surgeon closes the posterior rectus sheath and peritoneum as a single layer with running 4-0 Dexon. The thin, filmy omentum tends to pop out between stitches and must be carefully placed back inside before the final stitch is pulled up and tied. The anterior fascia is closed with interrupted 4-0 silk. The subcutaneous tissue, if thick enough, is closed with running 4-0 Dexon and the skin is sutured with running 5-0 nylon. A small dressing is used so as not to restrict breathing. If a gastrostomy was not left in place, a nasogastric tube should be inserted and placed to gravity drainage.

Lesions of the Urinary Tract

Most abdominal masses in the newborn originate in the urinary tract, and most are the result of obstruction. Essentially, all these lesions can be delineated with an intravenous pyelogram, but occasionally a voiding cystourethrogram, as an additional procedure, will further define the abnormality.

Masses in the Lower Midline

A distended bladder may account for a mass felt intermittently on physical examination. Transillumination can be helpful in outlining the distended bladder (Figure 18-1). Frequently there is no organic cause for the distended bladder, and the child does well without further treatment. However, in males a search for posterior urethral valves should be

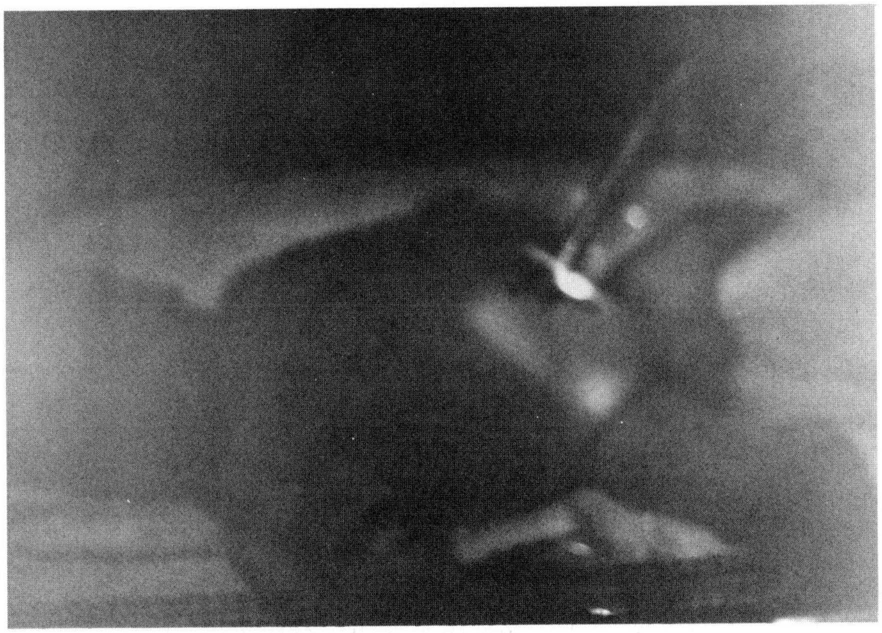

18-1

undertaken. Horseshoe kidneys or crossed renal ectopia should be apparent from the inferior vena cavagram and the intravenous pyelogram. Surgery should, of course, be avoided in these latter two conditions. The urethral meatus should be inspected because obstruction at this point can cause a large bladder and this can be cured with a simple meatotomy. Obstruction of the bladder neck was once a very frequent diagnosis, but at present, particularly in the newborn, this diagnosis is rare. Urachal remnants, which can be encountered in neonates, are discussed in Chapter 17.

Bilateral Masses of the Flank

Bilateral flank masses are worrisome when encountered in the newborn because the causes are serious diseases that affect both kidneys, with the resultant possibility of significant loss of renal function. Bilateral hydronephrosis and hydroureters should be suspected in a child when a mass is palpable in each flank. The intravenous pyelogram will greatly aid in delineating the lesion, but a 24-hour delayed x-ray film of the abdomen may be necessary because of poor excretion in patients with these problems. The use of fiberoptic transillumination will help differentiate hydronephrosis from distended loops of bowel. There are several different disease processes that can cause bilateral hydronephrosis.

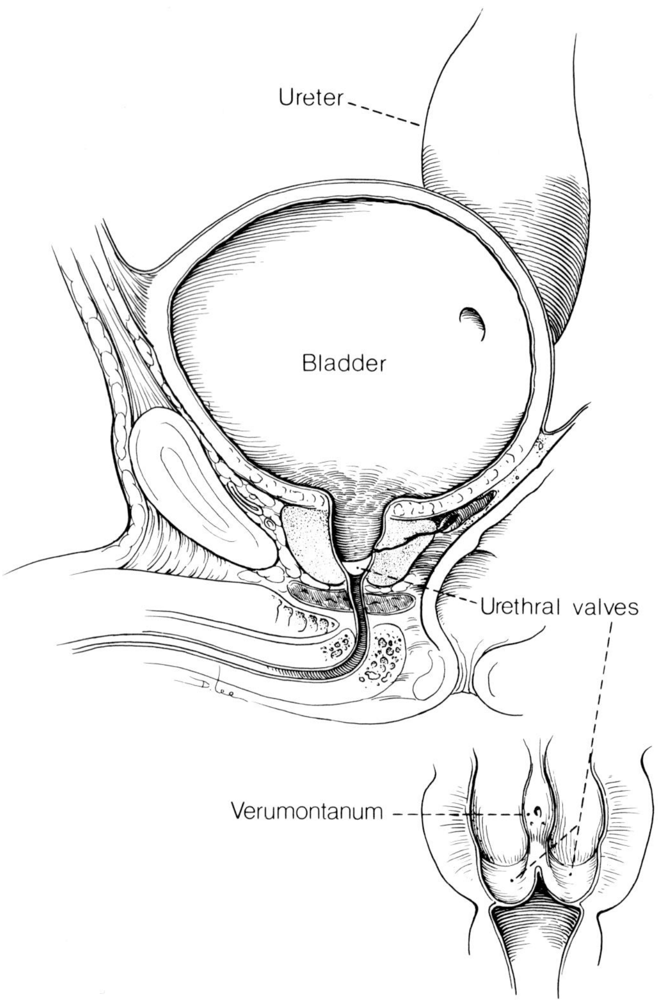

18-2. Thin, almost transparent valves appear like sails that obstruct the urethra at the level of the verumontanum. The proximal urethra, bladder, and ureters become dilated.

Posterior Urethral Valves

This problem is seen almost exclusively in males. When embryologic remnants of two valvelike structures near the verumontanum persist there is resultant obstruction at the area of the prostatic urethra, which causes dilatation of the proximal urethra, then of the bladder, and finally of the ureters and renal pelves (Figure 18-2). The degree of obstruction is in general related to the amount of permanent destruction of renal parenchyma. On the other hand, there may well be sufficient remaining renal tissue to allow for normal function if the diagnosis is made early and appropriate treatment is instituted. Logically it would appear that these patients should void infrequently and only dribble urine. This is not true. In fact, a good strong, long stream can occur in these male infants. The surgeon should not disregard this diagnosis just because a forceful stream has been seen in the examining room. Intravenous pyelography will reveal the dilated urinary system, and a separate voiding cystourethrogram (as in Figure 18-3) will occasionally demonstrate the saillike appearance of the valves one-third of the way down the urethra. More commonly, however, the clue to the radiologic diagnosis is the dilated posterior urethra.

When the diagnosis of posterior urethral valves is suspected, an indwelling catheter should be placed in the bladder. This will allow at least partial decompression of the urinary obstruction. The surgeon is cautioned to remember that there is a large reservoir from the previously dilated urinary system. It is not uncommon for these patients to go long periods without apparent urinary output because they store urine in their dilated system. A Credé maneuver may help prove that the child is continuing to make urine. To follow these children, renal function studies are necessary, including measurement of blood urea nitrogen (BUN), creatinine, and creatinine clearance as well as careful output with specific gravities. After it has been established that the child is in a stable condition, cystoscopy should be performed, and under direct vision the valves may be fulgurated with cautery. For some patients this may be all that is necessary to restore normal voiding, and, with careful follow-up, they may lead a normal life. On the other hand, many infants have a urinary system so dilated that peristalsis is ineffective and insufficient drainage occurs. Primary repair of the entire system in the newborn has been described by Hendren [10], but we prefer to delay this extensive procedure from six to twelve months and instead to perform bilateral high-loop ureterostomies, a vesicostomy, or bilateral skin pyelostomies.

Prune-Belly Syndrome

Prune belly, or congenital absence of the abdominal musculature, is another syndrome seen almost exclusively in males. The patient has a dilated bladder, dilated ureters, and dilated renal pelves, associated with absent or greatly di-

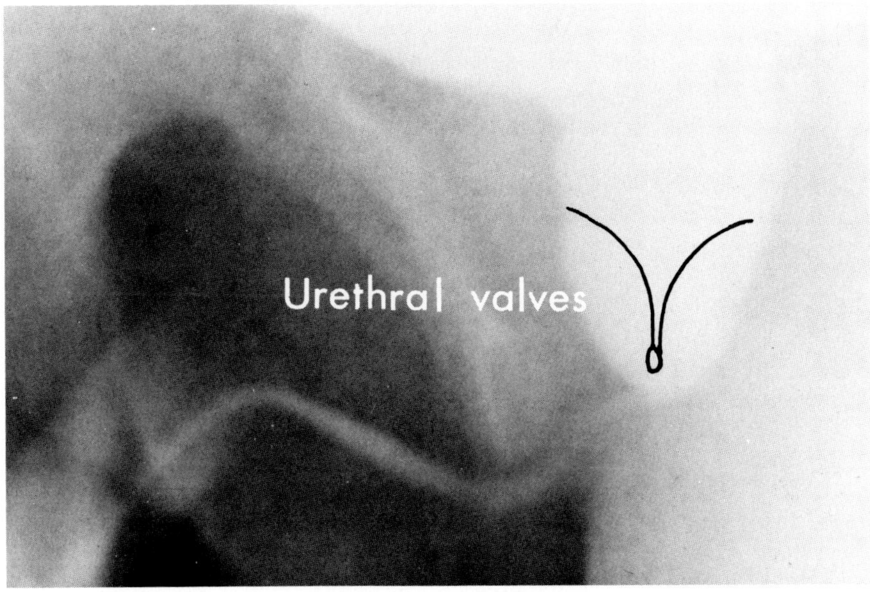

18-3. Voiding cystourethrogram in male with posterior urethral valves. Note the dilated proximal urethra.

minished musculature of the abdominal wall and bilateral undescended testes. The skin becomes redundant and has been described as resembling the skin of a prune (Figure 18-4). The diagnosis in the full-blown case is usually not difficult because the abdomen is striking in appearance. Not infrequently, however, there is some abdominal musculature present, so that the diagnosis is less obvious. An intravenous pyelogram and voiding cystourethrogram may help. Treatment for these patients is still somewhat controversial, but in the newborn an indwelling bladder catheter and an abdominal corset along with use of antibiotics may be all that is necessary. On the other hand, if renal function continues to deteriorate, high-loop ureterostomies, a vesicostomy, or bilateral pyelostomies may be necessary to provide adequate drainage of urine. At a later date, ureteral tapering and reimplantation can be considered to aid in the total care of these patients.

Ureteroceles

It is extremely unusual for ureteroceles to become clinically apparent in the first month of life; however, they can cause hydronephrosis in the newborn. Ureteroceles are seen more commonly in females, and frequently they are associated with ectopic or duplicated ureters. The resultant obstruction caused by the ureterocele is responsible for the hydroureter and hydronephrosis on the involved side.

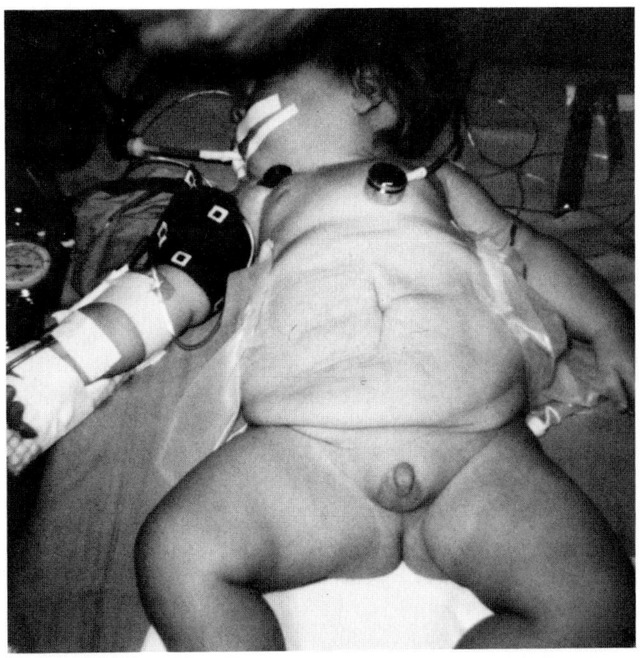

18-4. Male infant with prune belly. Note the absence of testes in the scrotum.

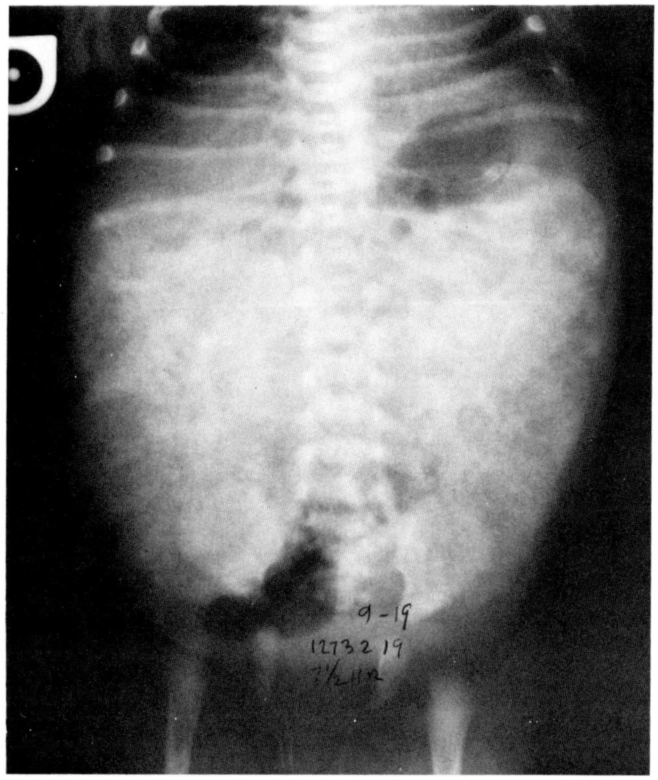

18-5. Intravenous pyelogram of infant with bilateral polycystic kidneys.

Polycystic Kidneys

Polycystic kidney disease occurs in both males and females and may show up as very large, firm, irregular masses in each flank. Intravenous pyelogram and inferior vena cavagram with a 24-hour follow-up should establish the diagnosis (Figure 18-5). The infantile form of this disease is usually fatal. There is no surgical treatment indicated in the first month of life. Renal transplantation may offer some hope, but this procedure in neonates is still not technically feasible.

Unilateral Masses of the Flank

Most masses seen in the newborn are single and lie on one side of the midline. The intravenous pyelogram with inferior vena cavagram can be extremely helpful in diagnosing these conditions. Rarely are other radiologic studies, such as arteriograms or retrograde injections, necessary to confirm the diagnosis.

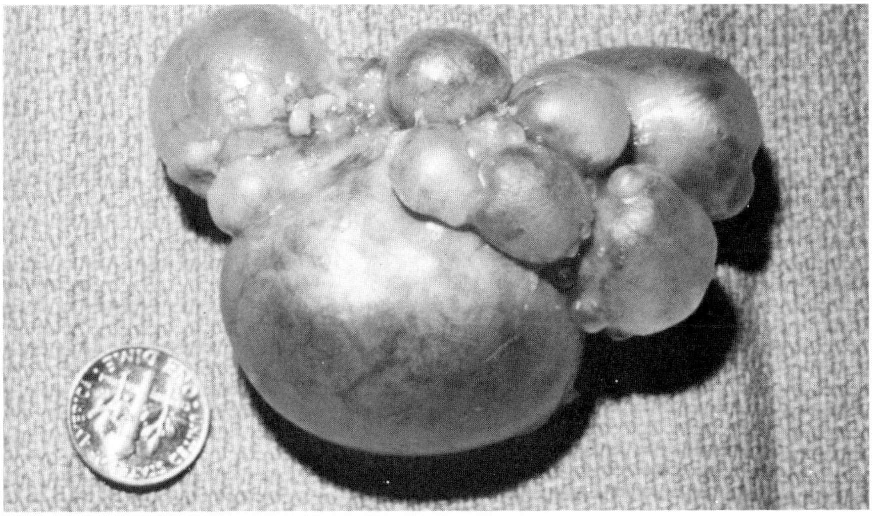

18-6. Multicystic kidney. No parenchyma is present, nor are the ureter and vessels seen.

Multicystic kidneys are unilateral and are more common on the left side (Figure 18-6). They are multilobulated, mobile, and cystic. Because there is no renal parenchyma, the intravenous pyelogram shows nonvisualization even on delayed 24-hour films.

Obstruction of the ureteropelvic junction (UPJ) occurs on either side and is usually unilocular; a small rim of renal parenchyma remains so that dye can be appreciated on the delayed films of the intravenous pyelogram.

Wilms' tumor, or mesoblastic nephroma, is an intrinsic kidney lesion that results in distortion of the caliceal structure on the pyelogram (Figure 18-7). Wilms' tumors are rare in newborn infants; they are treated with a radical nephrectomy and a paraaortic node dissection. Neuroblastomas are discussed later in this chapter.

Thrombosis of the renal vein as a cause of a unilateral mass in the flank in a newborn is exceedingly rare. It is mentioned here only for completeness, because the treatment is medical unless a nephrectomy is needed for a completely infarcted kidney.

Simple nephrectomy in the newborn with multicystic disease should be done extraperitoneally through the flank. The lesion can be sharply and bluntly dissected out with ease because large vessels are rarely encountered. The ureter is usually very small and, in fact, sometimes is absent. The wound is closed without drains.

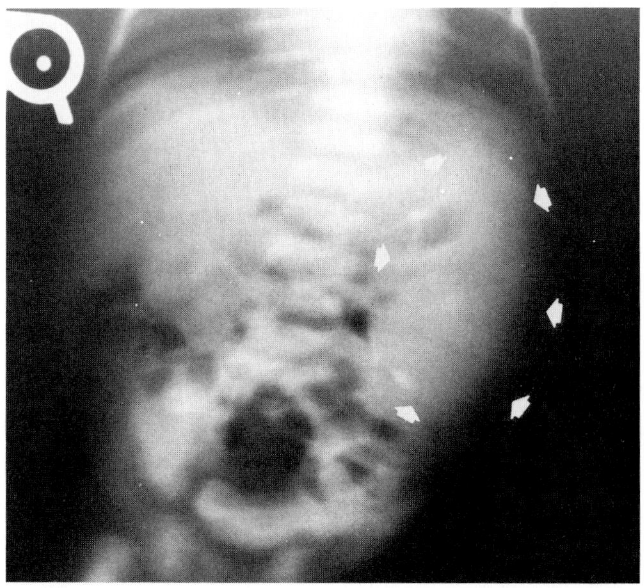

18-7. Intravenous pyelogram of infant with left Wilms' tumor that distorts the calices.

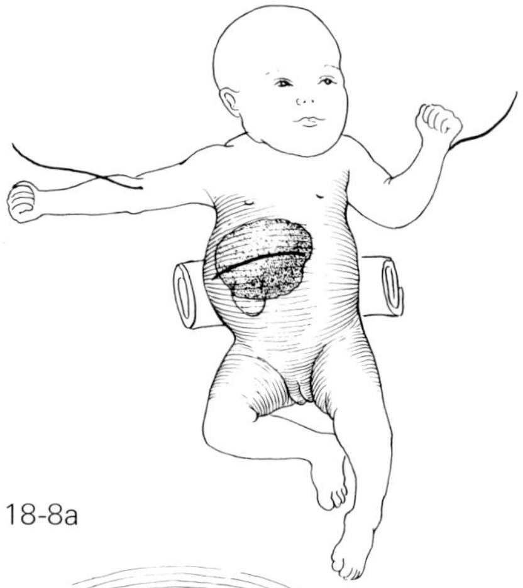

18-8a

Radical Nephrectomy for Wilms' Tumor

This procedure is done with the patient supine on the operating room table with the appropriate side elevated slightly. Because major blood loss can be encountered during this procedure, the intravenous line is inserted in an upper extremity. A supraumbilical transverse incision is made after general endotracheal anesthesia has been instituted (Figure 18-8a). This operation should be performed transperitoneally. Wilms' tumors rarely cross the midline but they can invade the liver or the colon, especially tumors on the right side. Fortunately, this local invasion is uncommon in children under one month of age. (Because a right radical nephrectomy is more complicated than a left, the discussion will focus on a right-sided lesion. Vascular control is simpler on the left.)

After the abdomen has been entered, the colon, which may drape over the tumor, is reflected medially. Care must be taken to avoid injury to its mesentery and to the accompanying colic vessels (Figure 18-8b). A Deaver retractor is carefully placed in the region of the liver, which is retracted cephalad. Because of the rapid hematogenous spread of Wilms' tumors, it is important to avoid handling the tumor until one obtains control of the renal pedicle, particularly the renal vein. Ideally, the renal vein should be ligated first.

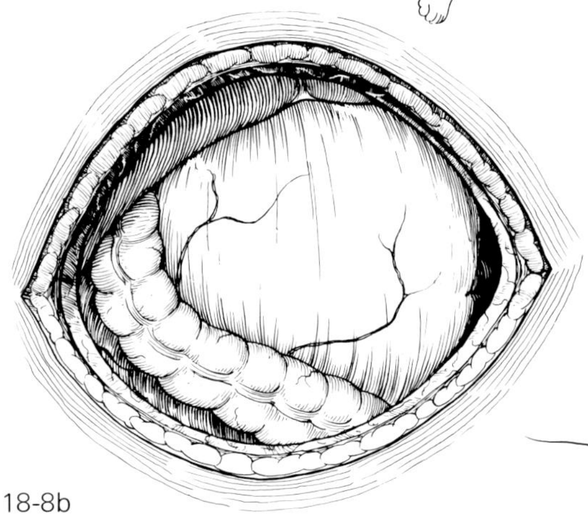

18-8b

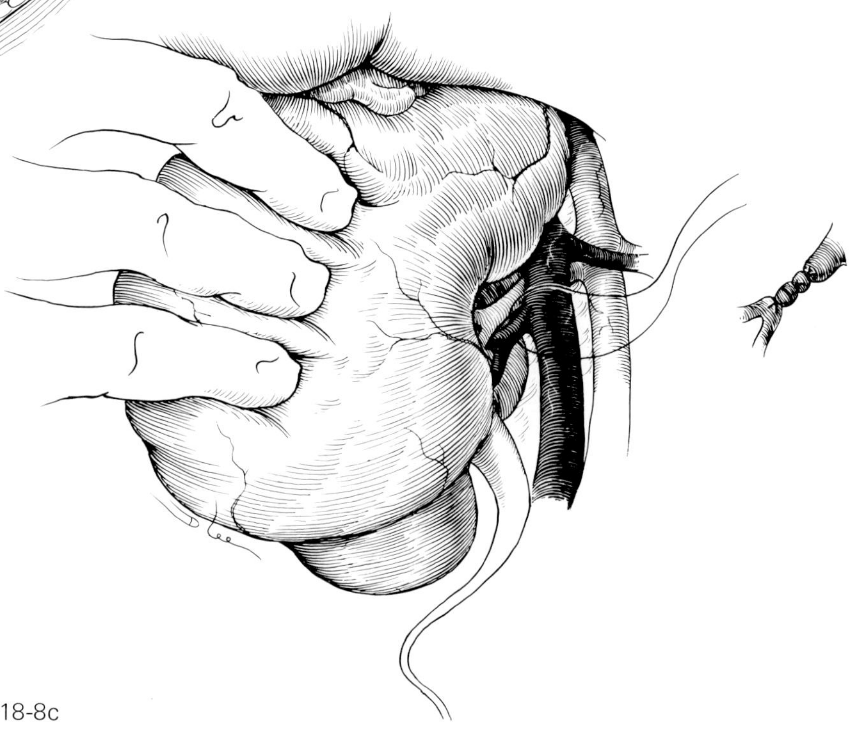

18-8c

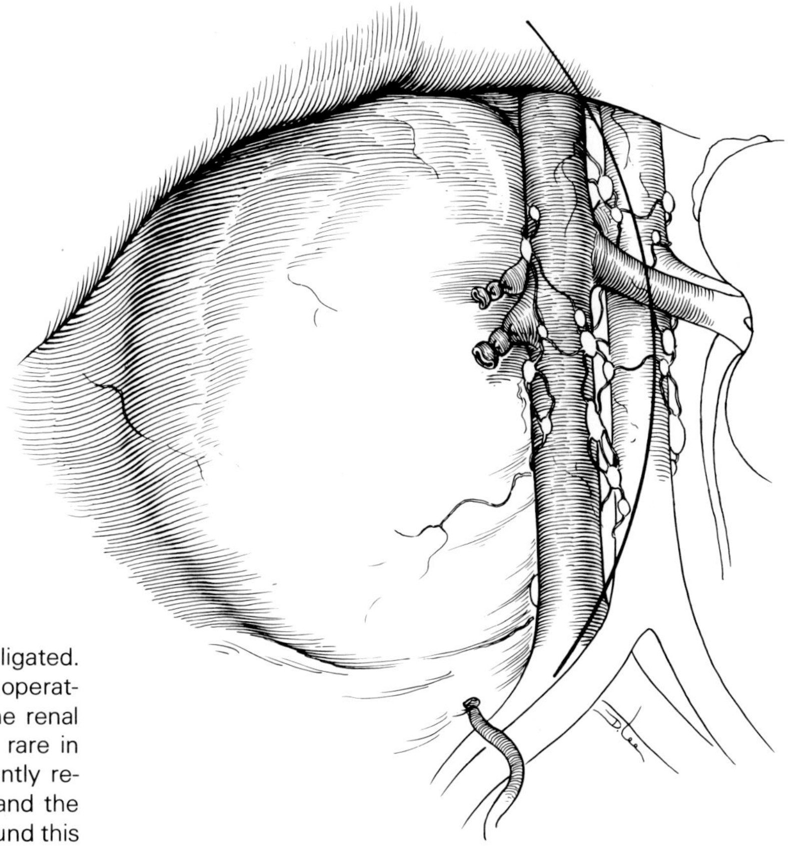

18-9. Bed of resected Wilms' tumor on the right side. Two ties remain on the vessels, and the ureter is ligated at the pelvic brim. The dark line marks the area to be cleared of lymph nodes.

The artery is palpated in the hilum and then doubly ligated. The vena cavagram, which should be available to the operating team, may suggest the presence of tumor in the renal vein and inferior vena cava, but this is exceedingly rare in patients under one month of age. The kidney is gently retracted laterally until the junction of the renal vein and the vena cava is seen. A right-angled clamp is placed around this junction and a 2-0 silk is placed around the vein but not tied (Figure 18-8c). The vena cava is further dissected free until the opposite renal vein is identified. Only when the surgeon is absolutely certain that he has identified the correct renal vein in the distorted abdomen of an infant with a large tumor should the tie be cinched down. A second tie is then placed proximally and the renal artery is identified and treated in a similar manner. If possible, the vein is ligated first.

After the vessels have been properly ligated and cut, sharp and blunt dissection with appropriate hemostasis is used to remove the tumor from the surrounding adventitia. The adrenal gland and its vein usually must be removed with the tumor but they may be spared if obviously not involved. The ureter is dissected down toward the pelvic brim until it disappears from view, at which point it is clamped and cut and the remaining end is tied with a 3-0 Dexon suture.

On right-sided lesions, after the specimen has been removed, a vein retractor is placed under the vena cava, which is retracted to the left. The adventitia surrounding cava and the tissue between it and the aorta is removed with sharp dissection as a separate specimen of paraaortic tissue (Figure 18-9). After a left nephrectomy, the left paraaortic tissue is removed (Figure 18-10). The authors have frequently been

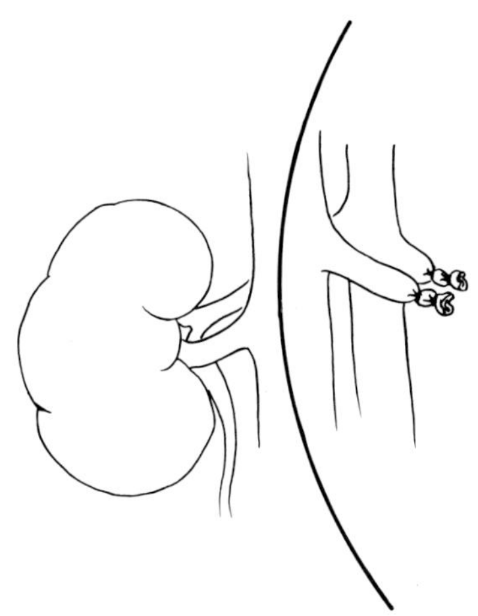

18-10. For a left-sided lesion, the node-containing tissue on the lateral aspect of the aorta is removed.

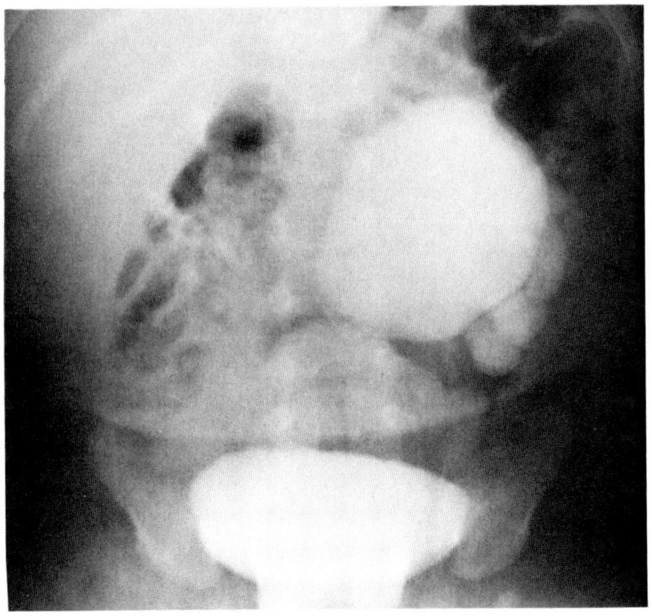

18-11. Delayed film of an intravenous pyelogram in a child with obstruction of the ureteropelvic junction. The amount of dye in the pelvis suggests that sufficient renal parenchyma exists to warrant an attempt at reconstruction.

surprised to find malignant tissue reported by the pathologist in lymph nodes removed in this manner. Despite the fact that this is not en bloc dissection of tumor and nodes, there appears to be no decrease in life expectancy when this technique is used.

At this point a careful inspection of the abdomen is undertaken, with special care taken to look for metastases in the liver. Palpation and visual inspection of the contralateral kidney are mandatory because there is a 15 percent incidence of bilaterality in Wilms' tumors, although not usually in patients this young. The posterior fascia and peritoneum are closed with a running suture of 3-0 or 4-0 Dexon, and the anterior fascia is closed with interrupted 4-0 silk and the skin with running 4-0 nylon. The patients are continued on antibiotics for five days postoperatively. They are usually ready to tolerate an oral intake within 24 to 48 hours and the intravenous infusion can be stopped at this time.

Only a limited number of cases of Wilms' tumor have been reported in the very young. In those whose tumors were definitely malignant and who subsequently died, metastases were present by four months of age. With this in mind, it is logical to consider a second-look operation three months postoperatively. We have had experience with one child with a malignant nephroblastoma with positive periaortic nodes at birth who was reexplored electively at 14 weeks, at which time no tumor was found. The child was given no radiation or chemotherapy and is well at 36 months of age, which is beyond the period of risk.

Hydronephrosis Secondary to Obstruction of the Ureteropelvic Junction

Some babies with obstruction of the ureteropelvic junction (UPJ) will not have sufficient renal tissue to make saving the kidney worthwhile. In these patients nephrectomy is performed in a fashion similar to that described for multicystic kidney, except that the renal artery, vein, and ureter must be located and appropriately tied. A greater challenge to the pediatric surgeon occurs in those patients where enough renal tissue is apparent at surgery to warrant plastic revision of the ureteropelvic junction (Figure 18-11). For these cases we prefer the Hinds-Anderson dismembered pyeloplasty.

Gastrointestinal Causes of Abdominal Masses

Lesions of the gastrointestinal (GI) tract leading to bowel distention are not often confused with true abdominal masses in the newborn. Malignancies of the GI tract are not seen in this age group, so that it becomes the surgeon's responsibility to rule out the more serious nonintestinal causes of abdominal masses rather than to search immediately for a cancer of the GI tract, as he would probably do in an adult. After chest and plain films of the abdomen have been reviewed, an intravenous pyelogram with inferior vena

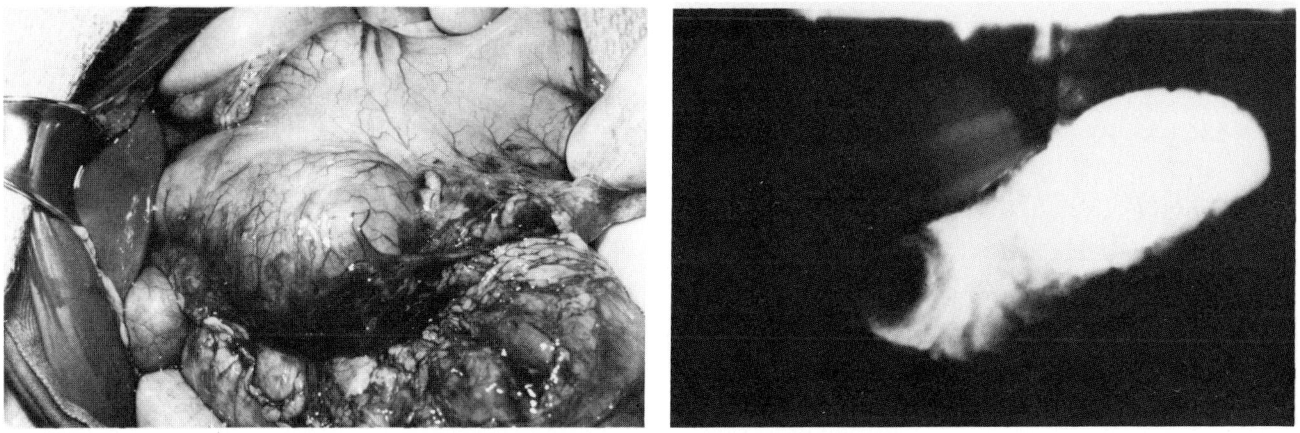

18-12. Operative and radiographic demonstration of antral duplication with partial gastric outlet obstruction.

cavagram is obtained. When it appears that the urinary system is not involved, x-ray films of the upper and lower GI tract are obtained as indicated. Intestinal duplications appear as extrinsic, space-occupying lesions or occasionally as a separate intestinal segment. Intussusception is exceedingly rare in the newborn but, if present, it should become apparent with appropriate contrast studies. Pyloric stenosis and lesions causing meconium buildup are each discussed elsewhere in this book.

Duplications

Duplications can occur anywhere in the gastrointestinal tract, from the mouth to the anus. Gastric, duodenal, and jejunal duplications are uncommon, however, while ileal and colonic duplications are seen with some frequency.

Duplications of the stomach usually occur in the region of the pylorus (Figure 18-12). They may present as gastric outlet obstruction and may or may not communicate with the lumen of the stomach. The treatment depends on the exact location, shape, and characteristics of the lesion. Complete excision may be feasible; partial gastrectomy with Billroth-I reconstruction may be necessary, or cystogastrostomy may be indicated if resection appears hazardous.

Duplications of the intestine usually occur in the ileum or colon; the treatment is essentially the same in any location. These lesions may be suspected on physical examination and the diagnosis may be supported by contrast studies, but almost invariably their presence is confirmed only at the time of exploration.

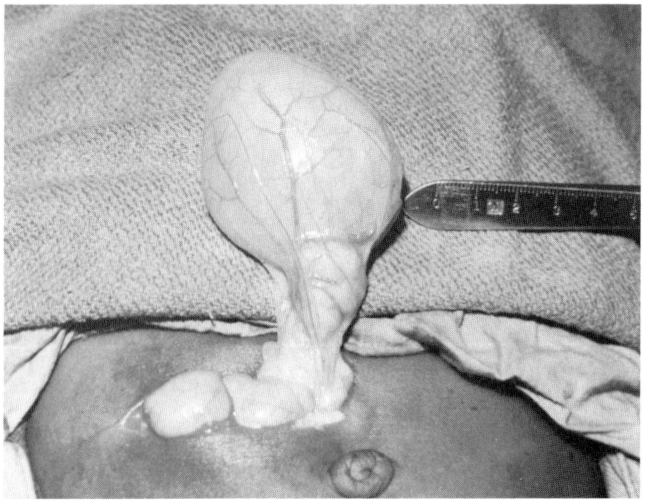

18-13. Ileal duplication on a pedicle.

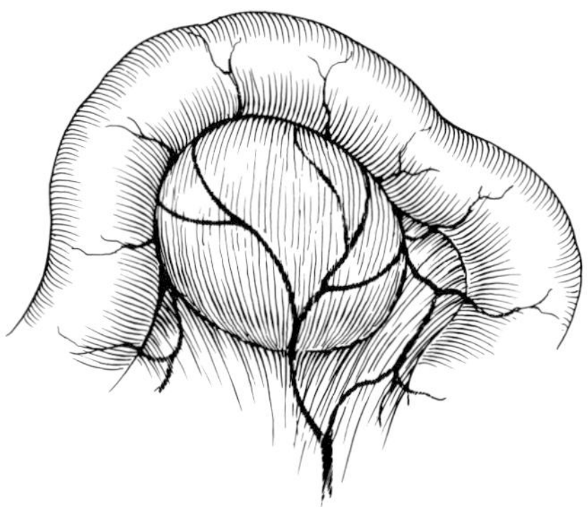

18-14. Cystic ileal duplication within the bowel mesentery.

Preoperative Preparation for GI Tract Duplications

In patients with duplication in the small or the large bowel, a nasogastric tube and an upper-extremity intravenous line are placed before surgery. Preoperative antibiotics and vitamin K are administered, and the child is operated upon on the infant warmer.

A right supraumbilical transverse rectus-cutting incision is made. Careful exploration of the abdomen is undertaken. A correct preoperative diagnosis of duplication is uncommon under one month of age; the intestine is therefore carefully examined and the area of duplication is assessed. Seen at laparotomy, duplications appear in one of two ways: as a single round cystic mass lying in the mesentery of the bowel or as a long tubular structure lying in the mesentery parallel to the bowel and even sharing a common wall with the bowel. The tubular lesions, in particular, may truly look like a second or duplicate intestine.

Procedure for Cystic Duplication

These lesions usually do not communicate with the intestinal lumen, so that their mucosal lining, as it secretes, causes the lesion to become progressively larger, resulting in compression of adjacent structures. Therefore, when encountered at laparotomy, the mass is in the mesentery and stretches the bowel supplied by that mesentery. The surgeon must decide if the lesion can be excised without injury to the bowel or the vessels that supply it. If the lesion is on a pedicle (Figure 18-13), simple ligation at the base will allow easy removal. If there is no pedicle (Figure 18-14), the peritoneum overlying the cyst is incised, and enucleation is attempted by using both sharp and blunt dissection. Cautery and silver clips can expedite this maneuver. If total removal is accomplished, the viability of the bowel is assessed and, if its condition is acceptable, the mesenteric defect is closed and the opera-

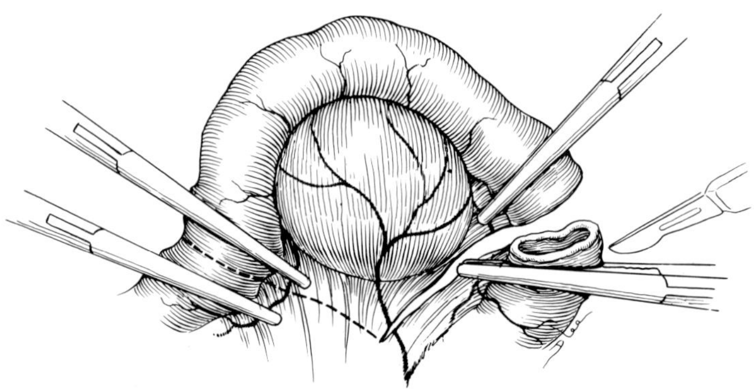

18-15a. A small duplication is resected along with its neighboring bowel.

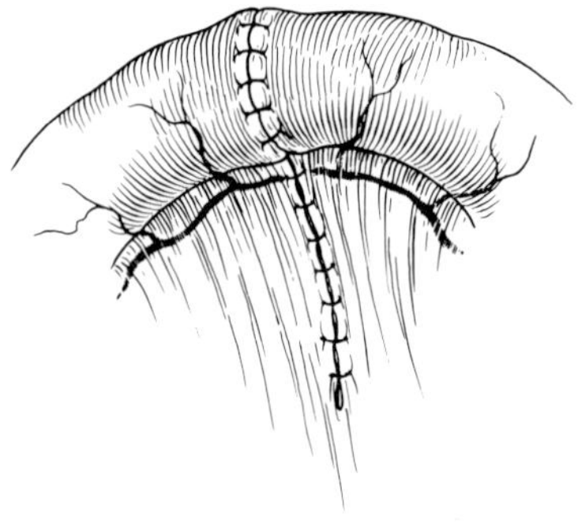

18-15b

tion is terminated. Unfortunately, in more than half the infants the mass cannot be safely removed without a wedge resection of bowel, mesentery, and duplication (Figure 18-15a). The divided intestine is reapproximated in one layer (Figure 18-15b). After the mesenteric defect has been repaired, the wound is closed without drains. A gastrostomy is rarely necessary.

Tubular Duplication

Tubular duplications often share a common wall with the intestine (Figure 18-16), thereby making enucleation difficult or impossible. If the lesion is small, resection of bowel, mesentery, and duplication is feasible, as described above; longer duplications, particularly of the colon, may mean sacrifice of excessive amounts of normal bowel, so that alternative methods must be considered. Correlation of the preoperative contrast studies and the operative findings will often suggest that the tubular duplication communicates with the intestinal lumen. If the communication is distal, then no further surgery may be necessary, because the lesion should drain. On the other hand, if the connection is proximal, an anastomosis of the lesion to the bowel distally is undertaken to create a double-channel lumen, which is usually satisfactory (Figure 18-17). An end-to-side, single-layer closure is performed with 4-0 silk with knots tied on the inside (Figure 18-18). Tubular duplications, regardless of size or location, may contain gastric mucosa, so that, with time, ulcer formation with bleeding or stenosis of the adjacent normal bowel may follow. It is our feeling that in neonates the risk of future ulceration is worth taking if extensive bowel resection is the only alternative, because future resection is always possible if complications arise years later.

Procedures removing the septum between the bowel and duplication or procedures in which the mucosa of the duplication is removed are hazardous and difficult. They are not recommended at the time of initial surgery in the newborn. However, they are useful in older patients.

Standard wound closure is undertaken. Gastrostomy may well be necessary in children who have extensive lesions. The postoperative recovery should be uneventful.

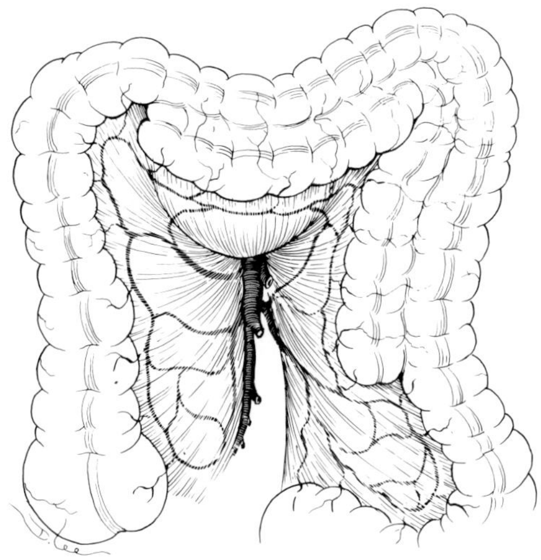

18-16. Tubular colonic duplication.

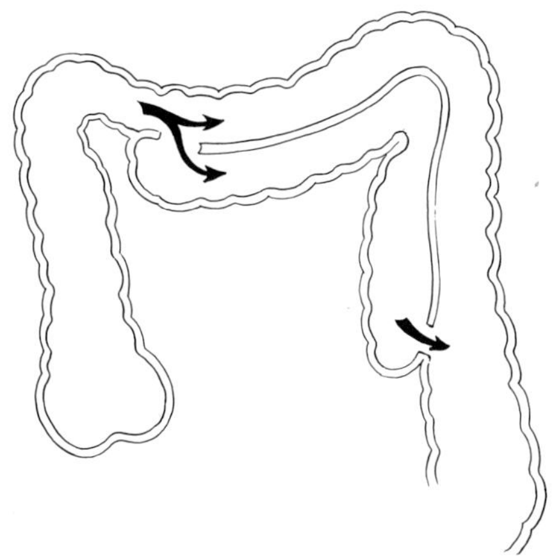

18-17. Schematic of a tubular colonic duplication. The lesion may open into the normal intestine proximally, distally, or both.

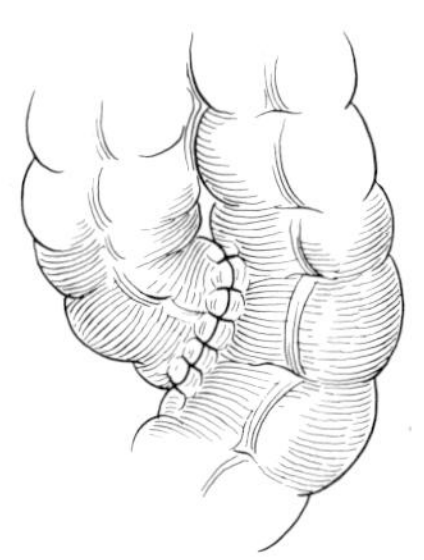

18-18

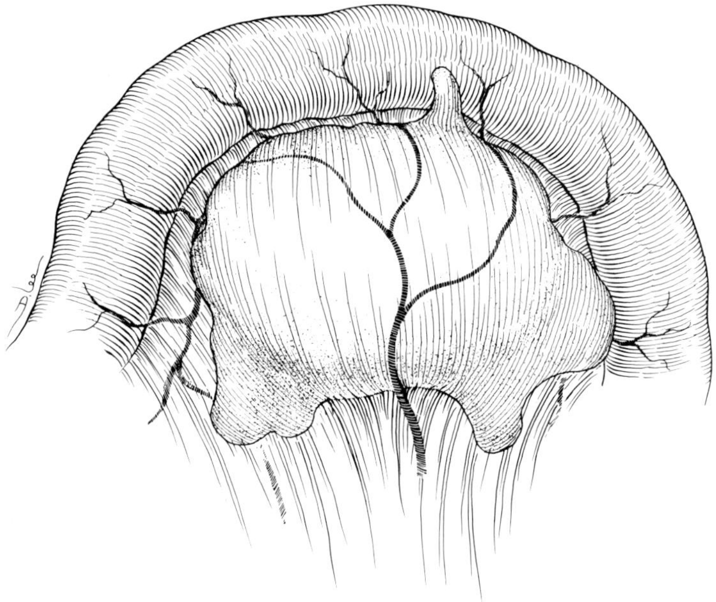

18-19. Soft, ameboid mesenteric cyst.

Mesenteric Cysts

Mesenteric cysts are thought to arise from embryonic lymphoid centers. These lesions enlarge slowly and infrequently appear as abdominal masses in small infants. They are thin-walled, single or multiloculated, soft, fluctuant masses (Figure 18-19) most often seen in the mesentery of the small bowel. They contain chylous fluid and at laparotomy are not difficult to distinguish from duplications. Surgical treatment is similar to that of intestinal duplications; however, many mesenteric cysts can be enucleated without damage to the adjacent intestine.

Genital Tract

Hydrocolpos

Hydrocolpos results from obstruction of the vagina by labial fusion, an imperforate hymen, or vaginal atresia (Figure 18-20). The normal female embryo secretes a mucuslike substance from the uterine glands as a result of stimulation from maternal estrogens. In female fetuses with normal genital tracts, this material is eliminated throughout embryonic development, but, if an obstruction exists, buildup occurs, causing vaginal and uterine enlargement. These babies then present with an abdominal mass in the lower midline. Physical examination of the perineum is extremely helpful. An imperforate hymen or membrane is visible as a bulging membrane just inside the vaginal introitus when the labia are separated.

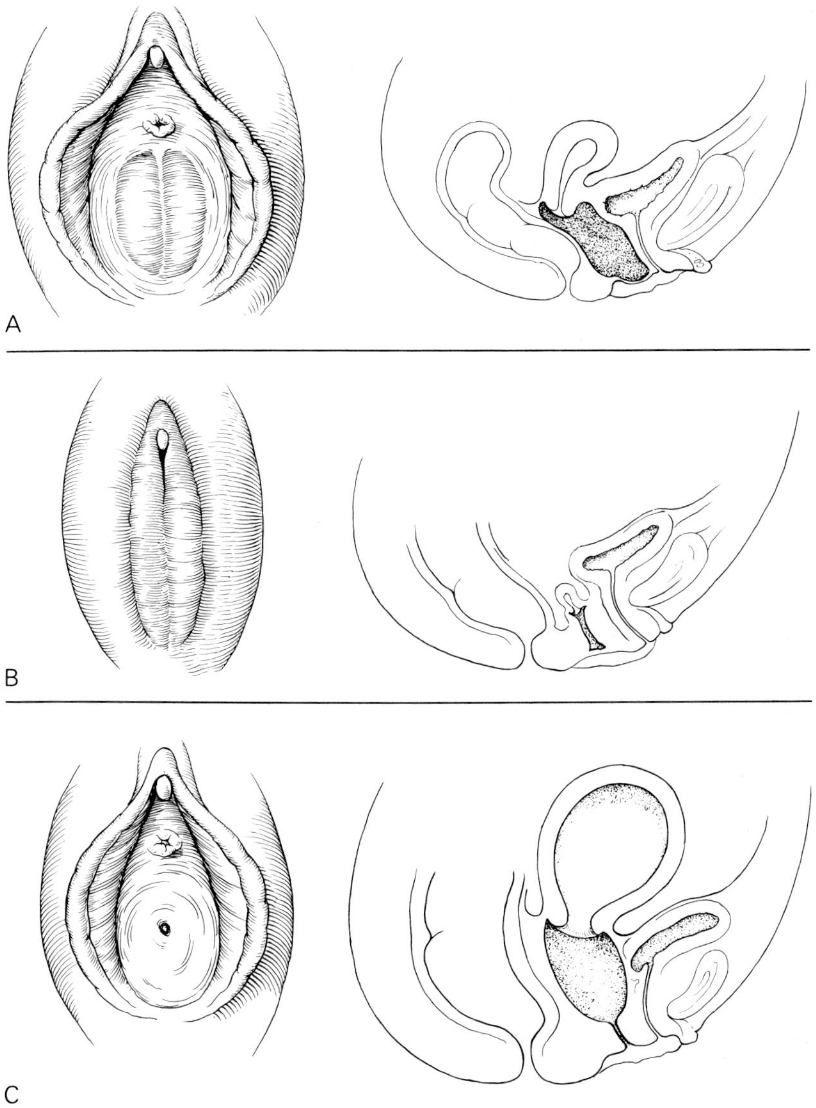

18-20. (A) Imperforate hymen; (B) labial fusion; (C) vaginal atresia with massive proximal distention.

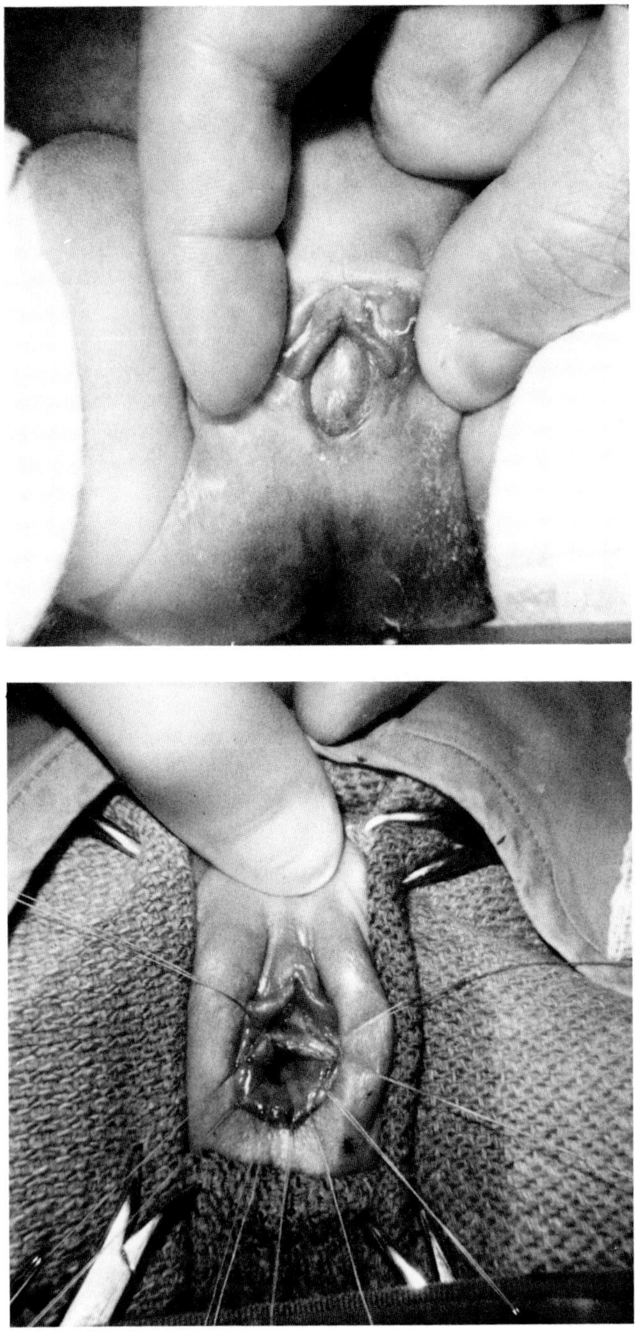

18-21. Imperforate hymen. After resection of the membrane, the edges may be sewn to control bleeding.

Patients with vaginal atresia do not have a bulging membrane but instead have a minute opening in the perineum where the vagina should be.

A cystogram by means of a number 6 or 8 Foley catheter will demonstrate anterior displacement and compression of the bladder. The mass may cause trouble with voiding or passing meconium. On rectal examination the enlarged vagina and uterus can be felt. An intravenous pyelogram should be obtained to search for upper-tract abnormalities, particularly agenesis of one kidney.

Operative Technique

A careful perineal examination in the frog-leg or lithotomy position is mandatory for proper evaluation of these infant girls. Frequently this part of the examination can be done in the operating room but without anesthesia. If not, appropriate intravenous fluids, antibiotics, and endotracheal anesthesia are instituted. Simple labia synechiae can be easily separated. If inspection of the perineum reveals a bulging membrane, a number 8 Foley catheter is placed in the bladder for identification of the urethra. Then a number 18 needle is inserted in the middle of the membrane and some of the whitish fluid is aspirated. Simple excision of the membrane is accomplished from below, and occasionally if there is bleeding the cut margin is oversewn with a 5-0 chromic suture (Figure 18-21). A number 16 soft Silastic catheter is inserted, and a slow injection of Hypaque is started while an x-ray is obtained to detail the anatomy. The cavity is then gently irrigated with saline, and the patient is awakened. Thrice-daily irrigations are continued for a week along with parenteral antibiotics. The child is then discharged and the cavity is followed weekly until the size returns to normal.

Abdominoperineal Repair of Vaginal Atresia

Infants with vaginal atresia have only a pinpoint opening visible just inside the hymeneal ring. Open abdominoperineal repair is the safest approach to this problem. In the frog-leg position the patient undergoes a Betadine scrub of the abdomen and perineum (Figure 18-22a). A Vaseline pack is placed in the rectum, and a number 6 or 8 Foley catheter is inserted into the bladder. A transverse incision in the lower abdomen is used; the top of the dilated uterine fundus immediately presents itself. The bladder is retracted anteriorly until the lower cervical region is exposed. A transverse hysterotomy is done at this level, and the mucoid fluid from the uterus is aspirated. A large clamp is placed through the hysterotomy, down the cervical canal, and into the dilated proximal vagina (Figure 18-22b). Attention is then directed to the perineum, where the small distal vagina is progressively dilated up to a number 8 Hegar dilator. A small nasal speculum is placed into the vagina to facilitate locating the tip

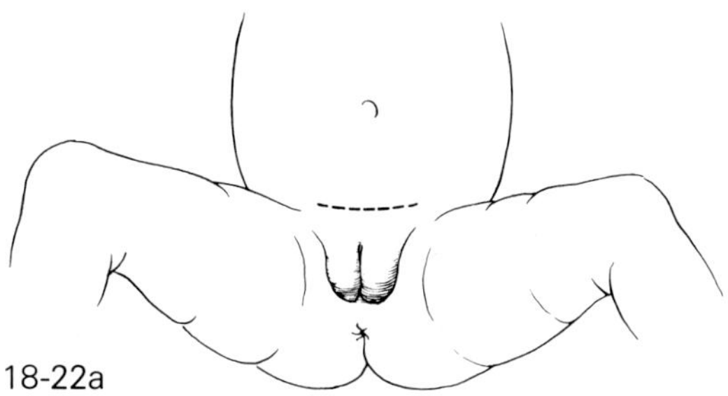

18-22a

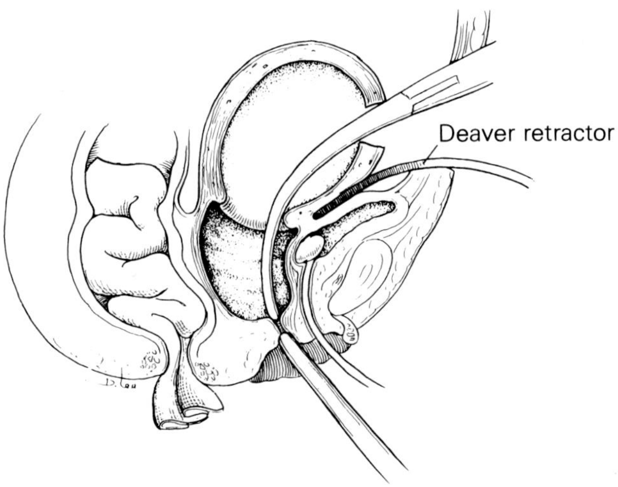

18-22b. A large clamp is inserted through the hysterotomy to the vaginal obstruction. A dilator is seen attempting to enlarge the vagina from below. Note the gauze packing in the rectum.

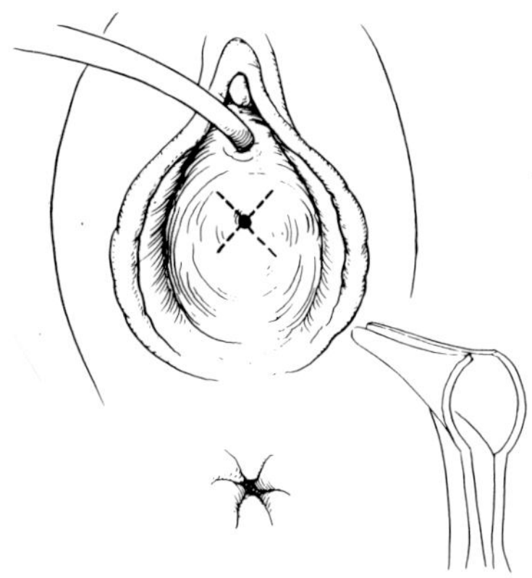

18-22c

of the clamp as it presses on the occluded vagina (Figure 18-22c). The atretic area is incised with a long-handled knife, and the clamp is brought down and out the vaginal orifice. A number 16 Silastic catheter is placed into the clamp and drawn up into the uterine cavity (Figure 18-22d). This catheter acts as both a stent and a drain. The hysterotomy is closed with two layers of 3-0 Dexon and the abdomen is closed without drainage. The infant is maintained on antibiotics and uterine irrigations for one week. The Foley catheter is removed after three days. The Silastic stent remains for six weeks and can be removed at an office visit. Further vaginal reconstruction can be carried out when the girl is pubertal.

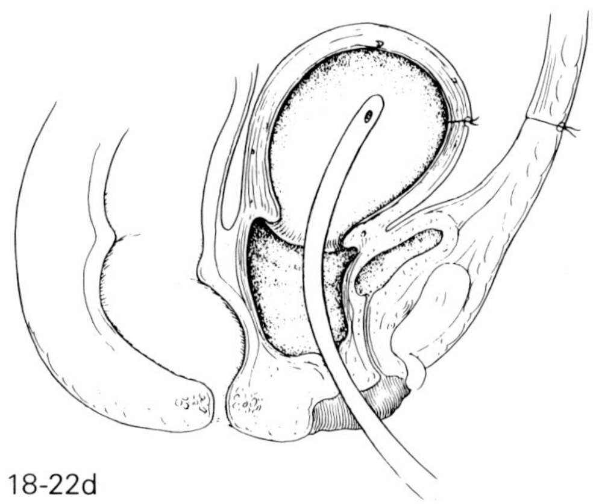

18-22d

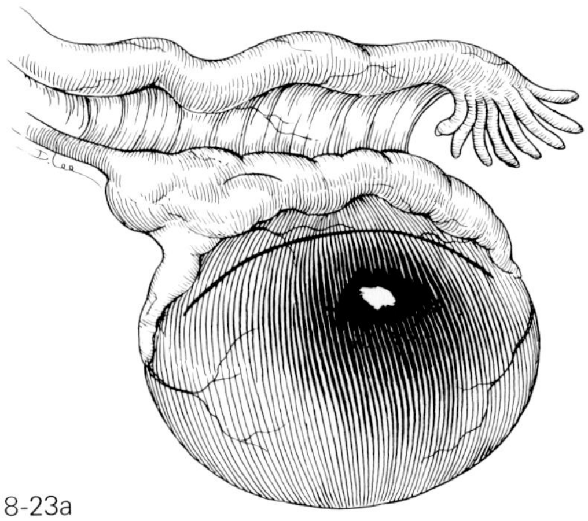

18-23a

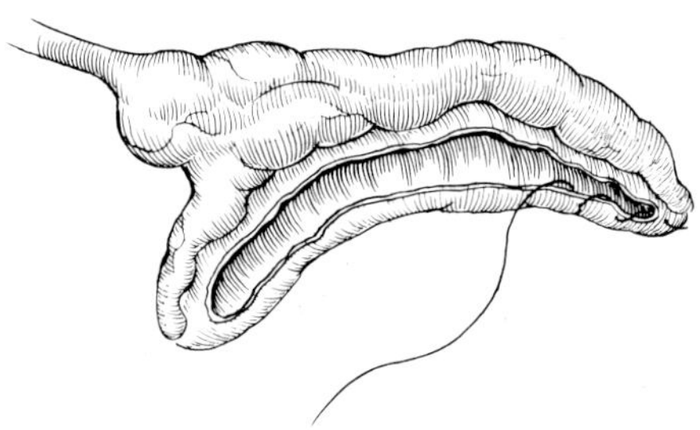

18-23b

Ovarian Cysts

Cystic lesions of the ovary are sometimes encountered in newborn infants. Female babies with abdominal masses undergo the entire work-up discussed at the beginning of this chapter. Because these cysts are mobile, the work-up is often inconsistent and nondiagnostic until celiotomy. These lesions are either simple cysts or cystic teratomas (commonly called dermoids). Every attempt should be made to preserve ovarian tissue during excision of these masses. Many cysts are bilateral. In the bilateral cysts it is mandatory to leave functioning ovarian tissue. It is not uncommon for these lesions to present with acute abdominal pain secondary to torsion with hemorrhage.

Operative Technique

At exploration through a transverse incision in the left or right lower quadrant, both ovaries are examined. The cystic lesions can be enucleated by incising the ovary longitudinally, avoiding the ovarian artery and shelling out the cyst (Figure 18-23a). With time, the thin shell of tissue left will resume normal function. The cut edge of the visceral peritoneum is closed with running 5-0 chromic suture for hemostasis (Figure 18-23b). The fallopian tubes and ovarian ligaments are often stretched by the mass but require no repair.

Postoperative problems are uncommon. Normal menses and normal fertility are known to have occurred in these patients in adulthood.

Intersex

Children with ambiguous genitalia do not really have abdominal masses but may require exploratory celiotomy for identification of internal sex organs. A Pfannenstiel's incision is used. If the gonads are not absolutely normal in appearance, they should be biopsied. Fortunately, modern biochemical and laboratory tests have all but eliminated the need for these exploratory procedures.

Some infants with ambiguous genitalia can present a complex picture and may require combined efforts by neonatologists, endocrinologists, geneticists, and pediatric surgeons to reach the correct diagnosis and treatment. A detailed discussion of these problems is not appropriate for this book; however, one common form of intersex does come to surgery in the neonatal period: Females with adrenogenital syndrome often have labial fusion and a hypertrophied clitoris, which needs removal, particularly for social acceptance by the family (Figure 18-24).

Girls with these conditions are tested endocrinologically to ascertain the biochemical defect present. This allows for proper steroid replacement before surgery, which is performed at about two weeks of age. Several different electrolyte abnormalities can be encountered because of the varying biochemical defects. These electrolyte abnormalities should be under good control before plastic revision of the perineum.

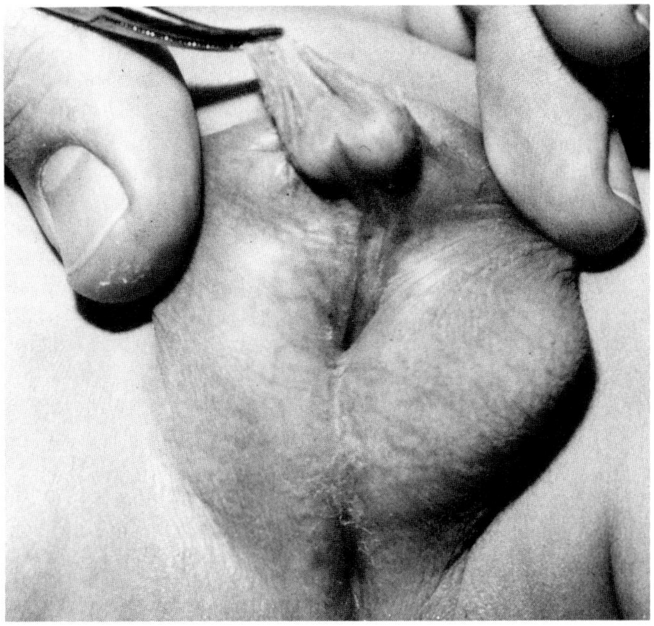

A

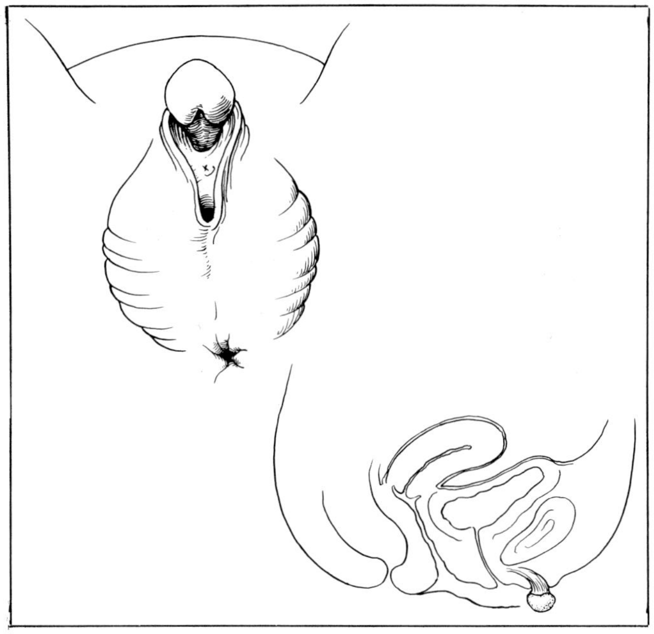

B

18-24. (A) Female with adrenogenital syndrome. The labia are fused, and the clitoris is enlarged. (B) Schematic of the infant in (A). The lateral view demonstrates the covering over the urethra and vagina.

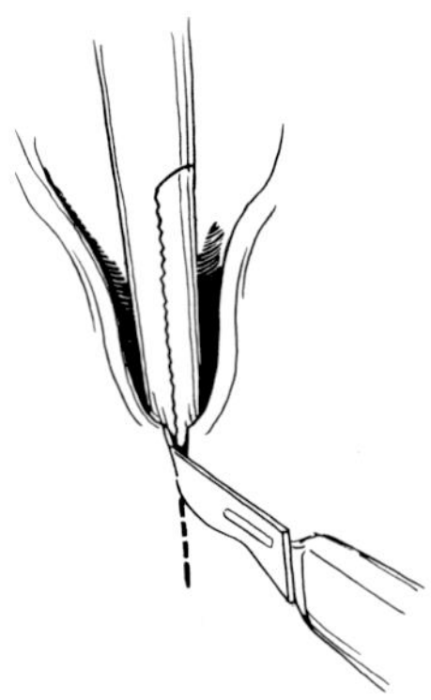

18-25a

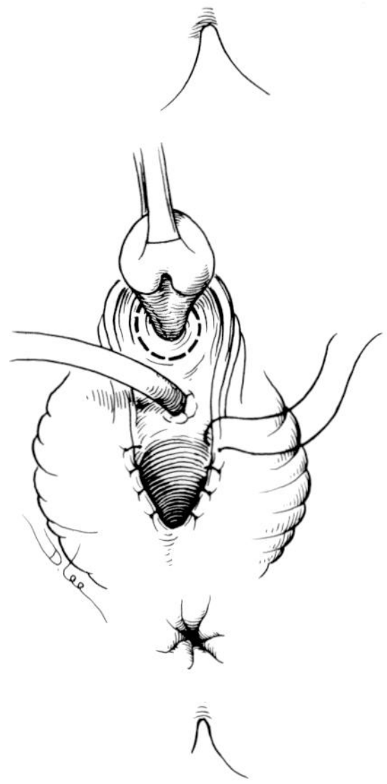

18-25b

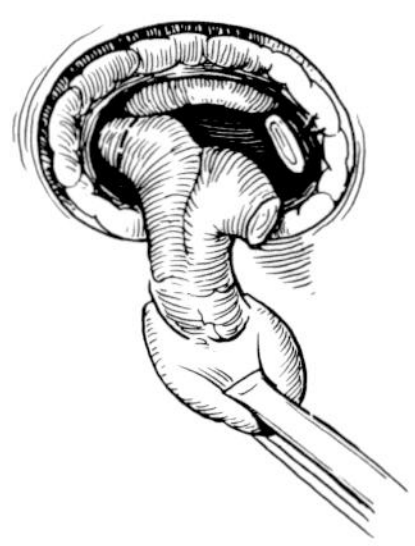

18-25c

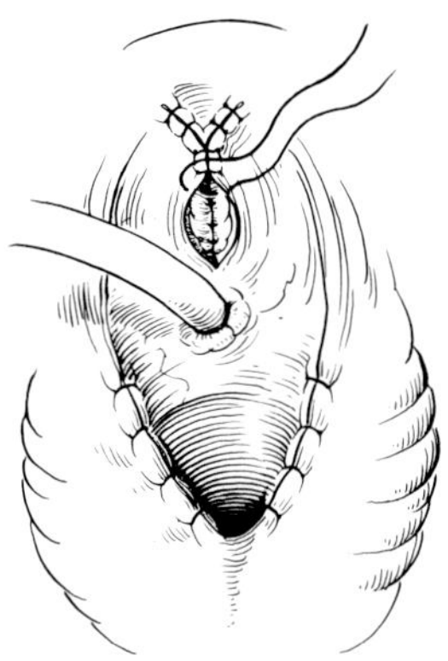

18-25d

Operative Technique

The infant is placed supine in the frog-leg or lithotomy position. A curved hemostat is placed into the urogenital sinus after appropriate preparation and draping. With the clamp used as a guide, the perineal skin is incised posteriorly to enlarge the opening (Figure 18-25a). The mucosa of the cut edges is marsupialized to the skin with interrupted 4-0 Dexon sutures. A number 6 or 8 Foley catheter is inserted into the bladder when the urethral opening becomes visible. A towel clip is then placed on the glans of the clitoris for traction. A circular skin incision is made at the base, and dissection is carried down the shaft of the corpora (Figure 18-25b). This plane of dissection is continued until the bifurcation of the corpora is encountered. This distance is often much longer than anticipated. A right-angled clamp is placed around each corpora. Then the two limbs are ligated with 3-0 or 4-0 silk sutures and the specimen is amputated (Figure 18-25c).

The wound is closed in layers with 4-0 Dexon sutures. Care is taken to build up tissue near the pubis with three or four layers of suture to create a mons veneris (Figure 18-25d). The skin is closed with 5-0 Dexon sutures, and collodion is used as the dressing. The Foley catheter is removed in four to five days.

In some centers clitoral recession is preferred to resection, but in our opinion this offers more disadvantages than advantages. The cosmetic results of resection are excellent, and sexual function later in life should be normal. Fertility, however, depends on the original genetic defect.

Hepatobiliary Causes of Abdominal Masses

Although the liver and biliary tree are rarely responsible for abdominal masses during the first month of life, liver tumors are occasionally encountered, as are hepatic cysts. In neonates the other hepatobiliary lesions listed at the beginning of this chapter do not occur with any significant frequency. Each must be treated on an individual basis.

A mass in the liver of a newborn requires essentially the same work-up as for an older child. Liver scans and echography are helpful in assessing the proper surgical approach to a mass. Liver function studies, coagulation studies, and alpha-fetoprotein assays are also performed. Angiography is often helpful but it carries a significant risk in the infant. The infants with vascular abnormalities are usually treated nonoperatively for several months before consideration of surgery.

A few significant differences between hepatic surgery in infants and adults deserve special mention.

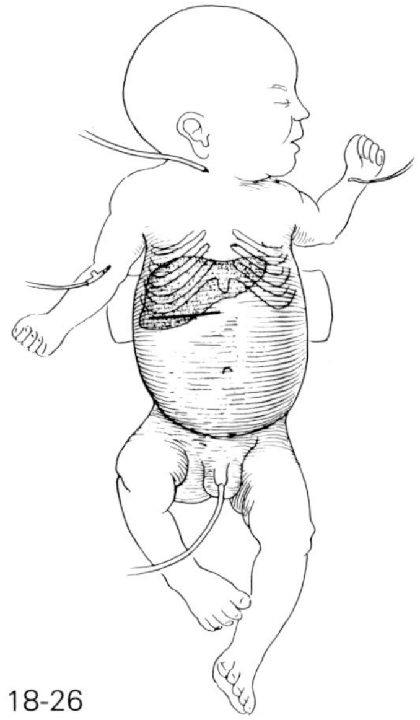

18-26

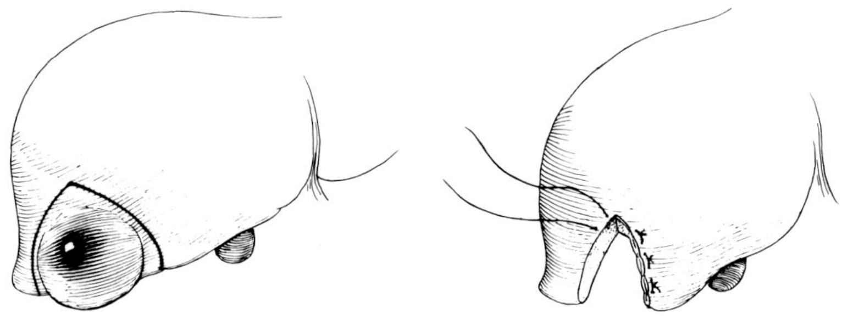

18-27

Special Techniques in
Hepatic Surgery for Infants

Major arterial and venous access in the upper extremities with monitoring of central venous pressure (CVP) and arterial pressure is mandatory. A Foley catheter is placed in the bladder, and the patient is positioned supine with a bump placed under the right costal margin. The entire chest and abdomen are included in the field. A generous transverse incision of the upper abdomen is used (Figure 18-26). Contrary to the case with adults, it is rarely necessary to enter the chest of an infant to obtain venous control before liver resection.

Hepatic cysts, when encountered, can be removed with a wedge resection of local liver tissue with closure of the edges by mattress sutures (Figure 18-27). Patients with primary liver tumors, however, require formal anatomic hepatectomy. Surgery offers the only real chance for a cure in patients with malignant liver tumors. Therefore a search for resectability is begun. The requirements for resectability are: (1) no evidence of distant metastasis on chest x-ray; (2) one hepatic vein free of tumor; (3) an uninvolved vena cava; and (4) an adequate amount of uninvolved liver tissue with good portal and arterial flow and bile duct drainage (Figure 18-28).

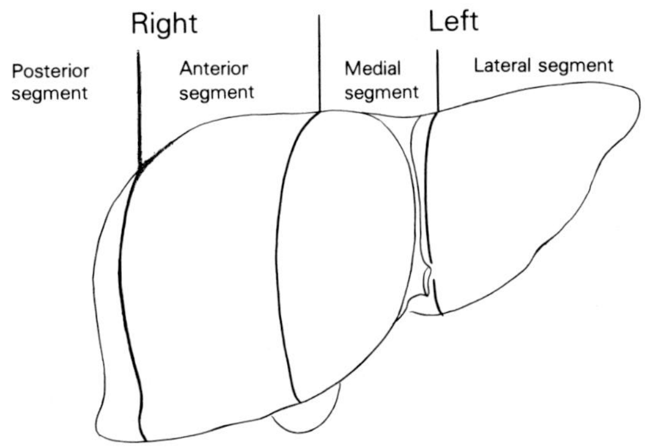

18-28. The left and right lobes of the liver meet on a line running from the gallbladder bed to the vena cava.

Resection is begun by carefully dissecting out the structures of the portal triad (Figure 18-29a). The hepatic artery, portal vein, and bile duct to the appropriate portion of the liver are isolated, ligated with a 3-0 silk, and divided. The liver is now completely mobilized by incising the triangular ligament. This mobilization allows isolation of the hepatic veins (Figure 18-29b), which are also ligated and divided, but special attention must be paid to preserving the hepatic veins that drain the liver segment to be retained. This dissection is possible in many children without opening the chest or diaphragm. The central hepatic vein should be preserved in a standard right or left lobectomy, but, in an extended hepatectomy the central hepatic vein is taken. In the small infant the hepatic veins are very short and therefore not readily accessible. If this is the case, the liver is finger-fractured and the veins are encountered directly as they enter the vena cava, where they are oversewn with 4-0 or 5-0 cardiovascular silk (Figure 18-29c).

After the artery to the lobe or segment to be removed has been ligated, a demarcation line becomes apparent between the perfused and the nonperfused, ischemic liver. The capsule of the liver is then incised along this line, which represents one of the anatomic planes between lobes or segments. Sharp and blunt dissection is used to transect the liver at this level. Major vessels and ducts are clamped and ligated with 3-0 silk. This is most easily carried out with the finger-fracture technique. This is the maneuver where the most blood is lost, especially in adults. In infants, however, the liver is small enough to allow excellent hand compression of the cut surface to control much of the bleeding (Figure 18-29d). When the specimen has been removed and the oozing has been controlled, an attempt is made to close over some of the raw surface of the liver. For this covering, omentum (Figure 18-29e) or adjacent liver capsule work well but are often not available in infants. The edges of the cut liver can occasionally be closed directly with 2-0 chromic sutures (Figure 18-29f). If the surface is dry, closure may not be necessary. Although the use of drains is controversial, one Penrose drain and one sump tube left in the right upper quadrant are effective in removing accumulations of blood and bile. A choledochotomy with T-tube drainage is never done in infants. The incision is closed in layers in a routine fashion.

Postoperative Care

Major hepatic resection is a great physiologic insult to the human organism. Although the liver is able to regenerate its mass and function rapidly, the first postoperative week is critical. Blood loss should be carefully assessed throughout the operation and in the postoperative period. Measurements of central venous pressure, arterial pressure, and urine output are of great help in monitoring volume replace-

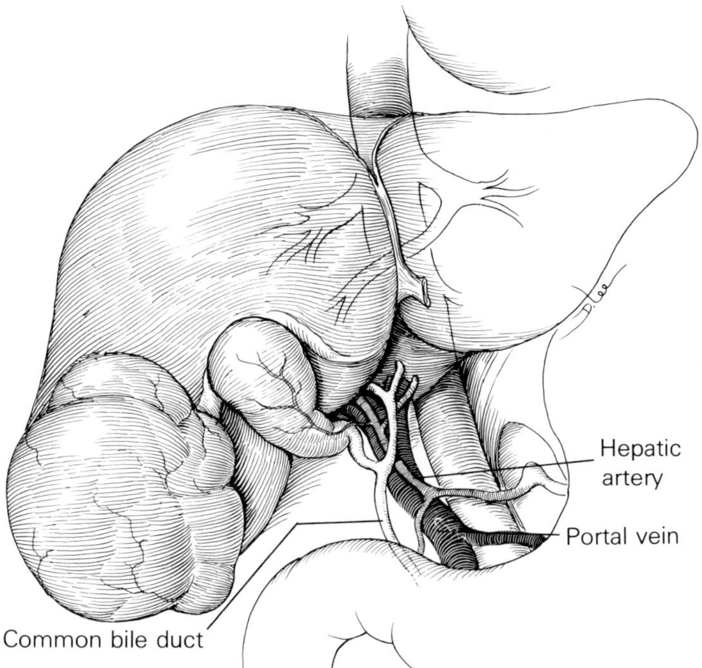

18-29a

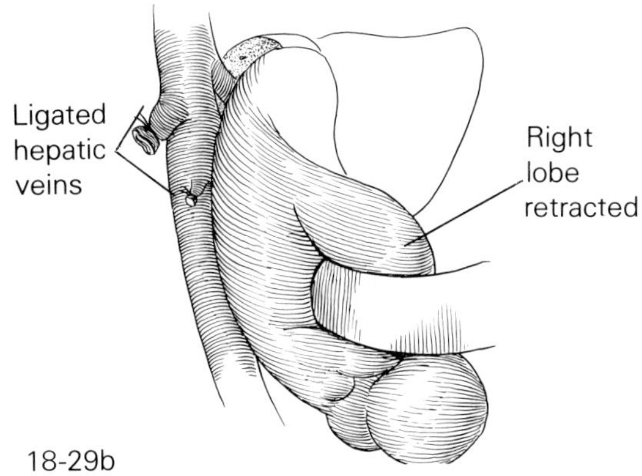

18-29b

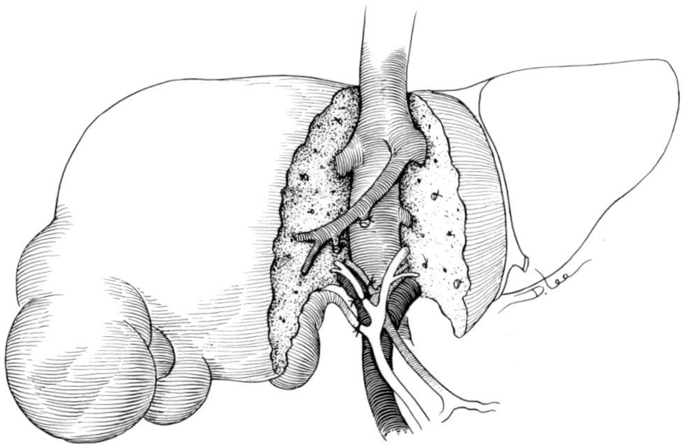

18-29c

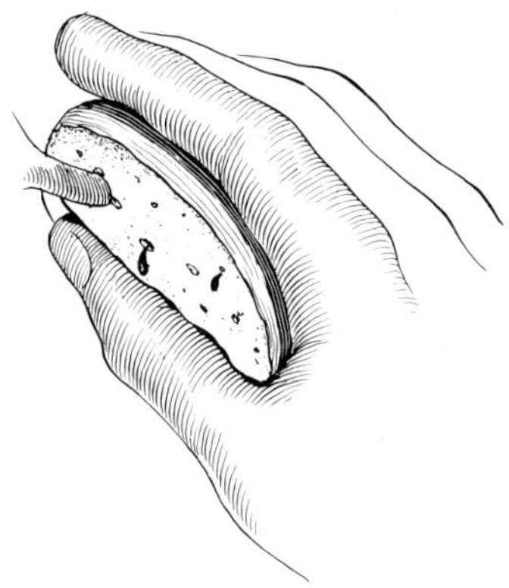

18-29d

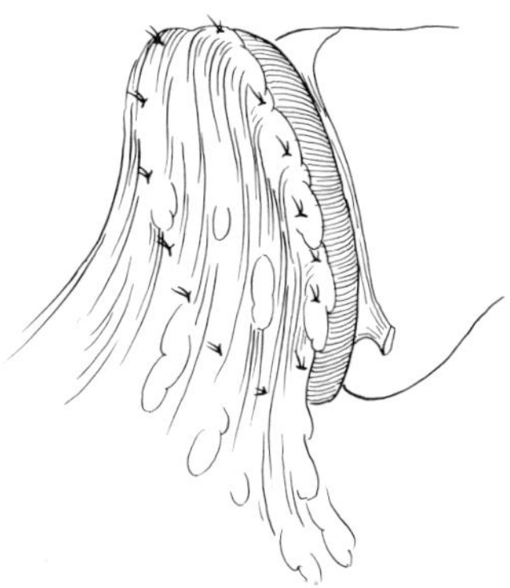

18-29e

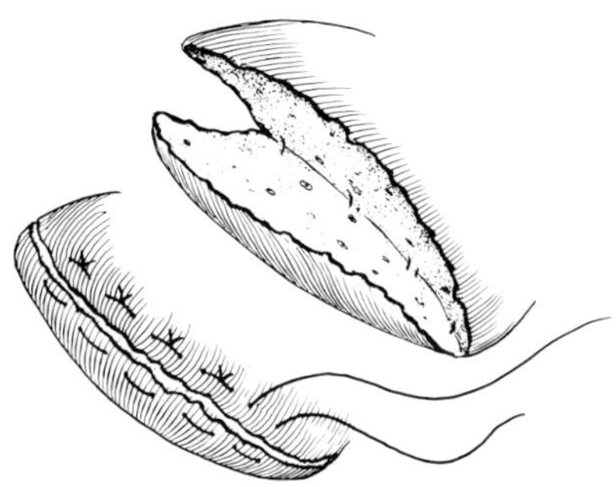

18-29f

ment. Hypoglycemia is common after hepatic resection, so that the patient should be maintained on 10% glucose solution, with appropriate electrolytes added as needed. Frequent measurement of blood sugar should be used as the guideline for glucose replacement. It has been our practice to keep the patient in 40% oxygen for at least the first 24 hours postoperatively to prevent hepatic hypoxia.

Albumin synthesis, which occurs in the liver, is decreased after liver resection; therefore albumin should be replaced intravenously at the rate of one gram per kilogram of body weight at least daily for the first postoperative week, with further doses added as indicated by laboratory or clinical findings.

Complications

Hypoglycemia and hypoalbuminemia should not be major postoperative problems if appropriate therapy is instituted during surgery and is continued in the postoperative period. Jaundice is routinely seen after massive liver resection but usually it slowly disappears. Continued jaundice after the first week should alert the surgeon to the possibility of infection, abscess formation, or mechanical obstruction of the biliary tree. The liver is also responsible for production of most clotting factors; fortunately, synthesis of these factors begins shortly after surgery. However, bleeding diathesis can be seen and should be treated with appropriate replacement.

Infection, particularly the formation of an abscess in the right upper quadrant, is an extremely serious complication seen after massive liver resection. This most often occurs near the resected liver edge. All patients should be placed on antibiotics preoperatively and maintained on them for at least one week postoperatively.

Results

The 30-day survival of patients undergoing massive hepatic resection is quite good. However, only 50 percent of patients with liver tumors are resectable at the time of surgery, and fewer than half of these will be cured of their cancer. In patients with benign diseases, excellent results are seen with surgical resection.

Postoperative follow-up of tumor patients should include alpha-fetoprotein assays at regular intervals. Chemotherapy and radiation therapy should be considered on an individual basis but should not be started for four to six weeks, to permit liver regeneration, which can be assessed by serial liver scans.

Other Causes of Abdominal Masses

A wide variety of other lesions can also cause abdominal masses in the first month of life. They are shown under Other in the list of causes at the beginning of the chapter.

Adrenal hematoma, splenic hematoma, and splenic cyst usually do not require surgery during infancy.

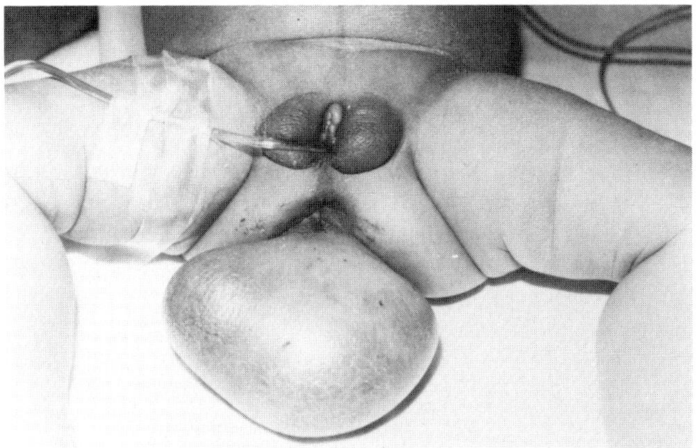

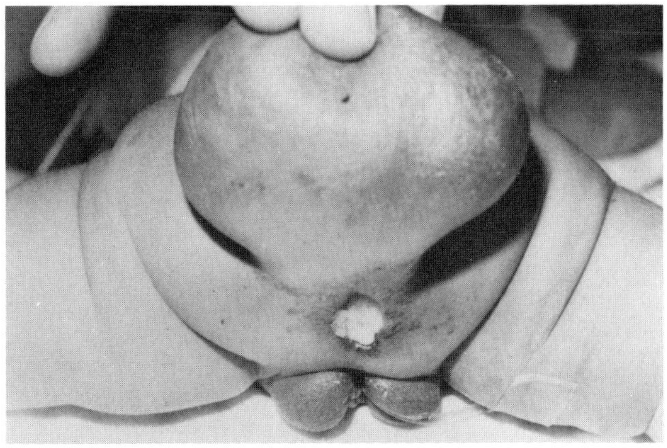

18-30. Newborn with large sacrococcygeal teratoma.

Anterior myelomeningoceles can show up as abdominal masses, but the neurologic abnormalities are usually apparent.

Neuroblastoma is uncommonly found under one month of age. An intravenous pyelogram showing a displaced kidney without distortion of the calyces should certainly make the surgeon suspect neuroblastoma. Treatment of this lesion is similar to that in older children. If the tumor cannot be safely excised, a simple biopsy is performed. Surgery is followed by simple observation or by subsequent chemotherapy and radiation therapy. A second-look procedure is often done some months later.

Neuroblastoma tissue bleeds easily when cut or when sutured. With this in mind, it is often easier to biopsy an involved adjacent lymph node than the main tumor. If total excision is possible, careful hemostasis and tissue identification are needed. The overall cure rate of neuroblastoma patients who are under one month of age is actually quite good (80 percent to 90 percent), even with widespread metastases, and is related to the immunologic aspects of this tumor. For this reason, chemotherapy and radiation therapy may not be necessary and may in fact be more harmful than beneficial.

Sacrococcygeal Teratoma

Sacrococcygeal teratomas can contain elements derived from all three embryonic germ layers. The diagnosis is usually apparent at the time of birth (Figure 18-30). The lesion is primarily posterior to the coccyx and extends externally above the buttocks. In one-half of the infants, varying amounts of tissue are found anterior to the coccyx, sometimes appearing as an abdominal mass (Figure 18-31). Despite the various presentations, almost all these tumors can be excised exclusively through the posterior approach.

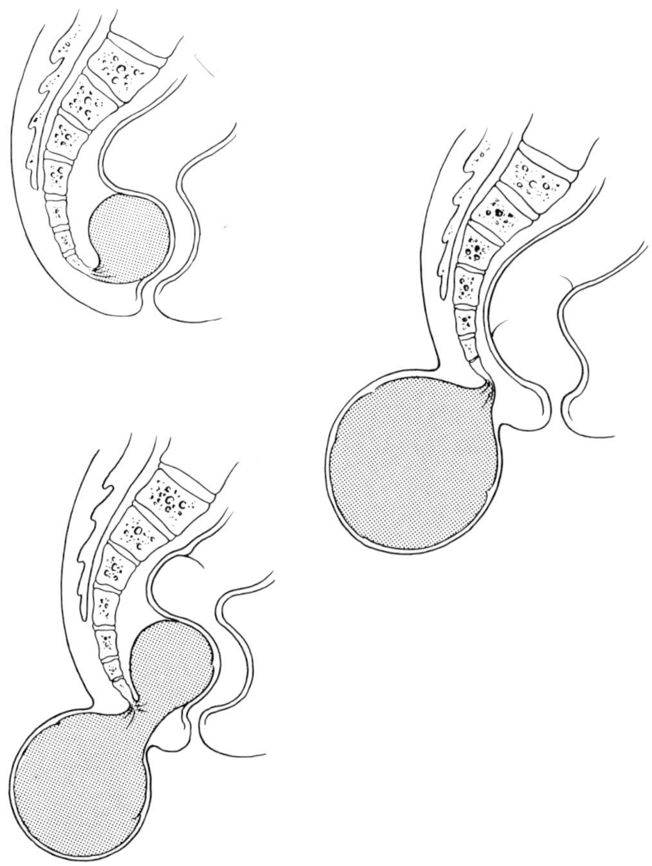

18-31. Sacrococcygeal teratomas may be chiefly anterior or posterior to the coccyx or they may be dumbbell-shaped.

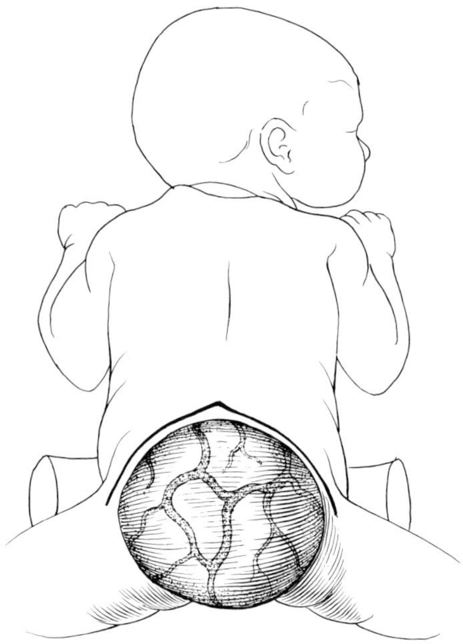

18-32a

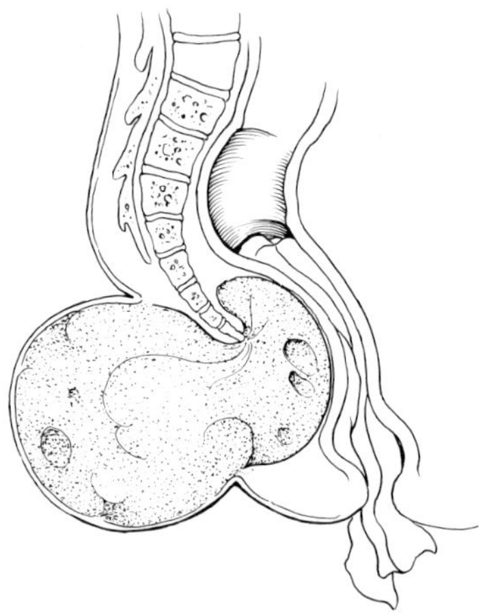

18-32b

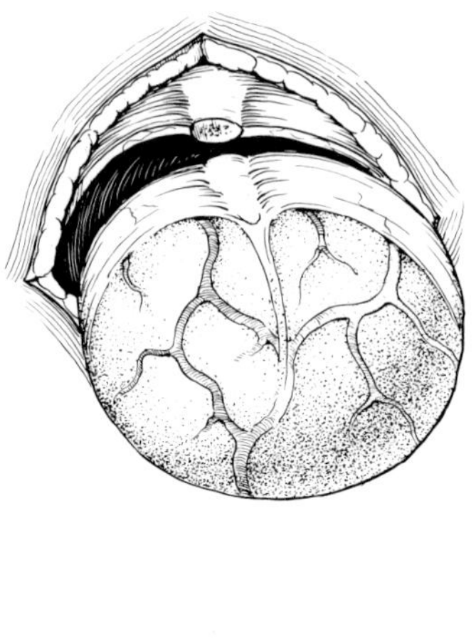

18-32c

The most important preoperative studies are the chest x-ray studies (to search for pulmonary metastasis) and the intravenous pyelogram (to assess the amount of mass anterior to the coccyx). The incidence of significant intraabdominal extension increases with age.

The principal differential diagnostic considerations in a newborn with a mass posterior to the coccyx are meningocele, chordoma, duplication of the rectum, neurogenic tumors, lipoma, and hemangioma. Fortunately, teratomas have a characteristic appearance that makes the diagnosis in the newborn relatively easy.

Operative Technique

The patient is placed prone on the operating room table with a towel under the pelvis (Figure 18-32a). An intravenous line is placed in an upper extremity and endotracheal anesthesia is used. A Vaseline gauze pack is placed in the rectum for future identification (Figure 18-32b). After the area is entirely prepared with Betadine solution, the field is draped in such a way as to exclude the anus from the operative field. This is most simply done by placing a suture from the drape to the skin just posterior to the anus.

An inverted-V incision is made well out along the side of the mass. The incision is carried down to the subcutaneous fascia until the capsule of the teratoma is reached. The dissection is then carried cephalad and laterally. The gluteal muscles will be encountered. Some of this muscle will have to be cut in order to approach the underlying tumor. However, the surgeon should attempt to go as inferiorly as possible so that the glutei can be retracted upward and outward with minimal loss of muscle (Figure 18-32c). This dissection is completed around both sides of the tumor.

The mass is then retracted inferiorly until the coccyx is brought into view. The coccyx is not ossified in infants and can be cut across with a scalpel. It is imperative that the coccyx be removed, because residual tumor in the coccyx has been reported as a cause of local recurrence. (There is usually direct microscopic extension of the tumor into the periosteum of the coccyx.) After the coccyx has been cut, it is retracted inferiorly along with the tumor mass, and the intraabdominal portion of the tumor is dissected. Usually a good cleavage plane is found between the mass and the anterior surface of the sacrum.

The mass is then dissected off the posterior wall of the rectum, where the cleavage plane is not so clear (Figure 18-32d). Direct extension of the tumor into the rectum is exceedingly rare, and the tumor can usually be dissected off the rectum. With continued sharp and blunt dissection, the entire mass begins to fall farther away from the abdomen. The rectum is easily identified because of the previously inserted gauze pack. After the entire anterior wall of tumor has been freed, the tumor itself is held directly up, so that an

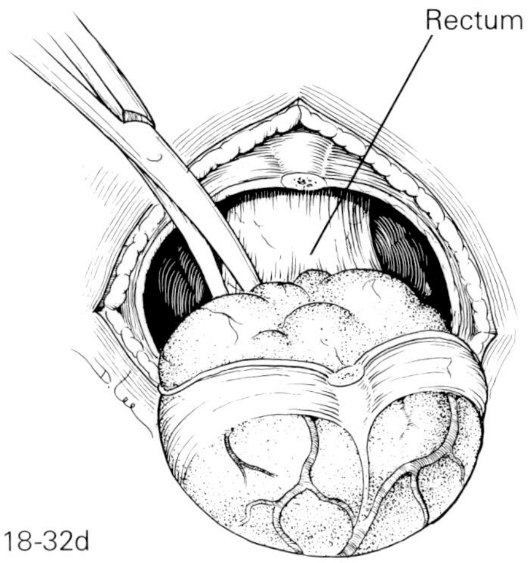

18-32d

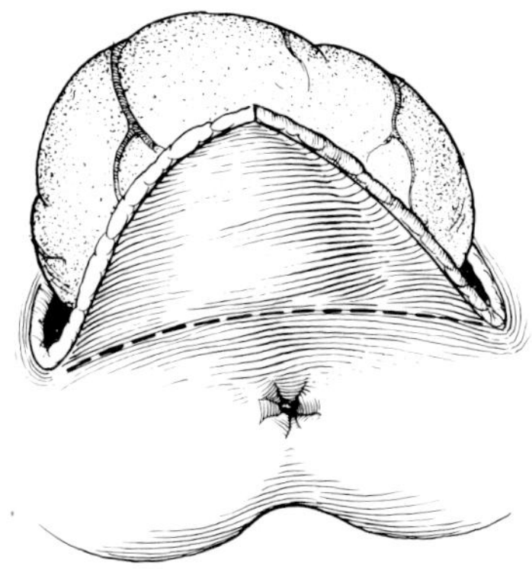

18-32e

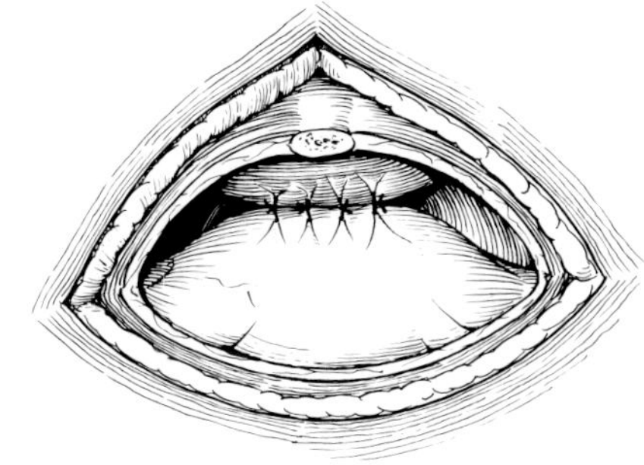

18-32f

appropriately placed incision can be made in the skin inferior to the tumor (Figure 18-32e). After this incision has been made, the specimen is removed. The tumor tends to displace the anus anteriorly; therefore, this final incision is made close to the anus so that the skin closure returns the anus to its normal position.

Since most sacrococcygeal teratomas are large and have grown slowly, they tend to stretch the rectum and perirectal structures. To correct this distortion, the rectum and levator muscles must be returned to their normal anatomic position. To accomplish this, sutures of 4-0 silk are placed in the presacral fascia superiorly and are sewn inferiorly to the superior and posterior parts of the levator muscles (Figure 18-32f). When these stitches have been tied, the perirectal structures are reapproximated into a more normal anatomic position. This decreases the rectal length and strengthens the sphincteric mechanism. The gluteal muscles are then resutured in the same direction in which they were cut (Figure 18-32g). There is usually excess skin remaining; and final trimming should be done on the upper flap to allow the anus to be in a normal position. A drain is often left in the sacral hollow and is brought out through the corner of the incision (Figure 18-32h). The subcutaneous tissue is closed with 4-0 Dexon sutures, and the skin is closed with running 5-0 nylon. At the end of the procedure the Vaseline pack is removed from the rectum.

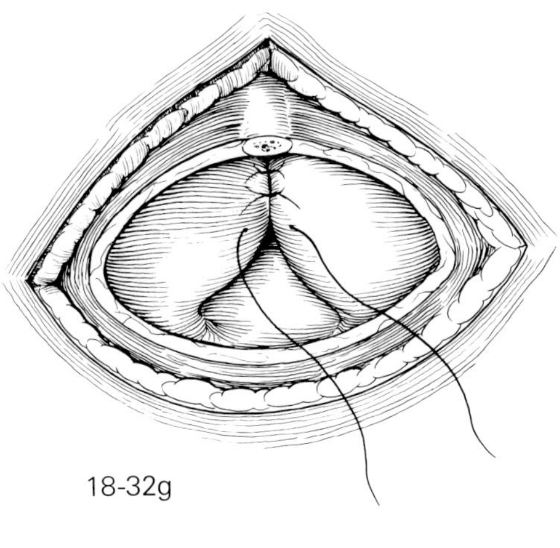

18-32g

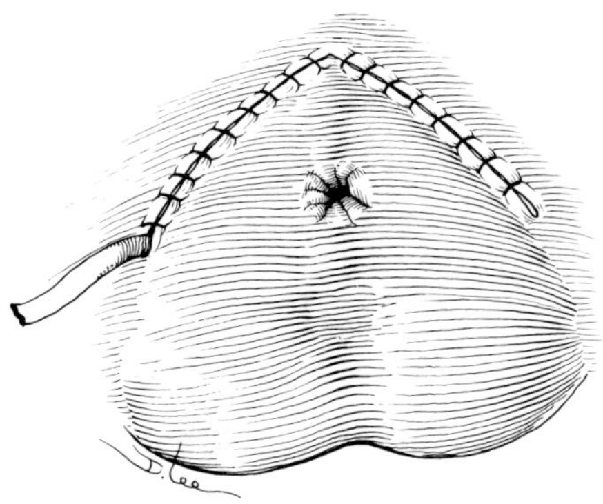

18-32h

Postoperative Care

The patient is kept in the prone position for the first postoperative week. This allows urine and feces to stay clear of the surgical wound if no diapers are used. These children usually have no difficulty in eating within 24 to 48 hours after surgery and thus do not need long-term intravenous therapy. The drain is removed the following day or as indicated, and the stitches are removed on the eighth postoperative day, just before discharge.

Complications

Wound infection is uncommon after this type of surgery, but, as in all other surgery of the newborn, broad-spectrum antibiotic coverage is maintained for five to seven days. Wound infections that do occur are treated no differently from those seen elsewhere in the body and should present no real problem. Urinary and fecal continence depends on the degree of nerve involvement and damage at the time of surgery and on the amount of levator muscle distortion. Proper repair of the levator muscle after tumor excision will result in minimal fecal incontinence.

Results

Approximately 20 percent of sacrococcygeal teratomas are malignant. Teratomas are more common in females, but malignancy is more common in males. The entire specimen should be sectioned by the pathologist to search for malignant elements. Radiation therapy and chemotherapy, particularly the use of Cytoxan, vincristine, and actinomycin, should be considered in patients when malignant elements are found. Unfortunately, there are almost no newborn survivors in whom the teratoma was malignant.

The number of deaths in children with benign sacrococcygeal teratomas should be minimal. In a large series surveyed by the American Academy of Pediatrics in 1973 [1], 2 percent of the patients operated upon for benign disease died postoperatively, half from hemorrhage and half from meningitis. There were other deaths in the benign group, but they were related to associated anomalies.

Selected References

1. Altman, R. P., Randolph, J. R., and Lilly, J. R. Sacrococcygeal teratoma. A.A.P. Surgical Section Survey, 1973. *J. Pediatr. Surg.* 9:389–98, 1974.
2. Bond, J. V. Prognosis and treatment of Wilms' tumor. *Cancer* 36:1202–7, 1975.
3. Burke, E. C., and Kallalis, P. P. Prune belly syndrome. *Am. J. Dis. Child.* 117:668, 1969.
4. Eagle, J. F., Jr., and Barrett, G. S. Congenital deficiency of abdominal muscles. *Pediatrics.* 6:721, 1950.
5. Ein, S. H. Benign liver tumors and cysts in childhood. *J. Pediatr. Surg.* 9:847–51, 1974.
6. Ein, S. H., and Stephens, C. A. Malignant liver tumors in children. *J. Pediatr. Surg.* 9:491–4, 1974.
7. Exelby, P. R., Filler, R. M., and Grosfeld, J. L. Liver tumors in children. *J. Pediatr. Surg.* 10:329–37, 1975.
8. Galviya, U. D., Howell, D. G., McMahon, M. H., and Mogg, R. A. Hydrocolpos. *Br. J. Urol.* 47:449–52, 1975.
9. Gebson, T. F. Hydronephrosis: Diagnosis and treatment of ureteropelvic obstructions. *J. Urol.* 75:1, 1956.
10. Hendren, W. H. A new approach to infants with severe obstructed uropathy. *J. Pediatr. Surg.* 5:184, 1970.
11. Hendren, W. H., and Crawford, J. D. The child with ambiguous genitalia. *Curr. Probl. Surg.* November 1972.
12. Koop, C. E. Abdominal mass in the newborn infant. *N. Engl. J. Med.* 289:569–71, 1973.
13. Lilly, J. R., Weintraub, W. H., and Altman, R. P. Spontaneous perforation of the extrahepatic bile ducts and bile peritonitis in infancy. *Surgery* 75:664–73, 1974.
14. Mahour, G. H., Woolley, M. M., Trivedi, S. N., and Landing, B. H. Sacrococcygeal teratoma. *J. Pediatr. Surg.* 10:183–8, 1975.
15. Somppi, E., Niemik, K., Ruuskanen, O., Arajarvi, P., and Lauslahti, K. Cavernous hepatic hemangioma in the newborn infant. *J. Pediatr. Surg.* 9:239–41, 1974.
16. Stone, H. Major hepatic resections in children. *J. Pediatr. Surg.* 10:127–34, 1975.
17. Towns, B. H., Mahour, G. H., Wooley, M. D., and Isaacs, H. Ovarian cysts and tumors in infancy and childhood. *J. Pediatr. Surg.* 10:311–9, 1975.
18. Vaage, S., and Knutrud, O. Congenital duplications of the alimentary tract with special regard to their embryogenesis. *Prog. Pediatr. Surg.* 7:103–23, 1974.
19. Waldbaum, R. S., and Marshall, V. F. Posterior urethral valves. *J. Urol.* 103:801, 1970.
20. Wedge, J. J., Grosfeld, J. L., and Smith, J. P. Abdominal masses in the newborn. *J. Urol.* 106:770–75, 1971.

19

Inguinal Hernia

Inguinal herniorrhaphy is the second most common operation performed in infants and children, exceeded in frequency only by tonsillectomy. Inguinal hernias in infancy are congenital in that they are present or potentially present at birth. The actual incidence of inguinal hernia in children under five years of age ranges from 0.8 percent to 4.4 percent. The largest number appear in the first year of life. Of those occurring during the first year of life, 80 percent are noted by the end of the third month of age. Although inguinal hernias are nine times more common in boys than in girls, the ratio is even higher during infancy. The incidence of bilaterality ranges anywhere from 15 percent to 50 percent, depending upon the series reported.

Preoperative Evaluation

An inguinal hernia is easily diagnosed in an infant when a bulge, which is easily reducible, is palpated or observed in the groin. In many cases, however, the hernia is not palpable during the surgeon's examination. Not even crying or any increasing of intraabdominal pressure can force the hernia to bulge out into the groin. In these situations, a definitive diagnosis can be made on the basis of a reliable history of a bulge either from the mother or from a referring physician. Usually the infant is asymptomatic unless there has been a previous episode of incarceration or strangulation.

On physical examination, if no actual hernia is palpated, the cord structures on the affected side will usually be found to be thickened, giving the sensation of silk rubbing together when the examining finger is rolled over the cord in the region of the external ring. During the examination one should always check the position of both testes and the presence or absence of a scrotal or cord hydrocele. The opposite side should be carefully examined for the presence of a hernia or for thickening of the cord structures to help in deciding whether or not to explore this side also at the time of surgery. Occasionally it is very difficult to differentiate an incarcerated inguinal hernia from a hydrocele of the cord. A rectal examination with palpation of the internal ring on the affected side will greatly aid in differentiating the hernia from a hydrocele of the cord.

The frequency of incarceration in childhood is surprisingly high. The highest incidence of incarceration, however, occurs within the first three to four months of life. These facts support the principle of surgical repair for inguinal hernias in infants upon diagnosis, regardless of age. Most, if not all, incarcerations can be reduced manually, obviating the need for emergency surgery to correct this condition.

The technique of reduction is important and involves sedating the infant with an appropriate barbiturate and then pushing the incarcerated hernia back through the external ring into the internal ring. This can be accomplished most easily by holding the baby by his feet and pushing the hernia initially caudad around the corner of the external ring and then pressing down cephalad to reduce the hernia into the area of the internal ring. This is a very effective technique and in almost all cases results in reduction of the incarcerated hernia.

Once the hernia has been reduced, the infant should be admitted to the hospital and given proper sedation, to minimize the risk of reincarceration. After about 48 hours in the hospital the baby should undergo elective herniorrhaphy. Only on rare occasions is the incarcerated hernia irreducible; this usually happens when the hernia has been incarcerated for a long time. In this situation an emergency operation is necessary to reduce the incarcerated hernia and to carry out a repair. Only occasionally does resection of the bowel at the time of the emergency herniorrhaphy become necessary.

One of the most common complications of hernia incarceration in infancy is hemorrhagic infarction of the testicle. If an infarcted testicle is found at the time of either emergency or elective herniorrhaphy, the testis should not be removed but should be placed back into the scrotum, so as to act at least as a prosthesis. In many instances this testicle will eventually atrophy. In male infants the incarcerated hernia usually contains intestine, whereas in female infants the most commonly incarcerated organ is the ovary.

Operative Technique

Almost all inguinal herniorrhaphies in infants are done as outpatient surgery at the present time, unless there are circumstances that require preoperative hospitalization, such as associated serious illnesses.

The infants are brought to the anesthesia department about half an hour before surgery, at which time they are examined and undergo a hematocrit and chest x-ray. They are then taken to the operating room and anesthetized.

The infant is placed on the operating table in the supine position and a small rolled towel is placed under the pelvis to extend the groin area slightly. Either mask or endotracheal anesthesia is used, depending on the preference of the anesthesiologist. An intravenous line is not introduced into the infant unless specifically requested by the particular anesthesiologist. The lower abdomen, groin, and perineum, including the penis and scrotum in the male, are then prepared and draped. A small incision, 1½ to 2 cm long, is made in a transverse fashion in the skin crease of the groin on the affected side (Figure 19-1a). The incision is then deepened to Scarpa's fascia by going through the subcutaneous tissue. At this point some small superficial vessels are seen and are clamped with mosquito hemostats on either side. The hemostats are left in place and held up by the assistant to tent up Scarpa's fascia. Scarpa's fascia is then grasped by the surgeon in the middle of the incision and cut so that dissection can be carried down directly through the

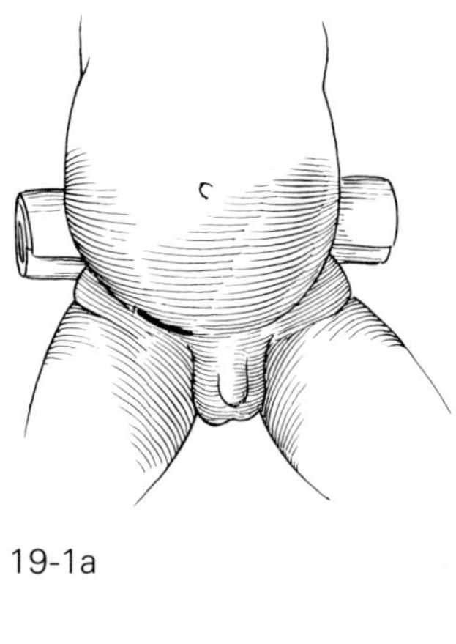

19-1a

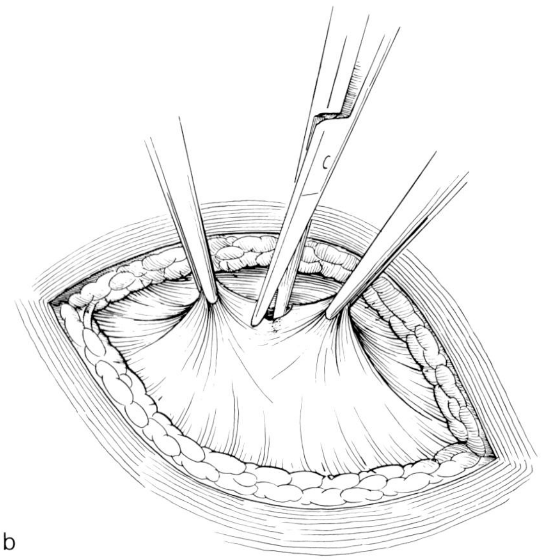

19-1b

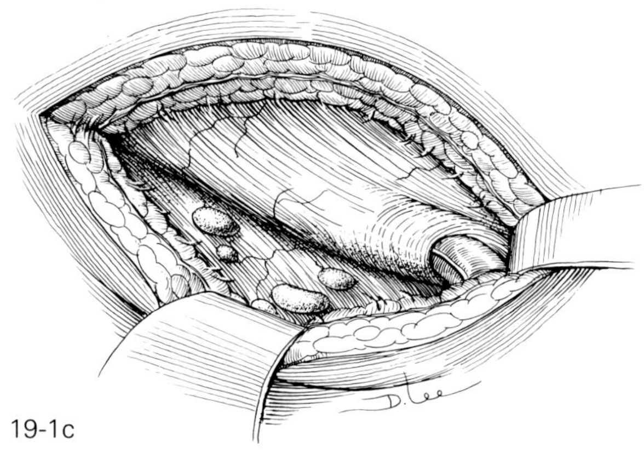

19-1c

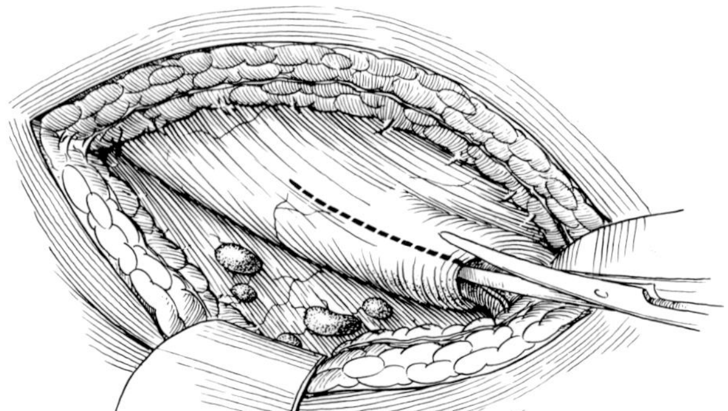

19-1d

small opening to the external oblique aponeurosis (Figure 19-1b).

Next, blunt dissection is carried out in a transverse direction, both medially and laterally between Scarpa's fascia and the external oblique aponeurosis. This is an important maneuver, because it is very easy to get lost and miss the inguinal canal in the small infant, especially if the patient is fat. At this juncture it is important to identify the external inguinal ring; often one misses the ring by dissecting too far down into the region of the inguinal nodes. This mistake can be prevented by placing two small vein retractors into the incision medially and inferiorly. This maneuver by the assistant will expose what is called the groove—the junction of the inguinal nodes and the surface of the external oblique aponeurosis as it curves around to form the shelving portion of Poupart's ligament (Figure 19-1c). This is a critical step in easily finding the external ring and the proper portion of the external oblique aponeurosis.

Next, the external ring is opened by hooking small Metzenbaum scissors underneath the ring and merely nicking the very edge of the external oblique (Figure 19-1d), to allow the ilioinguinal nerve to fall away and to prevent any damage to this structure. The cord structures are now gently grasped with two vascular forceps and are dissected free from the undersurface of the external oblique aponeurosis down to Poupart's ligament inferiorly and for a short distance superiorly.

Dissection is then begun in the middle of the cord structures by gently dissecting the cremasteric muscle and fascia from the hernia sac. This dissection should be carried out in the middle portion of the cord so that the testicle is not brought up into the incision and the procedure is not carried out close to the internal ring. As the cremasteric muscle and fascia are dissected off the sac, the vas deferens and spermatic vessels are seen along the undersurface of the sac (Figure 19-1e). A clear area is seen between the undersurface of the sac and the vas and vessels. Exposure of this clear area is often facilitated by having the operator place one finger underneath the sac while the dissection is being carried out. A hemostat is now placed through this clear area between the hernia sac and the vas and vessels. Then two hemostats are placed across the sac and the sac is divided (Figure 19-1f). The proximal portion of the sac is now dissected all the way back to the internal ring by gently freeing the cremasteric fascia attached to the sac and the vas and vessels. Once the base of the sac has been freed at the internal ring, it is twisted and suture-ligated with a 4-0 silk ligature (Figure 19-1g). The distal portion of the sac is now grasped and the testicle is brought up into the incision by gentle traction. The vas and vessels are then dissected free from the distal portion of the sac down to the level of the tunica vaginalis. This excess portion of the sac is then clamped and ligated at its base with a 4-0 silk, and the excess sac is excised (Figure 19-1h).

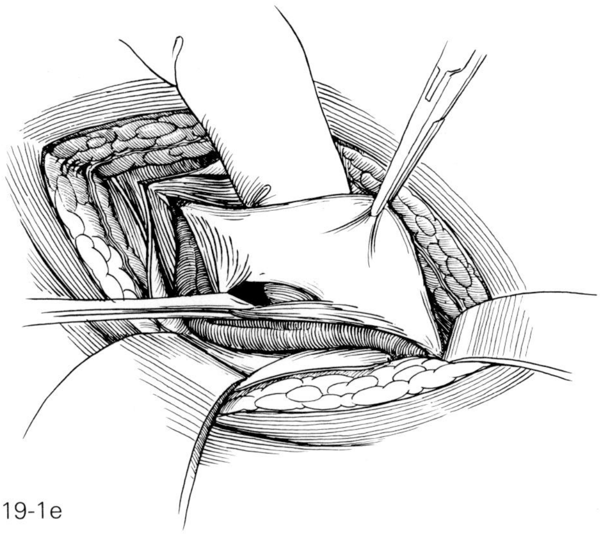

19-1e

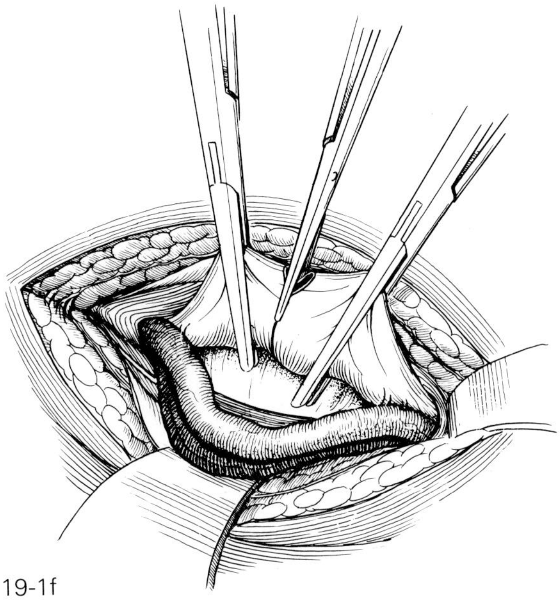

19-1f

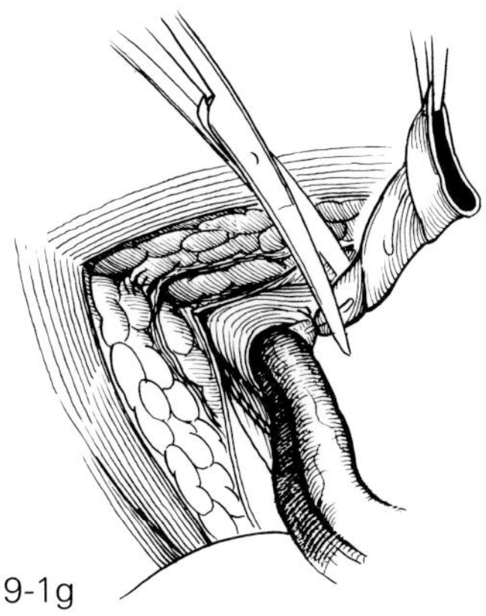

19-1g

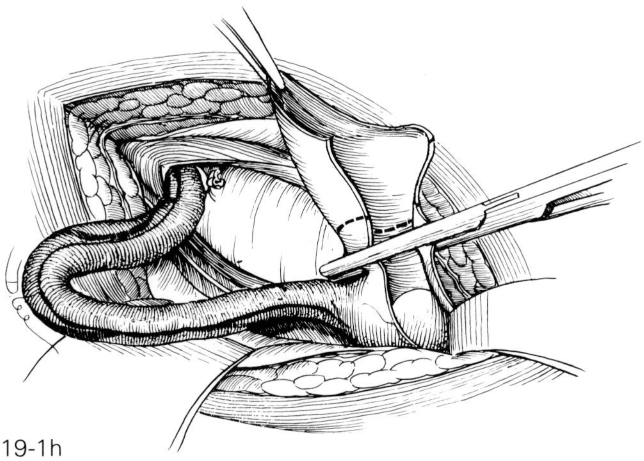

19-1h

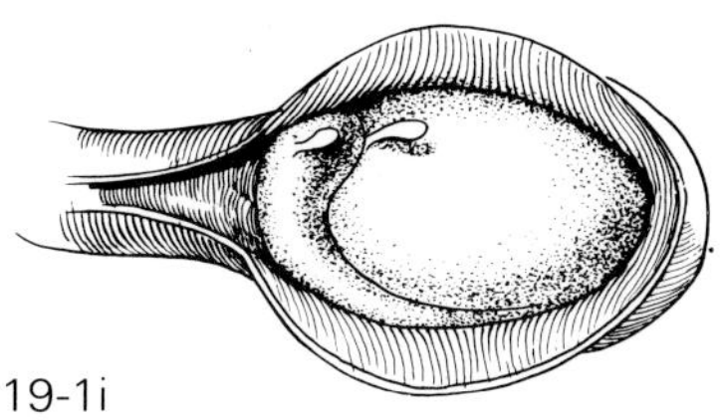

19-1i

The tunica vaginalis is now opened, and the testicle is exposed. The tunica should be opened wide to prevent the development of a postoperative hydrocele (Figure 19-1i). The testicle should be inspected for the presence of an appendix testis or an appendix epididymis. If either or both of these vestigial structures are found, they should be excised. The testicle is then returned to the scrotum in such a way that it is accurately replaced in its proper position. This is easily accomplished by grasping the scrotum on the affected side and pulling on the gubernaculum, which will always return the testicle to its proper location. The external oblique aponeurosis is then closed with a few interrupted sutures of 4-0 silk, and Scarpa's fascia along with the subcutaneous fat is closed with a few interrupted sutures of 4-0 Dexon. The skin is approximated with interrupted subcuticular sutures of 5-0 Dexon.

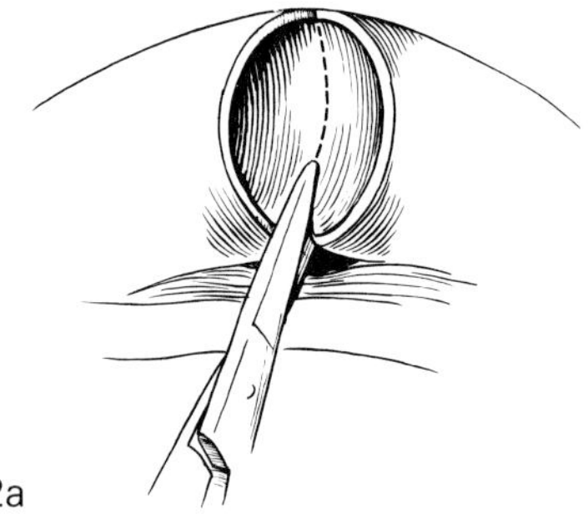

19-2a

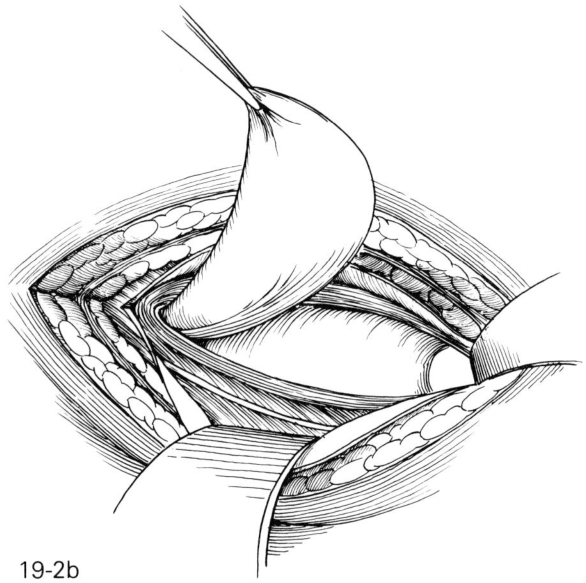

19-2b

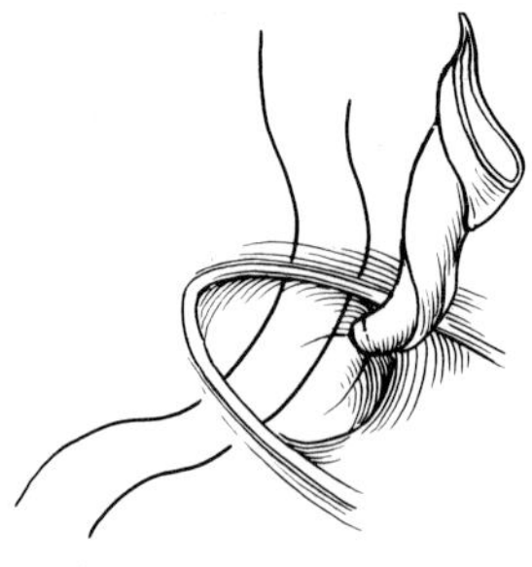

19-3

In all children two years of age and under, the opposite side is explored even though there is no clinical evidence of a hernia on that side. The operation is carried out in exactly the same way as on the clinical side. After the second incision has been closed, both incisions are painted with collodion. Before the patient is awakened from anesthesia, the perineum is checked to make sure both testicles are sitting properly in the scrotum. The child is then awakened from anesthesia and is brought to the recovery room, where he remains for the next half hour until fully awake. After this short recovery period the patient is discharged from the hospital to return home with his parents.

In the case of an incarcerated hernia, operated upon either when it is acute or 48 hours after reduction, the sac may still be quite edematous and much more difficult to dissect free from the underlying vas and vessels. In this situation it is sometimes safer to open the sac in its middle portion and then to dissect the sac from the underlying vas and vessels by employing a technique that is used for orchidopexies. This involves gentle blunt dissection of the undersurface of the sac from the vas and vessels with the tips of a baby Metzenbaum scissors and sequential division of the sac, as shown in Figure 19-2a.

In the female infant the inguinal herniorrhaphy is performed in the same way as in the male, with a few small differences. In the routine herniorrhaphy the round ligament on the affected side is included with the sac during the excision. Once the sac has been freed up to the internal ring, it should be opened and its contents inspected to determine whether or not normal internal female genitalia are present. The reason for this is that 1 to 2 percent of all inguinal hernias in females are associated with the testicular feminization syndrome. If normal internal female genitalia are detected at the time of herniorrhaphy, one can absolutely rule out the presence of this syndrome. If a testicle is found, the gonads should be returned to the abdomen and the hernia should be repaired. The bilateral gonadectomy is then delayed until feminization has occurred at puberty.

About 25 percent of female inguinal hernias are of a sliding nature. The broad ligament or vascular pedicle actually makes up part of the wall of the sac. In these cases the sac is simply ligated distal to the sliding portion, the excess of the sac is removed, and the stump is dropped back into the abdomen and retroperitoneum. The internal ring is then completely closed over, with some transversalis fascia used so that there will be no recurrence (Figure 19-3).

Postoperative Care

Postoperative care in these infants is negligible. As has already been mentioned, the babies are discharged from the hospital about half an hour after surgery. They are allowed to resume their regular diet and activities as soon as they return home. The mothers are instructed not to bathe the children by immersion for one week following surgery. The infant is seen in the office one week after the operation. At that time the child is discharged from the care of the surgeon. When the described techniques are used, the incisions are barely visible after three to six months.

Comments

Inguinal herniorrhaphy in the male infant can be one of the most difficult operations a surgeon faces, especially if the sac is quite large and thin. It is important to pay attention to the details described in this chapter and not to approach an inguinal herniorrhaphy in an infant by employing the same surgical principles and techniques used for inguinal herniorrhaphy in the older child or adult. It is easy to get lost during the initial part of the procedure and be in the region of the inguinal nodes or up higher in the abdomen, completely missing the shelving portion of the external oblique aponeurosis and the external ring. This mistake will be prevented by paying attention to the landmarks described. During dissection, extreme gentleness is required to avoid tearing the sac and causing irreversible damage to the vas deferens and the spermatic vessels. If attention is paid to these principles, bilateral inguinal herniorrhaphies can be performed in infants in less than an hour, thereby decreasing the risk to the baby of prolonged general anesthesia and tissue trauma.

Occasionally one encounters an infant with an obvious inguinal hernia who also has an obvious undescended testicle (not a retractile testis). In this situation it is perfectly reasonable to repair the hernia during infancy and at the same time carry out an orchidopexy. Contrary to the case with the older child, at the time of surgery the vas and vessels usually have adequate length after the hernia sac has been dissected free, so that it is usually unnecessary to dissect these structures into the retroperitoneum and take down the floor of the inguinal canal.

After the sac has been treated in the manner already described, the testis is pexed to the scrotum using the dartos-pouch technique. The scrotum on the affected side is stretched with one finger inside it. A ½-cm incision is made transversally in the midportion of the scrotum. The incision is merely carried down through the skin until the dartos muscle can be seen. Next, a subcutaneous pouch is dissected all the way around the incision so that the testicle will have adequate room to reside there (Figure 19-4). A mosquito hemostat is then placed through the center of the dartos muscle and brought up into the inguinal canal. The testicle, which has a 2-0 silk suture placed through the middle of it, is then grasped by the suture with the mosquito hemostat and is brought down into the scrotum. By gentle traction on the silk suture, the testicle is easily popped through the small opening in the dartos muscle into the subcutaneous pouch (Figure 19-5). The snugness of the dartos muscle around the top

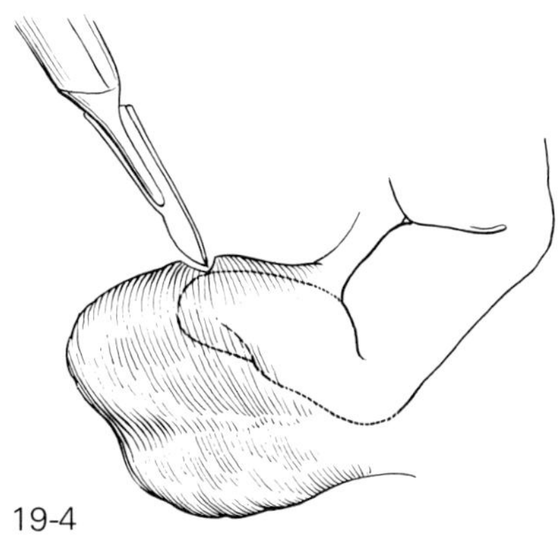

19-4

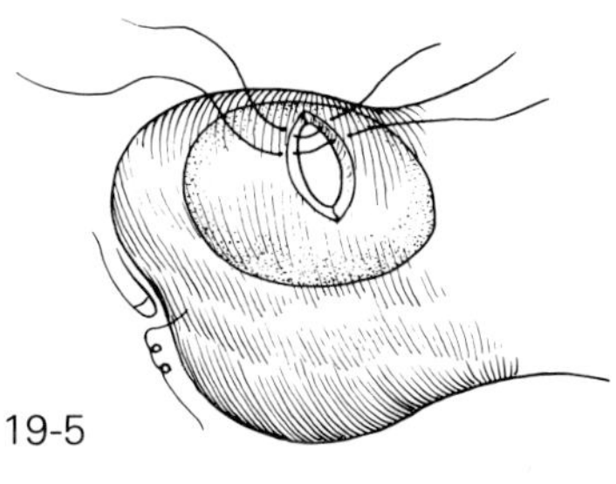

19-5

portion of the testicle and epididymis is usually sufficient to prevent the testis from retracting into the inguinal canal without in any way compromising the blood supply to the testicle. Occasionally the opening is larger than one would like; in this case, the testicle can be tacked to the surrounding dartos muscle with a few sutures of 4-0 silk put through the dartos muscle and the tunica albuginea. The small incision in the scrotum is then closed with one or two subcuticular sutures of 5-0 Dexon.

Selected References

1. Gans, S. L., and Rubin, C. L. Apparent female infants with hernias and testes. *Am. J. Dis. Child.* 104:114, 1962.
2. Gross, R. E. *The Surgery of Infancy and Childhood.* Philadelphia: Saunders, 1953.
3. Kiesewetter, W. B., and Parenzan, L. When should hernia in the infant be treated bilaterally? *J.A.M.A.* 171:287, 1959.
4. Mustard, W. T., Ravitch, M. M., Snyder, W. H., Jr., et al. *Pediatric Surgery.* Chicago: Year Book Medical Publishers, 1969.
5. Rickham, P. P., and Johnston, J. H. *Neonatal Surgery.* New York: Appleton-Century-Crofts, 1969.
6. Swenson, O. *Pediatric Surgery.* New York: Appleton-Century-Crofts, 1958.

20

Biliary Atresia

Jaundice in the newborn period can present a difficult challenge to the pediatrician and the pediatric surgeon. The importance of early differentiation of obstructive from hepatocellular abnormalities has been heightened by the successes of more recent operations in treating biliary atresia. Early diagnosis is critical because surgical procedures performed after three months of age are uniformly unsuccessful.

Differential Diagnosis

Infants who are jaundiced at four to six weeks of age should always be suspected of having biliary atresia. By this age physiologic jaundice should have cleared, leaving the differential between biliary obstruction and some form of hepatitis. The usual laboratory criteria for differentiating hepatocellular from obstructive jaundice in infants have not been very helpful. The serum bilirubin and hepatic enzymes are usually in the same range whether the cause is hepatocellular or obstructive; the stools may be clay-colored and the urine may contain urobilinogen in either situation.

The rose bengal I^{131} liver scan has been the most helpful single study for separating biliary atresia or obstruction from neonatal hepatitis. Infants with a patent biliary tree should excrete the radioactive dye from the liver into the intestinal tract within six hours (Figure 20-1). A child with obstructive biliary disease does not show activity in the intestinal tract at 24 or even 48 hours (Figure 20-2). Although children with neonatal hepatitis should excrete the dye into the intestinal tract, upon occasion the inflamed liver excretes poorly, so that the rose bengal scan may be indistinguishable from that seen in biliary atresia. Because of these inaccuracies, all children who fail to excrete the tracer at 48 hours should be suspected of having biliary atresia and should be scheduled for exploratory laparotomy. We have not elected to repeat the scan one week after administration of cholestyramine, which is reported to reduce the number of false positive tests, because we feel it is safer to operate on an occasional child who does not have biliary atresia than to delay exploration of an infant who has a potentially correctable lesion.

Operative Technique

During the past few years an increasing number of surgeons around the world have reported short-term and long-term successes using the portoenterostomy (Kasai procedure). Because there have been no reports of successful long-term results in patients operated on after three months of age, every effort should be made to identify children who need surgery before they are three months old.

The child is placed supine on the operating table with a nasogastric tube and an intravenous line in place. An incision in the right upper quadrant is made approximately one inch long just at the edge of the palpable liver and lateral to the

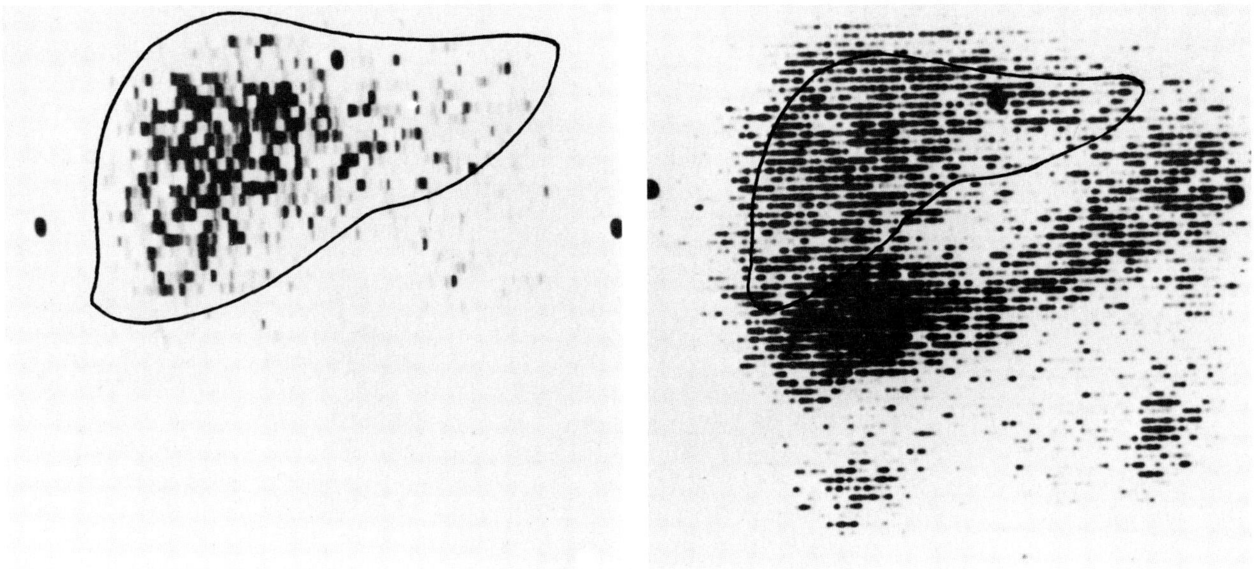

20-1. Rose bengal I^{131} scan at 0 and 6 hours, demonstrating prompt excretion into the intestine.

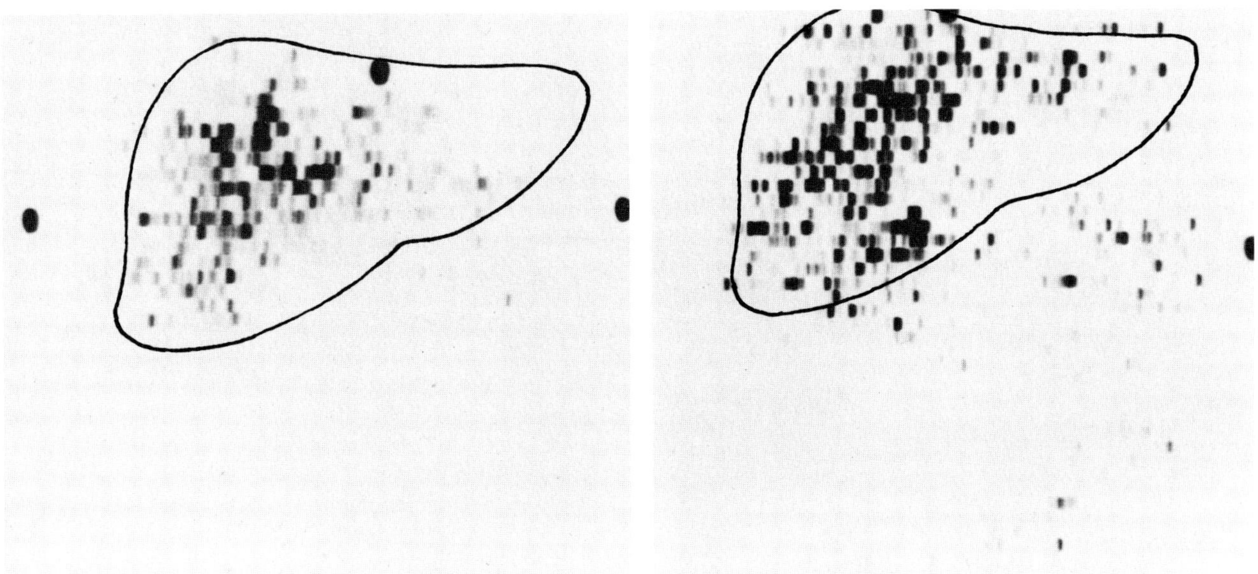

20-2. Rose bengal I^{131} scan at 0 and 24 hours showing dye only in the liver.

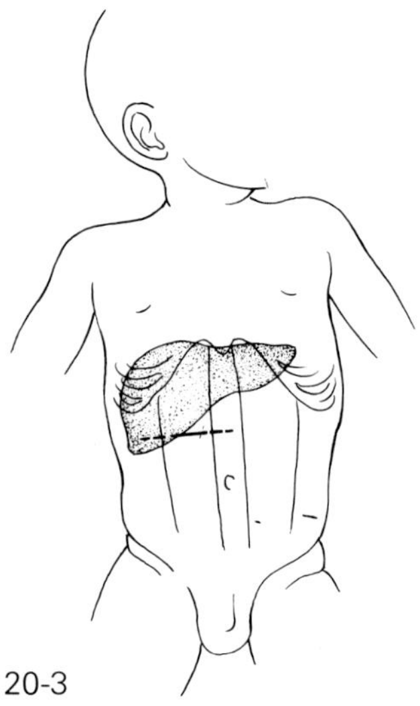

20-3

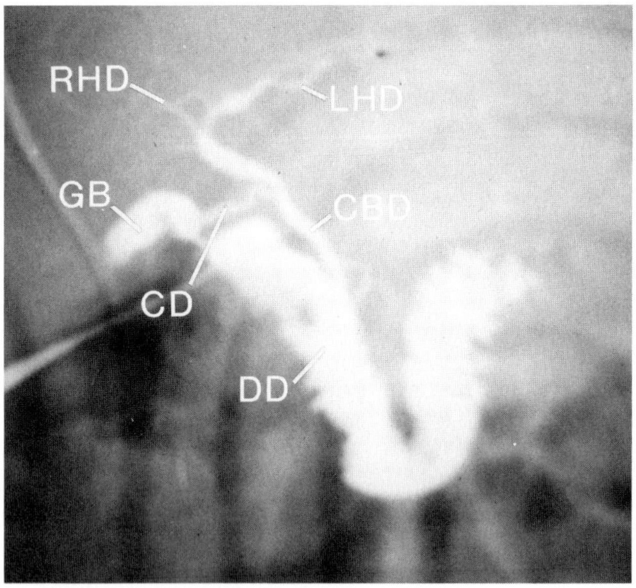

20-4. Operative cholangiogram done through gallbladder, proving the entire system is patent. *RHD* = right hepatic duct; *LHD* = left hepatic duct; *GB* = gallbladder; *CD* = cystic duct; *CBD* = common bile duct; *DD* = duodenum.

rectus muscle (Figure 20-3). The gallbladder is located, and a small polyethylene catheter is placed into the fundus in the center of a pursestring suture. Twenty-five percent Hypaque is injected into the gallbladder and an x-ray film is taken. If the x-ray demonstrates an entirely patent extrahepatic duct system with free flow of dye into the duodenum, and back into the liver (Figure 20-4), then a wedge biopsy is taken from the liver, and the incision is closed. These children usually have progressive clinical improvement. The histology will usually confirm a diagnosis of some form of hepatitis.

If dye does not leave the gallbladder or if the gallbladder is small or absent, the incision is enlarged and a full-scale portal dissection is carried out. At this point a thorough intraabdominal examination is performed because there is a high incidence of associated abnormalities in patients with biliary atresia. Multiple spleens and a preduodenal portal vein are among the more common lesions to be found; these should be carefully noted in the operative record.

Next, a methodical exploration of the hepaticoduodenal ligament is begun. Each filmy piece of tissue is carefully inspected and clamped, then cut and tied. It is important to ligate even the thinnest tissue because the lymphatic drainage through this area is extensive, and massive ascites may develop in the postoperative period. By using this approach, the major structures in the hepaticoduodenal ligament are skeletonized. If a structure resembling a common duct is found, it is obviously used as the focal point of the dissection; however, in only a few cases a remnant is found. In this circumstance, the dissection continues toward the hilum of the liver by tracing the hepatic artery into the liver. The normal bifurcation of the cordlike hepatic ducts occurs just inside the bifurcation of the hepatic artery (Figure 20-5a). In general, a cordlike remnant of the hepatic bile duct is found and can be traced up into the liver hilum. These landmarks should be carefully noted. With careful dissection, the small amount of tissue found in the crotch between the left and right hepatic artery is dissected free. A small nipple of this is resected and sent to the pathology laboratory for frozen section (Figure 20-5b). If the specimen does not contain ductules of 100 microns or greater in diameter, the Kasai procedure will not be successful.

If an appropriate-sized ductule is not found, further exploration and biopsies are undertaken until the appropriate area is exposed. If, after extensive dissection into the liver hilum, tissue with ductules of adequate size is not found, the operation is terminated after a liver biopsy has been taken. If the biopsy report is favorable, one should proceed with a portoenterostomy. A 30-cm section of proximal jejunum is used for the construction of an isolated loop. Jejunal continuity is reestablished with a single-layer end-to-end anastomosis using 4-0 or 5-0 silk with the knots tied on the inside. The mesenteric defect is closed with interrupted or running 4-0 silk sutures. A small hole is then made in the mesentery of

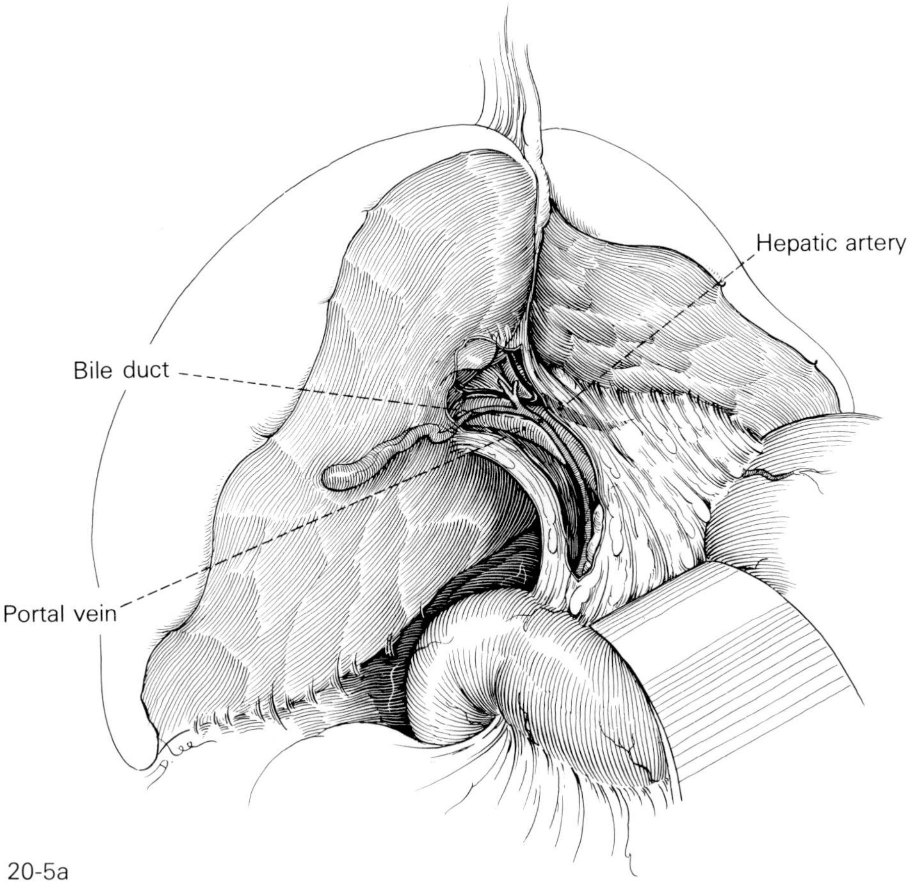

20-5a

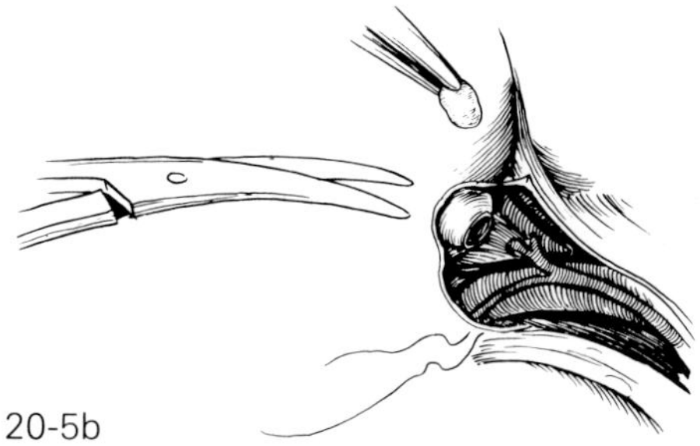

20-5b

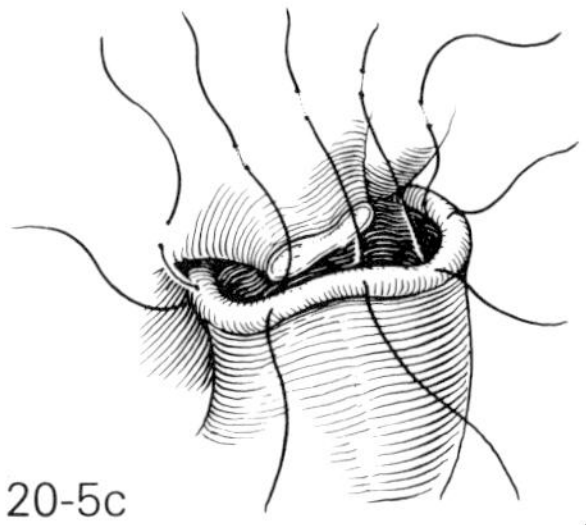

20-5c

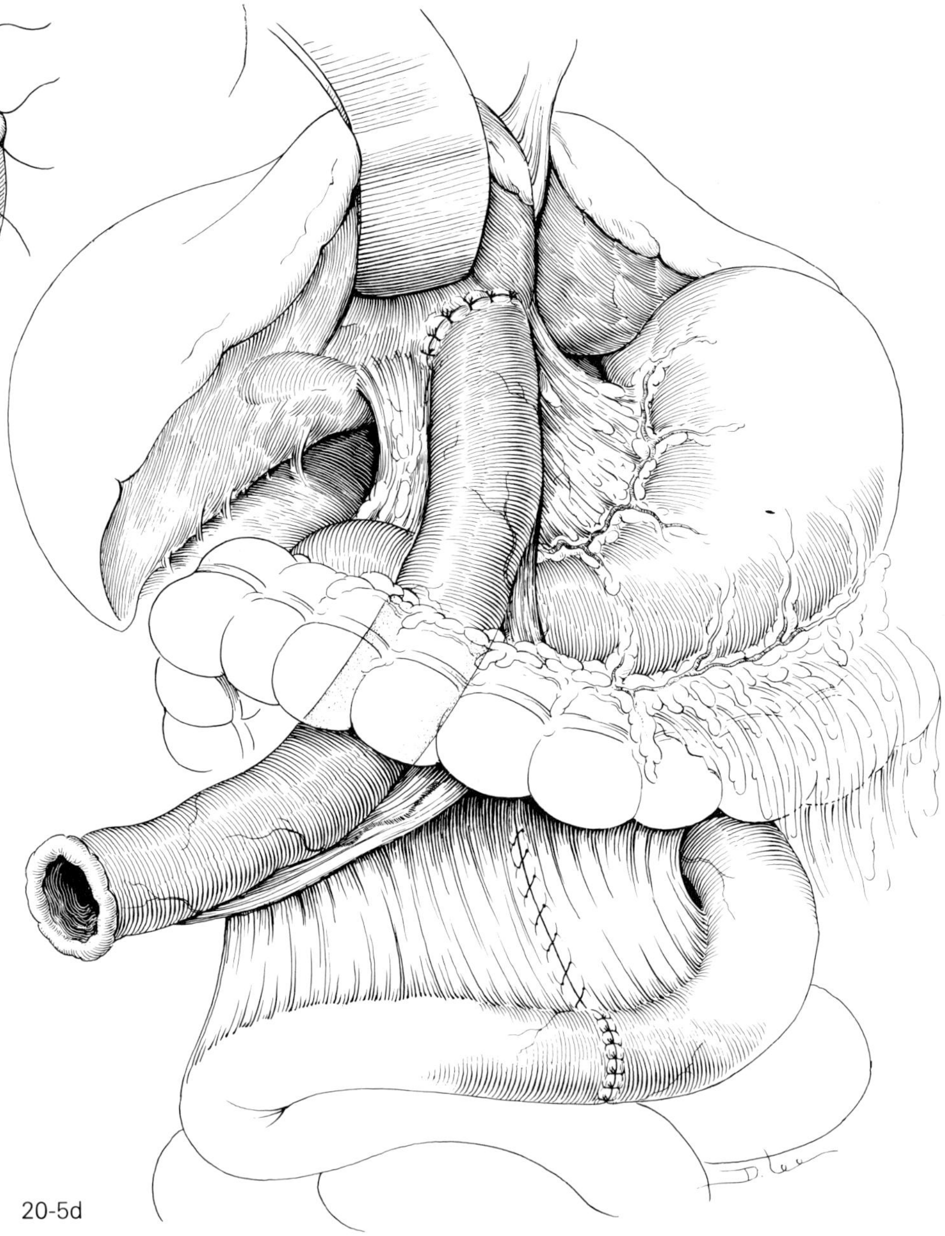

20-5d

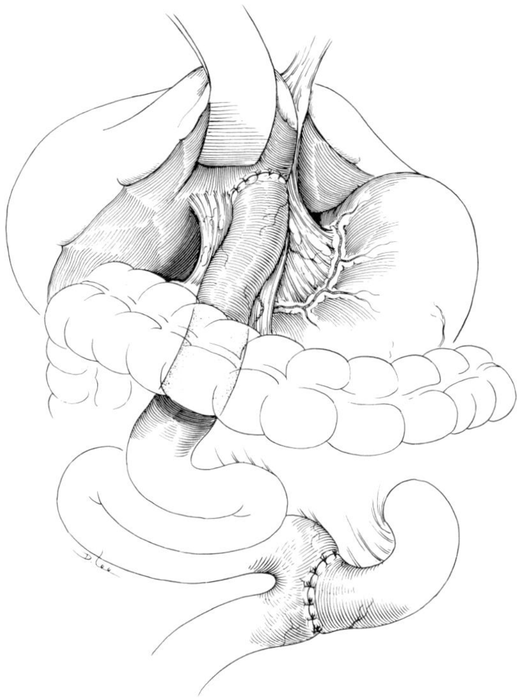

20-6a

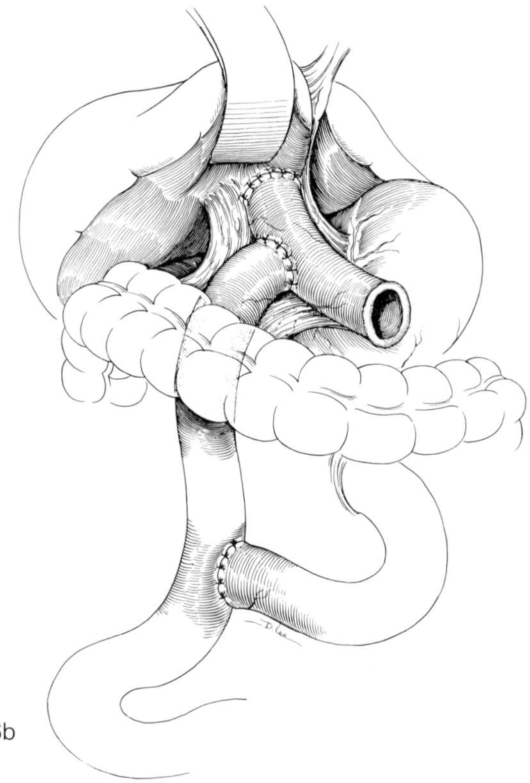

20-6b

the transverse colon, and the proximal end of the isolated jejunal segment is passed through this area up into the hilum of the liver. A single-layer anastomosis is then created between the end of this bowel and the capsule of the liver so as to place the intestinal lumen over the previously transected tissue (Figure 20-5c), using 4-0 silk sutures placed through all layers of the bowel wall. The other end of the jejunum is brought out lateral to the incision and matured as a cutaneous jejunostomy (Figure 20-5d). A liver biopsy is obtained, and a Penrose drain is placed near the foramen of Winslow and brought out through a separate stab wound. The incision is closed in layers.

In an attempt to reduce postoperative cholangitis, a number of different techniques have been tried. Roux-en-Y loops (Figure 20-6a), double Roux-en-Y loops (Figure 20-6b),

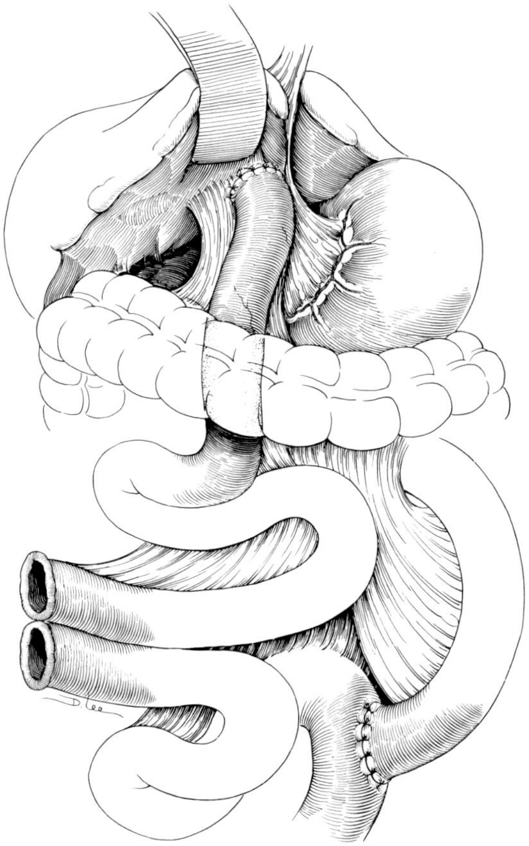

20-6c

and double-barreled enterostomies (Figure 20-6c) have been performed as part of the portoenterostomy. Each has advantages and disadvantages, and none has yet proved superior to the others. In a rare patient, the gallbladder and distal common duct are patent and are connected to the duodenum. In these infants the transected dome of the gallbladder can be used for the anastomosis (Figure 20-7).

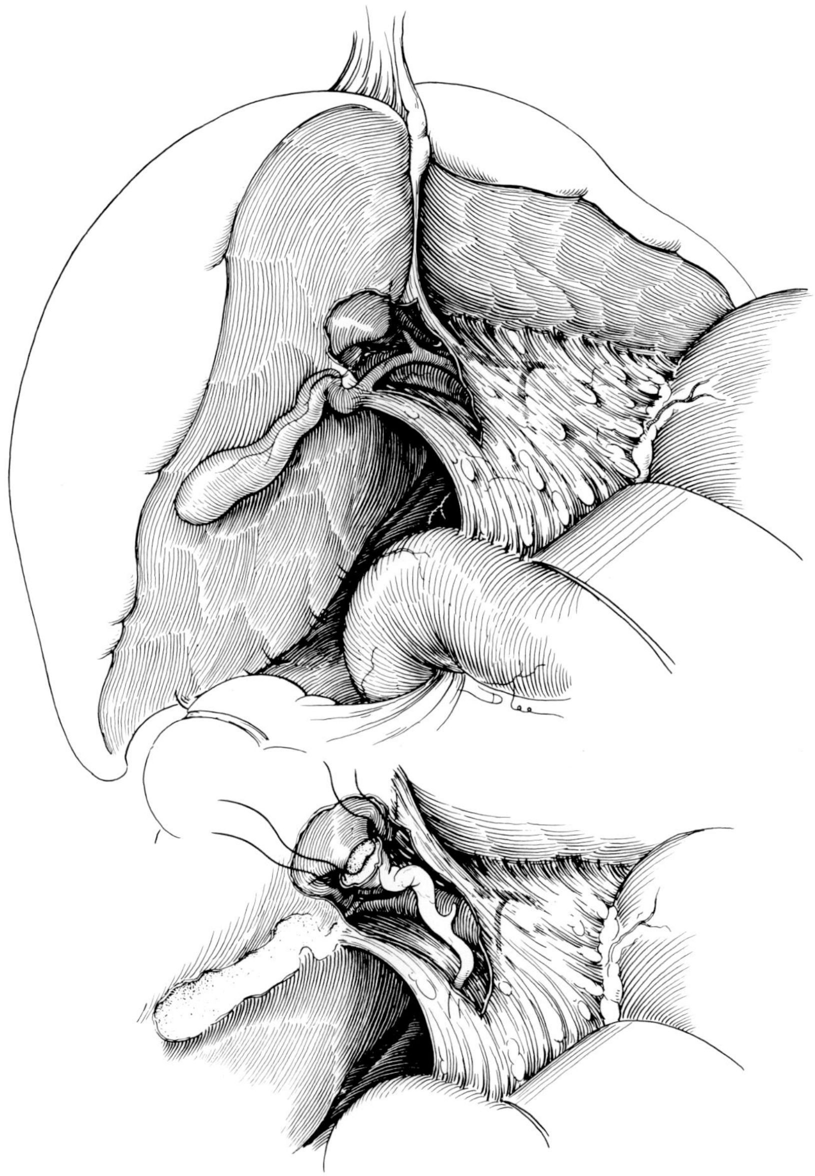

20-7. Patient with intact gallbladder and distal common duct but proximal atresia. The gallbladder is lifted from its fossa and sutured over the previously prepared tissue in the porta hepatis.

Postoperative Care

Children who have had operations for biliary atresia are maintained on parenteral antibiotics for 10 days. Intravenous feedings are continued for three to five days, after which time oral nutrition is begun. There is usually minimal drainage from the Penrose drain by five days, and it may be safely advanced after the drainage has subsided. To reduce the incidence of cholangitis, long-term prophylactic antibiotic coverage is started with trimethoprim and sulfamethoxazole (Bactrim) once parenteral antibiotics are stopped.

Complications

The most common complication of the portoenterostomy is failure to obtain biliary drainage. Infants who do not drain bile continue on the slow downhill course of biliary obstruction, which results in biliary cirrhosis, portal hypertension, and death from hepatic failure.

Recurrent cholangitis occurs in many of the patients who have had a successful portoenterostomy. The recurrent cholangitis develops whether the jejunal loop is in continuity with the intestine or is brought out as an isolated jejunostomy. Each attack of cholangitis should be treated promptly and vigorously, because stenosis or closure of the intestinal-biliary anastomosis can follow these infections. The frequency and severity of these attacks decrease with time; by one year of age, the risk of cholangitis drops markedly.

In patients in whom the portoenterostomy loop is exteriorized to the skin, massive loss of bilious fluid can occur. Many children put out from 300 to 1000 cubic centimeters of bile a day. This must be returned to the intestinal tract by one means or another. Some children will drink this fluid mixed with their formula. For others the fluid can be placed into the distal limb of their loop enterostomy or into a gastrostomy. Failure to return the bile to the intestinal tract will result not only in poor fat absorption but also in electrolyte imbalance and dehydration. At one to two years of age children with an exteriorized loop to the skin should be reexplored, should undergo a liver biopsy, and should have the loop taken down and the distal end placed into the jejunum, end-to-side, as a Roux-en-Y, so that the bile is returned directly to the intestinal tract. Recent studies have implicated bile salts as contributing to progressive biliary cirrhosis; in some centers the bile is not refed into the patient for this reason.

Results

Fewer than half the infants who undergo portoenterostomy develop true bile drainage into the intestinal loop; and of these, fewer than half have arrest of the progressive liver damage. Therefore, somewhere between 10 percent and 25 percent of patients with biliary atresia who undergo portoenterostomy achieve a long-term successful result.

Other Causes of Jaundice That Require Surgery

At exploration, a rare patient may have atresia localized to the distal common duct. The proximal duct is then massively dilated. (These cases were formerly called correctable biliary atresia.) A classic Roux-en-Y intestinal anastomosis to the proximal duct will correct the obstruction.

Choledochal cysts are rarely found in the newborn period, but, if they are encountered, surgical repair is feasible. Satisfactory results have been obtained with a Roux-en-Y intestinal anastomosis, but recently excision of the cyst with a Roux-en-Y jejunostomy to the end of the common duct has been used.

Choledochal cysts and distal common-duct atresias can indeed be corrected surgically, but in these patients the liver has been damaged by the biliary obstruction. Therefore, the overall outcome for these babies is affected by both the technical success of the surgery and the amount of permanent liver damage already present at the time of surgery.

Selected References

1. Altman, R. P., and Lilly, J. R. Technical details in the surgical correction of extrahepatic biliary atresia. *Surg. Gynecol. Obstet.* 140:952, 1975.
2. Kasai, M., Kimura, S., Asakura, Y., et al. Surgical treatment of biliary atresia. *J. Pediatr. Surg.* 3:665, 1968.
3. Kiesewetter, W. B. Choledochal cyst. In W. T. Mustard, M. M. Ravitch, W. H. Snyder, Jr., et al., *Pediatric Surgery.* Chicago: Year Book Medical Publishers, 1961. P. 747.
4. Lilly, J. R., and Altman, R. P. Hepatic portoenterostomy (Kasai operation) for biliary atresia. *Surgery* 78:76, 1975.
5. Pickett, L. K. Obstructive jaundice. In W. T. Mustard, M. M. Ravitch, W. H. Snyder, Jr., et al., *Pediatric Surgery.* Chicago: Year Book Medical Publishers, 1969. P. 732.

Index